The Forgotten Senses

Books by Donald E. Carr

THE FORGOTTEN SENSES
THE DEADLY FEAST OF LIFE
THE SEXES
THE ETERNAL RETURN
DEATH OF THE SWEET WATERS
THE BREATH OF LIFE

The Forgotten Senses

DONALD E. CARR

Doubleday & Company, Inc.

GARDEN CITY, NEW YORK

1972

Library of Congress Catalog Card Number 70–157578
Copyright © 1972 by Donald E. Carr
All Rights Reserved
Printed in the United States of America
First Edition

To Michelle and Angela

CONTENTS

Introduction

AT THE CORE of all philosophies, ancient or modern, there has existed a flaming little question: Do we perceive the universe *as it is?* There is obviously no answer to this question and there never will be. As advanced animals, we have highly developed eyesight—but not as good as the birds'. We have a subtle and crucial sense of hearing—otherwise we would not have made the enormous invention of symbolic language—but probably the dolphin exceeds us, certainly in sheer complexity of sound communication, although there is no proof that he uses *symbolic* signals. Our other senses are mediocre in comparison with those of many creatures with whom we share the planet. Furthermore, it is evident that various animals perceive sensual worlds that we cannot imagine. This is true of certain fishes who sense electrically and certain snakes who at a distance can distinguish temperature differences of a thousandth of a degree. It is becoming evident also that the *directional* instincts of many fishes, birds, turtles and others depend upon some inherited knowledge of the world and a way of surveying it which, as a young animal species, we can only imitate by instruments that are crude and clumsy in comparison.

It is the plan of this book to review in depth the various senses of animals, to compare their sensual worlds with ours and to speculate on how we might extend our repertoire of perception, but most importantly how we might adapt ourselves to a subtler *appreciation* of the meaning and the promise of a universe that pours out signals that now we either do not understand or cannot accurately translate into strategies of action.

We shall find one insistent theme in examining the senses of all animals: evolution designed them to perceive *only what is important to the life of the animal.* If a bird sees a star he may include it in a pattern that helps him to find his way home at night. He has no further interest in the star. The bird does not believe in astronomy. The remarkable automatic eye of the frog can instantly see and identify a *moving* insect, but he can be draped with dead flies and still starve to death. A mosquito may fly over a fierce artillery battle with nonchalance in pursuit of the tiny specific hum of his sweetheart, a sound so fairylike that we need special instruments to record it.

It is reasonable to suppose that human beings also perceive in this way. Evolution did not design man as an astronomer or as a designer of nuclear bombs, but as a predatory beast who is extremely interested not only in finding food but also in finding a mate. As an exercise in human optics, the miniskirt has had more concentrated eye power devoted to it (or what it discloses) than the distant sight of the beautiful blue earth from outer space. Even a dedicated astronaut is more interested in his wife and children than in the landscape of the moon.

What seems to me, in fact, most fascinating in the whole astronaut story is that from a hundred miles or so from earth various orbiting men were, *with the naked eye*, able to see dirt roads in Mexico, the wake of a water skier in the Salton Sea, the smoke from huts in the Himalayas, the street lights of forlorn little towns in Australia and other peculiarly *human things*. I have expounded a theory for this effect in the pages that follow. It is possible that the heightening of the sense of sight by weightlessness may be the greatest bonus of our space adventure. We need other adventures in the senses. The greatest of all would, of course, be the exploitation of those senses we do not understand and cannot describe anatomically. That they are possessed by certain other animals seems to me undeniable. That we possess them in residual or potential form seems to me possible. I have therefore devoted what to a Skinner-type psychologist may seem to be a scandalous amount of attention to "extrasensory perception," a term I heartily dislike since I believe what we have to explain is not "beyond the senses," but simply the unknown or the forgotten modes of perception and of communication which evolution tended to breed out of us when we climbed the critical plateau of symbolic thinking. I feel that we may before long be able at will to climb both up and down this plateau, and when we have learned to do this we shall find ourselves unexpectedly to be a new species of wiser animals.

CHAPTER I

The Eyes and the Beholders

THERE ARE two kinds of chemical reactions on our planet that depend on light, one of which (photosynthesis) is absolutely necessary to the survival of all animal life that consumes other life in making a living. The other photochemical reaction, although not entirely essential for all forms of animals, would if denied immediately result in the wiping out of whole animal classes (birds, for example). This is the chemical transformation that makes it possible for an animal to see. It is a very curious fact that once evolution discovered this single process, it used it to mold an enormous variety of eyes and it is still more curious that the process is so subtle yet specific that it is hard to explain it to anyone who has never studied chemistry, and in fact the familiar, precise elucidation of the photochemical process was delayed until only a relatively few years ago.[1]

What evolution found out, perhaps a billion or so years before that, was that the molecule known now as "11-*cis* retinal" when exposed to light forms the molecule all-*trans* retinal. This is a reaction of the type known as "isomerization" (that is, a change in the structure but not the atomic content of a molecule) and the structure change involved is so slight that it would have

[1] George Wald of Harvard shared a 1967 Nobel prize for work done earlier on the problem.

been impossible for the chemists of the last century even to detect it. Yet on this single, seemingly almost academic and trifling process, all the seeing that is done in the world depends. Man has invented various much more drastic photoreactive systems for making mechanical eyes of a sort, including the camera with the film emulsion that depends on the childishly simple fact that silver chloride, when exposed to light, will break down into metallic silver and chlorine, but for man, the beholder, to see his developed film, he must still depend on evolution's stubborn and weird selection of the 11-*cis* retinal to all-*trans* retinal gimmick. Biochemists are still trying to puzzle out why *this* and only this arcane process was chosen as the channel between every living individual (from a flatworm to Picasso) and the outside visual world of electromagnetic vibrations. But there it is. Until we are as good chemists as evolution (which may take a few millennia at the least) we can only wonder at this inscrutable specificity and try to answer further obvious questions, such as how does this reaction cause the sensation we know as sight?

First, we must have a little more chemistry. The molecular structure known as "retinal" is one of the so-called "carotenoid pigments"[2] and is invariably associated with a big protein molecule, opsin. The opsins vary in structure in different sorts of animals, just as the hemoglobin of the blood does. In humans, the combination of the pigment and the opsin is called "rhodopsin," and when "retinal" (the so-called "chromatophore" part of the rhodopsin) undergoes its isomerization because of light, it is no longer compatible with the opsin portion and the giant molecule therefore falls apart. What was a purple molecule becomes bleached. Retinal is actually vitamin A in slightly oxidized form (it is an aldehyde, while vitamin A is an alcohol), and regenera-

[2] Before the discovery of retinal as the crucial constituent of the eye-pigment cells of all eyes, various *cis-trans* isomerizations of vegetable carotenoids were familiar. A spectacular laboratory demonstration can be staged by extracting the carotenoid from the yellow tomato and exposing the extract solution to bright light in the presence of a trace of iodine. It turns suddenly to the brilliant dark orange of the all-*trans* compound of ripe tomatoes, called "lycopene."

tion of the protein-opsin complex, ready for another shot of light, is achieved in a number of ways, involving either the back-isomerization of the retinal or the oxidation of vitamin A in the blood to the 11-*cis* retinal. (The connection between vitamin A deficiency and night-blindness becomes apparent.) All the reactions that regenerate the initial rhodopsin are dark processes, although their speeds are very great. In some animals, after the essential light reaction has isomerized the 11-*cis* retinal, the opsin remains compatible with the all-*trans*-retinal, so that regeneration may be simpler or at least different. One of the reasons why opsins vary from one animal to another is that the color of light that is important to an animal's particular life habits may be different, and the color that is most important is absorbed most highly in his particular retinal-opsin molecule. Thus, as we shall explain later, blue is especially interesting to a frog and his opsin must therefore be so constructed that the absorption of blue light is assured.

Now with this excruciatingly important problem solved, as to how light could be made to carry out an effect of which an animal would be conscious or to which it would at least act out a patterned response, evolution proceeded to design all kinds of eyes, some of which were scarcely more than bent-over pigmented membranes with tiny hairs (cilia) playing a role. (It was not unexpected that in constructing a sight organ, evolution should use a cilium, for this primordial organ form goes back even to the protozoa.) The reaction to light does not require eyes in the head. In planarian worms photoreceptors of an obscure sort are distributed over the body. Sometimes the eyes are simply spots of pigment in the skin. Mostly in worms they are cups of pigment (ocelli), lying deep in the tissue beneath the skin or in the brain. In bristle worms there are usually more than six pairs of pigment-cup eyes and up to several hundred in some species. In land planarians there may be over a thousand ocelli. The primitive ocelli have from one to four sensory nerve fibers ending in an expanded knob, all inside a cup of one or more pigment cells. Needless to say, even in these coarse eyes, which can do little more than distinguish light from dark, or at best the *direction* of light, the active ingredient is 11-*cis* retinal. Eyes with lenses are a distinct luxury, but they are found in some bristle worms. Of nearly equal performance but of less elegance are the "camera-eyes" of many primitive creatures, whose operation depends on the well-known principle that a small hole in a dark box acts to refract light in much the same manner as a lens.

It must be confessed that we do not know precisely how the ancient and infallible retinal reaction results in the stimulation of a nerve fiber. Yet this retinal isomerization is the only case in which a *molecular* mechanism whereby a sensory cell detects the conditions surrounding it is known. Thus we know more about the eye than we do about far older organs and senses such as smell and touch, and we know more about the eye of *Limulus*, the horseshoe crab, an animal that was very old before the dinosaurs, than about any other eye. The reason for this is that the horseshoe crab has a compound eye which is nevertheless relatively simple and, *Limulus* being an animal of convenient size, its ocular apparatus has proved to be just about right for experimentation. The compound eye, as the name implies, is a whole colony of separate eyes. There are far more animals in the world equipped with compound eyes (perhaps 100 million times as many) than there are animals with the "simple" eyes such as ours. The notion of compound eyes appears to have occurred to evolution at least twice quite separately, since the insects do not seem to have inherited them from crustaceans but to have started out with the mixed ocelli and vague, not quite compound eyes of the millipede (or its larval form). On the face of it, the elaborate compound eyes of an insect (composed of several thousand "ommatidia," or facets or separate eyelets) with the incredible complexity of nervous organization behind them hardly seem worth while. For such a popular form of eye, however, there must be a cogent reason, since evolution seldom invents complexity just for the hell of it. Possibly evolution decided somewhat along these lines: If I am going to develop a small animal that is going to get around fast and be a good predator or scavenger and find his mate, he must be able to see instantly from a number of angles. But I cannot afford to give him too many muscles with which to turn his eyes and to accommodate their lenses. In the first place, muscle systems are tough to elaborate in such a small animal. My choice is between complicating the motor nerve system and making more eyes, which can co-ordinate well but don't have to be turned this way and the other. It is easier to elaborate the receptor nerves than it is to go through all that grief in designing the effector nerves and the muscles. So, let's try the immovable eye and see how it works out.

How it worked out can first be seen by analyzing the eye of the horseshoe crab *Limulus* by the methods applied by H. K. Hartline, who shared with George Wald the Nobel prize for his job. *Limulus* has some one thousand ommitidia, each of which contains about twelve cells. The receptor cells themselves, containing the photochemically active eye pigment, are arranged almost exactly like the segments of a peeled tangerine around the dendrite or shrubbery of a nerve cell, the nucleus of which is located in an eccentric off-center position peculiar to *Limulus* but irrelevant to the visual process. (Many neurologists believe, however, that the existence of the eccentric neuron means that the horseshoe crab's eye was also developed independently by evolution.) Now when the light reaction occurs (that is, the 11-*cis* retinal does its thing) something mysterious happens— exactly what we are not smart enough to know—that affects the dendrite of the nerve cell. The nerve cell develops a so-called electrical "generator potential" and, if this is large enough, the cell fires in the immemorial way of nerve fibers.[3] In the eyes of *Limulus*, as in all compound eyes, the activity of each facet is affected by the activation of its neighbors. (This was Hartline's fundamental discovery.) Mutual inhibition is brought about by the fact that the nerve fibers of each facet make synaptic contact with each other in a beltwork of fine connections behind the facets. When two neighboring facets are illuminated at the same

[3] One theory is that the act of production of all-*trans* retinal releases "transmitter substance" (like the materials that cross the cleft between nerve fibers in a synapse), thus profoundly changing the eccentric cell's membrane permeability.

time, each discharges fewer impulses than when one facet receives the same amount of light by itself. This applies to whole groups of facets. A more intensely lighted region of the compound retina exerts a stronger inhibiting effect on a less illuminated region than the latter does on the former. There is a clever reason for this. *Contrast* is heightened, and thus certain features of the retinal image—features that are important to the possessor of the eye—tend to be accentuated at the expense of the fidelity of representation. This is an immensely significant property of all really good eyes and goes to prove that the eye is not simply a passive optical instrument, like a camera, but is a purposive biological organ. The eye of an animal is designed by no means as an impersonal window to the universe but to detect such things as prey, mate and danger. (If we skip ahead for a moment to our own eyes we realize the importance of artificial contrast. Without the inhibitory accentuation which we share with *Limulus*, we would not be able to appreciate a cartoon or any drawing consisting merely of contours. Artists are thoroughly familiar with "border contrast" and may heighten it in their paintings.)

Compound eyes come in different sizes and the blueprints for their design are various. Two broad groups are differentiated: *apposition* eyes and *superposition* eyes. In the apposition eye the crystalline cone, or lens, is directly surrounded by pigment cells, while in the superposition eye the pigment cells are far from the cone, although attached by an optical thread or crystalline tract. In many crustaceans, such as crabs and lobsters, who have superposition compound eyes, migration of the pigment occurs under the influence of light (a hormone effect) and the facets are then isolated from each other optically. In the apposition eyes the image when formed in a single facet has no significance and with only one facet in operation the animal would not even detect the presence or absence of light.

In effect the compound eye, with its curious tangerine segments of retinular cells forming light tubes, has no obvious reason to be constructed the way it is, although the structure is nearly constant among huge classes, such as the insects. It may be, some have guessed, that this structure enables most possessors of compound eyes to detect the polarization of light. Perhaps we need to explain this matter of polarization. When a beam of sunlight is reflected off a bright surface, the reflected beam vibrates in one plane only—it is said to be "plane-polarized." The gleam of a water surface is polarized. But the rays of sunlight scattered by air molecules are also partly polarized and the amount of polarization varies throughout the sky. Different but predictable patterns of polarization are seen by the optically gifted as the sun moves along its path each day. If you take a piece of Polaroid film or a photographic polarizing filter and, while looking at the horizon through it, rotate your body around, you'll find that the sky darkens at right angles to the sun. This is an important thing to a small foraging animal, such as an ant or a bee, since with the ability to detect polarization, she has a sort of compass fix on her universe and a way of telling what time it is. Bees in fact can orient themselves and know which way the hive is if they can see only a small part of the sky. Mammals have no such ability and there is some doubt that birds do, in spite of their keen eyesight. In the ocean some marine arthropods guide themselves by the polarized light filtering down through the water. The sand hopper navigates by the polarized light of a waning day before switching to moonlight guidance during its inland wanderings among the dunes. In addition to the detection of polarization, many insects show that they have color vision by their behavior. Ants avoid violet light but seem not to distinguish red or orange from black. On the other hand both ants and bees are very sensitive to ultraviolet.

Thomas Eisner of Cornell University and his colleagues have shown how the world looks to a honeybee and to certain other insects by adding to an ordinary television camera (which by its nature picks up ultraviolet light) an ultraviolet transmitting lens. In looking through this instrument at a meadow in mixed bloom we suddenly are aware of the radiant cunning of flowers. Blossoms that looked banal and bashful now have ultraviolet-outlined nectar guides as blatant as a whore's paint. The meadow in garish bloom during daylight lures pollinators as the Ginza in Tokyo at night overpowers the imprudent tourist.

However, those few flowers that are pollinated by birds or bats do not of course exercise such general and specific ultraviolet seductions. Birds and bats are as blind as we are in the ultraviolet. A problem of strategy confronts certain animals with respect to ultraviolet camouflage. Should one hide from predators who cannot see ultraviolet or should one deceive insect prey who *can?* The crab spider has elected to hide from birds or lizards rather than to make herself invisible to bees—her chief diet. Although her visible color matches that of the floral heads upon which she stalks, her ultraviolet silhouette makes her conspicuous and terrible to a small insect so that the crab spider must make up in muscular blitzkrieg what she lacks inherently in hunting stealth.

Several differences in insects may show up only in the ultraviolet. In certain butterflies, for example, we ordinarily cannot tell a boy from a girl, but with the ultraviolet TV camera the difference is dazzlingly obvious. As usual, the male has more sexual paint.

Let us briefly note some other incidental features of compound eyes in the gigantic arthropod phylum. Not all of them are especially acute. The eyes of most male dayflies are different from those of the females (as is proper, since this male's only brief mission is to locate a female and impregnate her). His eyes are enormously enlarged and in some species are bipartite, so the insect has four instead of two compound eyes, called "turban eyes." They do not give him especially keen sight, but they do enable him to detect swift movements in the dusk. The male is aware vaguely of his surroundings and of the watchful swarming of his fellow males, but even in the dim light his eyes focus instantly on the flight of a female—a non-participant in the male swarm. The signal of femaleness is measured by zigzaggedness of flight. Since his turban eyes register only movement without any clear image of source, he may make a grotesque error and try to mate with another male breaking out of the swarm, or even with a flying insect of another species.

The splendid, ancient dragonfly is one of the only insects which has *rotating* compound eyes. His head is a sort of cockpit from which the eyes allow him to see on all sides. So compelling is his sense of vision that, as he consumes a victim in flight, he may drop the cadaver half consumed and swoop in a different direction after a new prey. The eye of the dragonfly has as many as 28,000 facets, the upper ones being fitted for distant vision and the lower ones for nearby vision. Although bionics scientists who would like to develop new optical instruments have always been interested in the dragonfly, he proves a little too complicated. The Radio Corporation of America, however, has invented a new radar device imitating the compound eye of the housefly. This instrument has a multi-element-phased array which produces simultaneous ability of "looking" from one direction to the other, as does the fly's compound eyes. Lacking such bionic equipment, even when two or more conventional radar sets are operated together for reinforcement, each separate set can still only report the presence of objects in one small segment at a time. It must search by successive sweeps of individual antennae through small and slow changes of azimuth and vertical deflection. RCA's new radar apparently gives scanning in all directions and simultaneous tracking of many targets.

There is another way in which any advanced fly's eyes are quantitatively different from ours. Movies and television are based on the principle of flicker-fusion in the human eye. When a number of closely similar images are flashed before our eyes, a critical speed of flashing is arrived at when the brain perceives no distinct flicker. Although the fly also experiences flicker-fusion, it is at a much higher rate of flicker than ours. Supposing that a fly were interested in a movie, he would see it as a distinct series of slides, like somebody's tedious projection of the still shots taken on a vacation trip to Mexico. Since the adjacent frames would be so similar to each other, however, the fly would probably go to sleep or die of boredom.

The color vision of insects is a matter of some importance to plant life. Originally European flowers did not develop red colors because the European bees were blind to red. On the other hand, hummingbirds are peculiarly sensitive to red and most of the flowers they pollinate, especially in tropical America, are red. There are no hummingbirds in Europe. Since most flying insects are *not* strongly attached to yellow, yellow light bulbs are often used in outdoor lights.

Some insects see quite differently from different regions of the compound eye. A horsefly behaves, for example, as if he wore bifocals. In the aquatic whirligig beetles (*Gyrinus*) the upper and lower parts of the compound eyes are actually separated. The upper part is designed for vision above the surface of the water and the lower for below the surface. The side part of the eye is dominant in most insects but not in the formidable praying mantis. The mantis follows the movement of a fly she is about to seize by two kinds of head movements: quick jerks or slow continuous turning, according to the fly's distance. In either case she is trying to keep the image near the center of her compound eyes. Since a crab or an insect cannot tell us if it has seen something, all conclusions are based on behavior. For example, crustaceans wave their antennae when they have recognized something and usually this is something that has moved. Form vision is sufficiently developed so that the individual can distinguish display from threat. (In other words, it can distinguish the messages "Hi" from "I'm going to pull your leg off.") One of the most popular laboratory procedures is putting a crustacean or an insect inside a cylindrical enclosure and then rotating a banded drum around the animal. In most cases, the creature will follow the rotating figures with its body. Since it will not respond to a black or white rotating drum, it is often possible to tell by its response or lack of response whether it has color vision or not, although one must be careful to avoid effects due to the perception of ultraviolet or polarized light. Some very advanced insects, such as the honeybee, can even detect a difference of *phase* in the rotating bands (for example, if a sequence of blue-green-black-yellow bands is changed to a sequence of blue-black-yellow-green). In the honeybee drone (the male), the receptor cells all have the same spectral sensitivity, peaking in the blue part of the spectrum, but in the worker (the sterile female), a much more subtle creature, there are at least two peaks of sensitivity, one in the ultraviolet and one in the green.

Perhaps the most astounding of all eye performances is that by which the honeybee worker transfers information about the distance and direction of a source of food into a so-called "waggle-dance" in the hive, in which the angle of the direction to the vertical of the main course of the dance signals the outside direction of the food source as measured from the direction of the sun, and in which the frequency of the waggles signals the distance. This honey-dance language, discovered by the Austrian Karl von Frisch, has been one of the most remarkable and highly publicized of all phenomena in the animal kingdom, yet there are signs that it may turn out to have been misinterpreted. Two Californian entomologists, Adrian M. Wenner and Dennis L. Johnson, have shown that it may be odor or sound that conveys the message. Let us review what the worker bee does on returning to the hive with a full belly. She makes a short run about twice her own length while *shaking* her nice full belly. At the end of the run she turns back to the starting point, then repeats the waggle run. The number of turns per unit depends on the distance of the food. The shorter the distance, the more runs. If the wagging run is directly downward, this is supposed to mean that the food is directly away from the sun; if directly upward, the food is directly toward the sun. If the wagging run is at an angle of 60 degrees left of the vertical, the food is to be found in a direction at 60 degrees to the left of the sun.

Now when all this is read in a textbook we visualize a lot of eager recruit bees standing around staring carefully at the motions of the full-bellied bee taking notes. Unfortunately a hive is not like that. It is a great mess of bees, as crowded as maggots in a piece of rotten meat, and furthermore the hive is pitch dark. There is a dance all right, but it can be followed only by the bees who are close enough to the forager with the full belly to follow her movements with their antennae. With rather compelling evidence, Adrian Wenner has presented a theory that the actual message is, in fact, conveyed by sound and we shall discuss this possibility more fully in Chapter 2.[4] Far from making the performance less remarkable, however, this would make it almost incredibly sophisticated. For there is hardly any doubt that the bee in her foraging *does* record in visual memory the location of the food, and if she reports this location in terms of the frequency of sound vibrations (as Wenner believes) then she is in effect *telling* what she has seen, using one modality— sound—to translate numerically another modality—sight. No other animal except man, carrying a compass, can do this. It is true that the noble dog, after little Agnes has fallen into the well, can come back and make a frantic hullabaloo, but as a signal this is no more significant than the return of a riderless horse. Suppose the dog, because of some incapacity, was unable to lead its master back to the well to rescue poor little Agnes? The bee, on the extremely unlikely assumption that she could interest herself in such matters, could report that Agnes is now located at 410 yards from here at a direction to the right of the sun of 26 degrees. If Agnes were a source of honey, every bee worker that heard (or saw) this statement would be descending upon Agnes within less than a minute.[5]

As a machine the bee is just too much for us. So far the bionics engineers who have interested themselves in the optical system of arthropods have been content to study less complex animals. In addition to the RCA radar device that simply records more data, in effect imitating the scope of the compound eye, the ability of this organ automatically to intensify contrasts has been roughly duplicated in an instrument developed by David

[4] As we shall see in that chapter, Wenner and his associates later abandoned even the sound-communication hypothesis. The history of biology is full of gallant theories destroyed by additional facts.

[5] Bees in different parts of the world appear to have different languages and dialects. In some cases, when a swarm is on the move, shutting up its hive for the winter, scout bees report back and appear often to disagree on where the swarm should go. These disagreements commonly end in a deadlock, with the cluster simply remaining on a limb of a tree and being killed by the frost.

Hildebrand of General Electric's Advanced Electronics Center. The numerous photoreceptive cells of this gadget influence each other just as we have seen in the case of the eye of *Limulus*. In Germany, years of studying a beetle's reaction to moving light patterns have convinced a team of entomologists, physicists, electrical engineers and mathematicians at the Max Planck Institute for Behavioral Physiology that a beetle in flight determines its speed by patterns seen in the environment. In this case, only two facets of the eye are necessary and a two-facet ground-speed indicator for airplanes was invented on this principle.

Some arthropods not only have compound eyes but use accessory eyes of a simpler sort for special purposes. For example, the crayfish has a pigment-cup (ocellus) kind of eye in its tail which it uses when it wants to back up into a dark crevice. (The operation of this organ has been of interest to IBM.) Only the short-lived male winged ants have ocelli, yet many day-flying insects lack them. The daily rhythm of cockroaches is apparently determined by their pigment cups, accessory eyes which may serve as an input stimulus to a neurosecretory (gland) system. The compound eyes of this ancient, mysterious insect are attuned to things that move and flicker, while the ocelli probably are able to measure automatically the total time spent in darkness. Many of the larval forms of arthropods have simple pigment-cup eyes on their sides, which then either disappear or migrate, usually to the back, upon metamorphosis. The primitive simple eye of the nauplius form of many crustaceans is often retained as an accessory eye in the adult, even when new, splendid compound eyes suddenly blossom.

Throughout the animal kingdom evolution has decided that living creatures, particularly the more helpless ones, should not only be able to see their predators, but should also have some means of avoiding being seen by them. A subtle extension of this principle is that if the animal is caught by the predator, this villain must remember the act of capture with horror and never attack such an animal again. Let us examine some of these techniques of evasion and of forced contrition. Many crustaceans can change colors by an act of will (or if this sounds too anthropomorphic, call it a conditioned reflex). The shrimp *Hippolyte varians* will rest upon either red or green seaweed and be invisible in either case. (One change that all shrimps, whether young or old or whatever their "everyday" color is, make every night is turning blue.) On the leaves of sea grass one can, with sufficient care, detect shrimps and isopods which follow in their bodies the seasonal change of the grass from green to brown. In the case of isopods we have, however, a noteworthy exception to the rule that the eye of the creature rules its changing coloration. The dark pigment spreads over the animal surface on a dark background and contracts on a white one, even if the eyes are covered or destroyed. This seems therefore to be a color conversion older than the eyes and older than the brain. The little amphipod *Hyperia galba* travels around attached to the umbrellas of jellyfish and in this condition is colorless. However, when it can find no jellyfish to bum a ride on, its color changes to yellowish or brown like the bottom of the sea. In an aquarium fitted with a choice of strips of colored paper, crabs will always choose the pieces most nearly approximating their own color. The coloration of the young green turtle suggests that of free-swimming deep-sea fishes, dark above and white below. Viewing it from below one finds it hard to see against the brightness of the sky, while from above its dark shape merges with deep water, hopefully to hide from carnivorous water birds.

Probably the most advanced animal still capable of changing its color is the dibranch cephalopod (octopus or squid). These vivid, complicated and rapid color changes come from the muscular expansion and contraction of pigment cells all through the top layer of skin and are made by direct command of the brain after conference with the eyes. The change of color to correspond with the background is thus an internal reflex. Unfortunately such animals are highly emotional and, like men, they express these emotions by color changes. They turn pale when frightened, flush a dark color when angered and such trans-

formations override the camouflaging reflex. An octopus would
be a very poor poker player.

Fishes, especially those subject to the scrutiny of bigger fishes,
have sophisticated color-change systems. The flat fish are especially adept and it may have something to do with the curious
typography of their eyes. *Sinistral* flat fishes, such as the turbot,
have both eyes on the left side, when swimming. *Dextral* fishes,
such as the halibut, flounder and plaice, have both eyes on the
right. Yet as fry (small hatchlings) all flat fishes have eyes on
each side of the head. One of the eyes (always the same one in
the same genus) travels, as the fish grows, all around the head
to join its companion. With the flat fish the color mimicry varies
according to the season and the environment. It is not exactly a
duplication of background color but, to use a painter's expression, it is *adaptation of values*. This tonality in the turbot is remarkable. Georges Pouchet, the French biologist, showed that a
blind turbot no longer reacts in this way and takes on a uniform
grayish color. Cutting the sympathetic nerve cord makes the fish
gray in the region serviced by this nerve. The pigmentary cells
of fishes or of animals with variable tonality are called "chromato-
phores." The pigment is concentrated in the center of the
cell but can spread, when the cell is nervously excited, through
the whole protoplasm. It is the pigment itself that spreads to the
limits of the cell under some rather cryptic kind of centrifugal
force, perhaps involving the formation of a streaming of protoplasm. How these color currents are controlled by the sympathetic nerve fibers is a question whose answer eludes us. It is certainly much more mysterious than our mechanism of blushing at
a dirty joke, where messages are given, not to the chromato-
phores, but to the blood capillaries. The plaice, when put in a
narrow tank, the bottom of which is half covered with charcoal
and half with chalk, will color itself half black and half white.
When the floor is covered with pebbles, the skin develops a
pebblework surface. This form of mimicry is purely protective
since the flat fish does not want to be spotted by a conger, a ray
or an angler fish. In many cases, however, the tonality of the
environment is adopted to fool the prey. This is the case with

aggressive predators such as the wrasse, the scorpion fish and the grouper.

Some fishes change color in a spectacular way when they die. The ancient Romans used to exploit the kaleidoscopic display of dying mullet to give an edge to their appetites. At posh banquets the jet-set hosts would have the still-living mullet brought in, swimming around in a crystal vase. The water would be removed and the mullet left to gasp their lives out, while the guests slaveringly watched the patches of red, ocher, green iridescing under the pearly skin until finally, pale in death, the fishes were returned to the kitchen. Even Seneca disapproved of this. He said, "Now the orgy of tongue, teeth and belly is not enough. They are now gourmets with their eyes."

One of the most concrete examples we know of adaptive evolution is seen in the phenomenon known rather pompously as "industrial melanism." This is when insects, such as moths, change to black in order to match the changing hues of air pollutants. As a result of the Industrial Revolution in England vast quantities of soft coal soot settled in the wooded areas around cities, killing the light-colored lichens which used to cover the tree trunks, thus blackening the bark. In Darwin's day a few of the moths that frequented these areas had black wings, now almost all of them do. Quantitative experiments by H. B. D. Kettlewell have shown that where the trees were still lichen-covered, the birds found and ate at least three times as many black moths as those with peppered wings. In woods where the tree trunks were black with soot, the results were precisely reversed. The black-winged forms originate by gene mutation—an exquisite example of natural selection in action in a sequence of about fifty generations.

However, there is another color mechanism by which insects, especially butterflies, can protect their race if not their own lives. This is to develop a highly noticeable color, usually white, which is perceived even by color-blind predators, and then to make oneself so nasty to eat that the creature that has swallowed one will never forget it. Usually this taste is due to a bitter plant alkaloid, or it may be histamine, developed internally. Experiments with feeding such unpalatable species to ducks show that the memory of this awful taste caused the ducks to avoid any white butterflies through the rest of their lives. (The white butterfly *Pieris* is hardly ever attacked by any predator.) Other edible insects take advantage of this heroic martyrdom to imitate the colors of the poisonous or evil-tasting forms. (These are known as "Batesian mimics.") Obviously this is the same evolutionary psychology that is used by the honeybee, who dies as she stings but impresses her predator with the fact that honeybees are not to be attacked with impunity. (Unfortunately some attackers, such as bears, are not in the least impressed.)

In many cases the colors of animals seem to have little significance, except the obvious one of sexual attraction or the related one of intimidation of rivals of the same species. When you see plain-colored fishes and fishes of the same genus that look like Spanish posters, the chances are very good that the plain ones are timorous schooling fishes and the poster-colored ones are fierce owners of territory. The coral fish is poster-colored in youth and dull-colored at sexual maturity, a curious inversion that shows up in behavior, since the young ones, both male and female, are ferocious adherents of the "territorial imperative" and apparently divest themselves of their terrifyingly lovely color and of their wild temper in order to make possible a friendly contact between the sexes. The fact that such behavior is observed far from rarely in the animal kingdom must give us pause before we accept broad and implacable rules based on a supposed master instinct for the defense or acquisition of territory. But what is one to think of the most gorgeous colors seen among animals, those of the mollusks? What are the wonderful, intricately filagreed, delicately hued shells of some pelecypods for? Why not just a plain sand-colored shell, like a clam, with no classical sculptured flourishes? Is it significant that the scallop with a row of jeweled eyes also has a shell with fancy frills? Or, still more puzzling, consider the radiantly pulsing rainbows of the mantles of certain mollusks *inside* the shell, only to be seen when a brutal predator gorges himself or when a philosophic malacologist excavates such beauty, hidden otherwise more securely from the observing universe than any flower "born to blush unseen." (After all the flower is *not* unseen. Whether in a desert or an impenetrable forest, it is an object of intense and businesslike interest on the part of the color-conscious compound eyes of hordes of flying insects. In fact, the flower was born for this attention and not for the edification of romantic poets.)

The questions raised are at present insoluble but the future answers are more likely to be chemical than esthetic. Perhaps, just as an oyster manufactures a pearl consisting of nacreous calcium carbonate to cure a lesion, the other lovely hues may be based on the behavior of molecules containing copper, iron or vanadium, which the mollusk requires to make a living and which tends toward beauty, just as the march of light through inorganic aerosols tends toward the glory of the setting sun. Still one must admit that many members of the huge and alien phylum of *Mollusca* have eyes and can see each other. Here we are far away from the arthropods, and the compound eye is not even considered as a possibility. Probably all pelecypods (clams, oysters, etc.) have at least light-sensitive cells at the ends of their siphons. The eyes of the scallop (*Pecten maximus*) are about sixty in number, each about one millimeter in diameter, and peep out on the edge of the mantle. Each eye has a lens and a retina, but behind the retina there is an accurately spherical, highly reflecting layer, the argenteum. This reflects an image onto the outmost layer of the retina, which is concentric with the reflecting mirror and is composed of cells with fibers connecting to the optic nerve. There is a separate inner layer of retinal cells. The optical system is thus a highly sophisticated combination of a concave mirror and a lens of long focal length (as if designed by an astronomer). Probably the fine resolution is limited to the central region of the retina. This may be why *Pecten* has so many eyes, which can scan some 300 degrees of its surroundings. It is significant that the retina is inverted (that is, the light-sensitive nervous structures point *away* from the source of light) and that this is the case in all vertebrates, including man. That a practically immobile mollusk can develop an eye so similar in this respect to that of a member of another wholly dissimilar phylum is one of those cases of "convergent evolution" that at one time served as one of the talking points of so many lectures and books by philosophers such as Henri Bergson. Bergson, like George Bernard Shaw, believed in "creative evolution," that is, in the notion that animals create, by a sort of inner urgency, the organs that they need, rather than falling heir to them as a result of random shuffles of the genes. Since there are only so many ways to trap light and to take account of it, Bergson argued that the scallop simply wished harder than other pelecypod mollusks and therefore attained sixty clever eyes. The fact of the matter is, however, that the scallop does not make very good use of his eyes and is not an exceptionally successful animal. It is always possible, of course, that hundreds and hundreds of millions of years ago the scallop was a pretty big operator and that he found things too easy and relapsed into degeneracy. However, the absolutely whimsical way in which evolution has distributed good eyes to one genus or species and denied them to their close relatives, who presumably could wish just as hard during a billion years, argues against the doctrines of Bergson and Shaw. It is certainly true, nevertheless, that there *are* only so many ways to trap light biologically and, in fact, there is only one that we know of and have already discussed. There are many ways in which the trapped light can yield nervous repercussions.

The double retina of the scallop is especially interesting in that the nerve from the innermost retina carries impulse bursts at the onset of illumination while the outer retina only responds when the light is turned down. Such "off-receptors" are otherwise known only in vertebrates. *Pecten* gives a response to only 0.3 per cent decrease in light intensity, which is probably more than you can detect. The optical nerve fibers in *Pecten* go to his "stomach brain" rather than to the so-called "cerebral ganglion," which may explain why the scallop spends most of his time staring, in wait for a change of light indicating that it is time to eat or defecate. However it must be admitted that for a shellfish *Pecten* is a good swimmer and some of his eyes may be useful in nautical maneuvers. Something rather similar to the lateral-inhibitions effect in compound eyes can be detected. If you put a scallop in the test cylinder and try the revolving drum trick that has taught us so much about the optical systems of arthropods, he will respond by turning *some* of his eyes to follow an eight-striped pattern, but in order to get this response most of the edge of the mantle has to be blocked off by a screen. What this seems to mean is that, faced with a socially meaningless movement, some of the eyes tell the others to pay no attention and thus when all eyes are uncovered the fully visible drum is ignored. The central nervous system in this animal has no effect on regeneration of lost or damaged eyes, possibly because the optical nerves go to the stomach ganglion, which is not so much like a gland as is a brain in the "head."

The eyes of advanced mollusks such as the octopus and squid are in many ways similar and even superior to those of the higher vertebrates. We find a transparent cornea over the front, a pigmented iris, a spheroid crystalline lens, a large vitreous chamber behind it and a retina. There is even a cartilaginous sclerotic coat as in birds. The eye is accommodated to distance by sensitive and complex muscle systems. The appreciable difference is that the retina is *not* inverted. With two-eyed creatures such as these, capable of learning, we meet with one of the strangest and least understood of all evolution's puzzles— the crossing over of the nerve fiber from the right eye to the left side of the brain and vice versa. In the octopus and squid this cross-over is only partial, as it is in mammals. Discrimination and tricks learned by one eye are, however, promptly transferred to both optic lobes of the cephalopod brain, since the trick is not forgotten even if the optic lobe of the trained side is removed.

As we ascend the various stages of the creatures of the vertebrate phylum we see only minor changes in eye structure from fish to man, but we also see some fundamental distinctions in the way the optical information is routed to and used by the brain.

Fishes tend to be nearsighted and there is a good excuse for·

this, since the water is more often turbid than not. If we lived in a world of continuous heavy fog we should be nearsighted—and as a matter of fact we usually are, but for other reasons. What myopia means in mechanical terms is that the lens structures of the eye are more or less frozen into spherical shape and cannot accommodate by flattening out. In order to develop far-sightedness the spherical lenses had to be flattened, reduced in size and moved back from the cornea in order to focus a long-distance object accurately on the retina. Certain fishes have adipose eyelids in which a cartilaginous growth partly covers the eye and contains a small circular opening for light. More primitive types, such as sharks, have the same kind of eyelid as a frog—a nictitating membrane that goes up from the lower part of the eye, like a curtain. In the abysmal depths of the oceans one usually finds fishes with radiating organs to light their way, but the grenadiers, or rattails, which feed on the luminous fishes rely solely on their eyes. They follow the moving lights and swallow them. The eyes of the family of Giganturidae are telescopic, attached to the front end of protruding cylinders which can be directed forward and upward, like the stalked eyes of a crab. The eyes of fishes that have almost decided to spend their time out of the water are naturally rather ambiguous in nature. The skipping gobies, for example, have gone so far as to develop aerial vision and one of them (*Periophthalmus*) has perhaps the most grotesquely versatile pair of eyes known. With one eye he can look upward while with the other he scans the terrain by partly rotating the eye as a periscope turns in a conning tower. The skipping gobies have unfortunately forgotten how to hear, at least on land, since you can put a gunshot close enough to spatter them with mud without in the slightest degree disturbing their foolish gambols. Two kinds of fishes, *Dialommus fuscus*, one of the blenny family, and *Anableps* are loosely called "four-eyed." Actually they have only one pair of eyes, but each eye is divided into two distinct units, one for seeing in air, the other in water, and at the surface both can function simultaneously. The lower pupil is shielded by the double shade formed by the projecting parts of the iris and can be expanded and contracted to cut out surface reflections from above, which might otherwise blind the fish or obstruct its view in water.[6]

There seems to be no doubt that many fishes have color vision and practically all fishes, with or without perception of color, seem to be attracted to bright lights. The fishermen in the Sea of Galilee used torches to attract fishes to their boats at night. The commercial herring fishermen on Puget Sound use mercury vapor lamps. The herring sleep on the bottom during daylight, so fishing is done after dark when they rise to the surface to feed. A startling new lure, consisting of a phosphorescent plastic worm or some other tempting form, has been commercialized for sports fishermen and appears to be highly successful, although its use is banned in certain states. Nigel Daw has taken advantage of the color response of the goldfish to study the actions of separate nervous cells in the ganglion behind the retina. Certain cells respond to contrasts between red and green in the field of vision. However, other cells will only respond when the whole field is first red, then changed over to green or vice versa. Since the response of *individual* cells to the simultaneous contrast of red and green is also noted in nerve fibers in the monkey, this is a kind of optical cell that seems to be common in every color-conscious vertebrate.

Now we must emphasize that in all vertebrate eyes there is a principle which pervades the whole system in the same way that it was shown to do in the case of the compound eye—the principle of lateral inhibition. In the vertebrate retina there are outgoing fibers that pass along the optic nerve to modify the response. There are also intraretinal circuits that depress elements around a strongly stimulated spot. The advantage of this for purposes of contrast and for focusing attention is obvious. A change in sensitivity activates the whole organism for predation or for flight. But for an animal who wants to know

[6] It should be noted that certain birds, such as the penguin, have almost reverted to the life of a fish. They spend so much time under water that they are notoriously myopic on land, to which they must return to nest.

about the world, the accuracy with which the central nervous system is informed depends on whether it "knows" by how much it has changed the sensitivity. If you don't have this information, as a man you may see ghosts; as a frog, you may starve with dead flies all around you.

The frog is, in fact, a famous case and his optical system has been not only intensely studied but imitated in electronic devices. In the laboratory of Dr. Jerome Y. Lettvin of MIT a series of crucial experiments were started in 1959 on the optic nerve of the leopard frog (*Rana pipiens*) in which the nerve fibers were "tapped" and the frog's responses to various images projected on a screen were recorded in the most minute detail. The investigators concluded that the frog's eye language is a classification scheme. There are cells that are edge detectors, convexity detectors and cells that respond only to the motion of little dark spots, that is to say, "bugginess" detectors. The frog will jump at an insect only if it moves. As we have said, he will starve to death in a cage filled with dead flies, because his bug-detector has been set only to fire in the biologically normal case of a *moving* fly. One type of optic fiber responds only to the sudden darkening of the frog's whole field of vision, such as might happen when a hawk swoops down upon him. Another fiber notices only the edge of an object. In the tectum (or optical brain) of the frog the images are projected to four thin layers of nerve cells. The top layer is the contrast, or edge, fiber. The next is the bug-detector layer, followed by the motion layer and the dimness layer.

It must be emphasized that in the frog eye, as in all vertebrate eyes, there is a kind of funneling process in which a number of nerve fibers pass from the retinal cells to a relay layer called the "bipolar cells," then to a still smaller number of ganglia cells which then proceed to hook up with the optic nerves on their way to the central nervous system centers. Thus there are many more light receptor cells in the retina than fibers in the optic nerve. The retina is more filter than photographic film. In the frog (and as later proved, in other lower vertebrates such as the pigeon and even the rabbit and the ground squirrel)

the sorting and discrimination is done in the retinal system rather·
than in the brain. The eye itself decides what is important, what
should be played up by the method of lateral inhibition, what
should be ignored. Each fiber reports not simply whether illumination is present but whether some rather complex situation
—such as the appearance of a bug—exists in a given part of the
visual field. On reaching the optic tectum in the brain, the optic
fibers project a *selective* map of reality, the fibers of the
tectum being arranged, as mentioned, in layers. But not all the
optic fibers go to the tectum. W. R. A. Muntz of the University
of Oxford found that some go instead to a secondary visual
center in the back of the thalamus. This system is the forerunner
of the internal visual system in higher animals, including man.
(In man the tectal network is small and trivial. Most of the
fibers go to the so-called "lateral geniculate nucleus" of the
back of the thalamus before being relayed on to the cerebral
cortex.) Muntz found that all the optic fibers in the frog's
thalamus were sensitive to the onset of illumination ("on"
signal) and to no other stimulus. But they are not only sensitive
to the presence or absence of light but to the *color* of the
light; and most strongly to blue. Why should this be? It is
understandable when you imagine yourself as a frog. He lives
near a pond, but is surrounded by green vegetation. When he
is attacked, his best bet is to jump for the pond over which the
blue sky has more chance to shine. These are the little built-in
panic buttons that evolution has made handy for the small and
the helpless. So sharp indeed is the frog's preference for blue
as compared to the neighboring green of the spectrum that his
thalamus responds much more strongly to pure dim blue than·
to a bright unsaturated green that actually contains more blue
wave energy than the dim blue.[7]

In making an electric replica of the frog's eye M. B. Herschner
and his associates at RCA were not interested in that part of

[7] An unsaturated color is reflected light containing all wave lengths
but peaking slightly at the dominant wave length of the apparent color.
Thus the light from a dazzling green dress may actually contain more
blue energy than the light from a faraway bluebird.

the frog's optical equipment that urged him to jump into the pond. What fascinated them was the single-minded properties of abstraction of the retina and its back-up neural shrubbery that made the frog concentrate on a moving bug. This is the kind of brooding sentinel that defense departments need to cut down the costs of vigilance—an automatic eye that is on the look-out for just one patterned thing. The very large RCA model (including over 32,000 individual circuits) duplicates in a rough way the anatomy of the various neural layers of the frog's optical system. Since the frog's optic ganglion cells are sensitive to both speed and size of the image, this sensitivity was incorporated in the model.

Note also a further distinction. A fly is important to a frog, but a fly traveling away from the frog is not. The eye automatically discards this information and the frog's brain never sees the departing fly. A *sudden* shadow may be important. The frog's retina tells this to the brain. But the frog learns nothing from the shadow of a cloud leisurely crossing the sun, even though the eye sees it.

The RCA model of the frog's eye similarly abstracts such features from the scene before it, beginning with 1,600 photocells in the first layer. Red lights on the final panel beneath five layers of screening and processing circuits show edges, green lights show the moving convexities or corners which the "eye" decided were going in the right direction to merit attention, yellow lights show the leading and trailing edges of such a moving object and white lights show the effects of quick dimming from the hawk or the Russian missile swooping down. Instead of the conventional computer logic, the frog's eye model uses "neuron logic," which is of the voting type. A majority of circuit components expresses opinion about what is seen, and whether it is worth putting up on the display board. Also this is the first electronic optical instrument that works by parallel processing instead of serial processing. This is an important distinction that separates the television principle, for example, from the way the biological eye works. A TV camera breaks up a picture into lines strung out end-for-end in relation

to time. It is only because it works so fast that it is able to con
you into believing you are seeing all these things in "real time"
(that is, simultaneously). In this sense there is no such thing as
a "live" TV picture. This is serial processing. However, if you
look at a small square on a piece of paper, information about
its corners, sides, thickness and color reaches your brain at the
same time and through different receptors and different nerve
fibers. There is no scanning and no waiting. This is parallel
processing.

Although reptiles are regarded as a step upward in evolution
from amphibians such as the frog, the reptile whose eyesight
has been most urgently studied, the sea turtle, was originally
a land animal who returned to the sea. Thus, like the penguin,
his eyes do not work especially acutely in comparison with
those of terrestrial birds which are designed to work on light
rays in the air. However, it had been hoped by studying the
sea turtle's ocular system to learn something about this animal's
extraordinary gifts of navigation and, as a hatchling just out of
the egg, to waddle unerringly toward the ocean. The water-
finding process seems to be the same in marine and fresh-water-
species and all studies indicate that the main sense is sight,
that there is some quality or quantity of light over the water
that leads the hatchlings in the right direction. They can find
the sea by day or at night, in all weather except extremely
heavy rain, with the moon or the sun hidden or shining brightly
in any part of the sky. One thinks immediately of polarized
light, since the reflected light from water is always in this
condition, whether it reflects the moon or the sun. David
Ehrenfeld of the University of Florida tested this possibility
by putting spectacles containing depolarizing filters on turtles,
but this made no difference at all. This is not the way they
find the water. Ehrenfeld used various filters in the spectacles to
find out which color of the spectrum was most effective. It
appeared to be mainly green. Filters that allowed the turtles
to perceive only blue caused a little trouble but not much.
However, when the turtle could see only red, he meandered
around in a confused way and took a long time to reach the

water. Nicholas Mrosovsky, a British psychologist, working on the beach with powerful colored lights gave baby turtles a choice between heading in the direction of the sea or turning at right angles to it to go toward the lights. He found that the blue and green light could compete with the light from the sea in attracting the hatchlings. From other experiments it seems that whatever the guidepost may be it is not high in the sky, but low over the horizon, since the hatchlings do not raise their eyes to the sky.

As to the incredible navigating ability of turtles on the open sea, Ehrenfeld and Arthur Koch, in a general study of the eyesight of both fresh-water and marine turtles as well as tortoises, have made it seem impossible that eyesight has anything to do with the uncanny accuracy with which mating green turtles, for instance, return for nesting to Ascension Island from the shores of Brazil. Fresh-water turtles, because they have very well-developed ciliary and iris muscles and a highly flexible lens, are able to accommodate their eyes over a wide range and they see very well in both air and water. Tortoises on the other hand, like humans, cannot overcome the loss of corneal refraction under water, although they see excellently in the air. The great sea reptiles, such as the green turtle and the hawksbill turtle are very handicapped in seeing through the air. The ciliary muscles do not even connect directly with the body of the lens and there is no apparent way in which they can accommodate the iris. Navigation by the stars now seems utterly impossible for them. They probably cannot even see the stars when they are swimming on the surface. Theoretically they might be supposed to see the stars, when submerged, but this also seems unlikely except in exceedingly calm water—a condition that practically never occurs, at least during the period of their exact, two-thousand-mile odysseys. We shall re-examine this exasperating problem in connection with other famous navigators of the animal world in Chapter 5.

The eyes of other reptiles are of special interest only insofar as they foreshadow the remarkable eyes of their descendants—the birds. Snakes stare at you unblinking, because they have no way to blink. They have no eyelids. The eye is permanently protected by a transparent cap which is shed periodically along with the skin.[8] Instead of the glassy eye of the snake, lizards have a variety of eye curtains. The lizards may look out between well-developed lids, the lower ones being movable. They may peek through a transparent disk in a fixed lower lid. They may stare like a snake through a permanent transparent covering of the whole eye or, in specialized burrowers, they may peer through beetling scales which all but shut out the light.

In general design, the bird's eye resembles that of a lizard, as it should, but it has been glorified and superstructured beyond a lizard's imagining. A lizard of the same weight as a perching bird has a brain only one-tenth as big, and most of the bird's brain is concerned with its specialties—flying and seeing. Furthermore, the avian optical apparatus does not vary very much in fundamental anatomy throughout the whole gigantic class. In all birds, without exception, there is complete cross-over of the optic nerves, one of the features that prevent most birds from having stereoscopic vision. For their purposes, they do not need it. Birds have very large eyes. Hawks, eagles and owls often have eyes larger than a man's. The ratio of eye weight to head weight is less than 1 per cent in a man, while it is 15 per cent. in a starling. The eyes are indeed so large that the sockets meet in the middle of the skull. Most birds have strange powers of near-and-far accommodation, but to tell the truth we do not know for sure how this accommodation is brought about. Ciliary muscles apparently act on the sclerotic ring surrounding the cornea and on the so-called "annular pad" to bring pressure on the lens and thus change its shape. (In the human eye the ciliary muscles act to release a stretching tension on the lens, allowing the elasticity of the lens itself to determine its shape. This is not a very trustworthy mechanism, as too many of us know.)

[8] The foolish notion that snakes can hypnotize their prey is probably a literary deduction from their unblinking stare. That the same "hypnotic" effect could probably be exerted on neurotic humans by a toy snake with buttons for eyes was suggested in a famous short story by Ambrose Bierce.

Nocturnal birds, such as the owl, usually have tubular-shaped eyes and the retina is full of rods (light-detecting pigment cells) rather than cones (which are specialized for daytime color vision). Owls in fact are unable to focus their eyes on close objects. They must back away from any food offered them in order to fix it sharply before they pounce.

Two notable features of the eyes of most birds are the pitlike fovea (center of the retina, such as we have in less exaggerated form) and the pecten, about which we shall have more to say later. The steep sides of the fovea magnify extremely slight movements of the image. But for light from a point source to reach into such a narrow pit, the eye has to be turned *exactly* toward the source. This very deep fovea is characteristic of hawks, kingfishers and other birds of prey. The density of cones in daytime birds is far greater than in man and in the fovea of hawks and of the European buzzard it reaches the incredible number of one million per square millimeter. (This is the area covered by a small o in newsprint.) Condors and vultures incidentally have, like all birds, little or no sense of smell so their perceptions of the deadness of a body is pure optical deduction.[9]

Some birds that need especially sharp eyesight to catch flying insects on the wing (for example, purple martins) have a second, temporarily placed fovea in each eye to provide binocular vision. Many birds (hawks, eagles, ducks, shore birds) have a horizontal streak or central area across the retina, usually for a fovea at each end. This allows sharp economical scanning of the horizon without eye or neck movements. In many daytime birds of prey the sensory cells are more numerous in the upper hemisphere of the eye (which perceives images on the ground) than in the lower hemisphere (which views the sky). The goshawk, when it wants a good look at the sky to see whether a rival

[9] Conservationists, trying to attract the attention of the rare and disappearing California condor, have been known to put on a "ham-actor" show of having a heart attack, clutching the air and falling on the ground. If the condor is anywhere in the vicinity, he will sail down to investigate this promising pantomime.

or a mate is in sight, inverts its head over its back or down near its belly, so that it can use the more acute upper part of its retina. Even birds that have no pronounced foveas, such as barnyard chickens and doves, make a brave attempt to keep a steady flow of visual information coming in by accompanying each walking step with a sudden forward jerk of the head. The head then remains fixed in space as the body moves forward until the end of the step. This gives sharper vision since the moving head cannot see important moving objects, such as the lurk of a fox, as clearly as a head fixed even temporarily in space. If you watch perching birds on a waving twig or a telephone wire you will have noted that, as they sway, they twist so as to keep the head and therefore the eyesight relatively stable.

Many shore birds, although clearly their eyes are not designed for binocular vision since the eyes are located too far apart, manage to achieve a sort of distance discrimination by manipulating the head. This is the reason sandpipers, for example, continually bob their heads up and down. Raising and lowering the head quickly causes the object viewed to shift its relative position against the horizon, which enables the bird to judge its distance. The parrot can achieve a certain stereoscopic effect by cocking its head and looking at the same object from two slightly different angles. Cocking the head is surely one of the most ancient of vertebrate official gestures, since even in advanced mammals, such as dogs and men who have stereoscopic vision, one sees the quizzical cocking, which in these animals is usually a reflex no longer expressing the need for a better look but for a better understanding of what is seen or heard. When a woman cocks her head, it is usually to express some such feeling as "Oh, these men! What next?"

In precocial birds (who are ready for action immediately after hatching), such as domestic chicks, it is found that not only is form vision well developed but the preference for things to peck at is logical. Refuting John Locke's naïve notion that the brain at birth starts out as a blank slate, Robert Fantz has shown that newborn chicks, presented with eight different-shaped objects will peck ten times as often at an object that is roughly spherical, about the size of grain or seeds, than at forms with no resemblance to the things chickens have eaten from the beginning of the species. (As we shall mention later, Fantz also found certain preferences in the things that very young babies prefer to look at.) Built-in form perception in baby birds is also dramatically illustrated by the panic that is aroused by the moving silhouette of a paper goose flying *backward,* in which case the goose's head looks like the tail of a hawk. If the paper silhouette moves forward the chicks show no concern.

We have mentioned the optical novelty in birds' eyes called the "pecten." This is a heavily pigmented, vascular, comblike projection which fingers out into the vitreous chamber from the retina at the point where the optic nerve leaves the eye. There have been more fist fights among stout-hearted ornithologists about what the pecten is good for than there have been brawls between biologists and Southern Baptists. The most plausible theory (to me, anyway) is that in some way the pecten makes possible the detection of extremely minute movements within the field of vision. Hawks, which detect the motion of mice obscurely scrabbling around in the grass a thousand feet below them, have particularly well developed pectens. It has recently been suggested that the pecten enables birds to determine the position of the sun in the sky, thus possibly contributing to the almost magical gifts that some birds have for precision world travel. Conservative sages of ornithology, such as Joel Carl Welty, will admit that of some thirty theories about the pecten, the only one that has solid proof is that it helps in the nourishment of the eye by diffusion of substances through the vitreous body.

In diving birds, such as certain ducks, loons and auks, there is a third eyelid, or nictitans, which in its center has a clear lens-shaped window of high refractive index that serves the bird under water as a "contact lens." This membrane has on its margin a fold so slanted that it cleans the under surface of the eyelids on the reverse journey of each sweep, working like a windshield wiper. Although the majority of birds close their eyes, like lizards, by moving the bottom eyelid upward, there are some dissenters, such as owls, parrots, wrens and ostriches, who use the top lid. Owls in fact use the upper lids. to wink and the lower lids to close the eyes in sleep. The acuity of night vision of an owl can be appreciated if one realizes that an owl can see its prey at a distance of six feet or more under an illumination of only seven ten-millionths of a foot candle. A man needs a hundred times this much light to see his hand in front of his face. Unlike snakes, however, no. bird appears to respond to infrared (heat radiation).

Another puzzling novelty in the bird's eye is oil droplets, one droplet for each cone in the retina. Daytime birds have droplets of various colors (red, orange, green, etc.) Crepuscular or nocturnal birds have colorless or pale yellow oil droplets. Presumably these are chemical filters of some sort that serve to increase contrast and contour. For example, if a red insect in green foliage is scanned by a bird having red oil droplets in some of its cone cells, the image of the insect will blink on and off as it sweeps across the cones that do or do not have red oil droplets, so that the message "red insect" becomes more positive. The droplets may also act as haze-piercing camera filters do, by holding back some of the glaring short wave lengths. By adopting a checkerboard sort of red filter, birds can probably see farther in hazy weather. Most of this is speculation, since although we are a highly eye-minded race of animals, we cannot pretend to have solved all the secrets of the marvelous avian eye.

A valiant attempt has been made, nevertheless, to simulate the eye of one of the simpler birds, the pigeon. (We shall see later that this animal is by no means so simple as was once assumed.) What appealed to the bionics experts of Douglas Astropower Laboratory was that the pigeon's eye, like that of the frog, is a pre-processing machine, but where the frog's eye rejects the outward motion of a fly, the pigeon eye follows. closely any directional movement. As modified into a radar device, this kind of eye would be splendid for detecting aircraft flying in a single direction, perhaps inbound. In the Douglas pigeon-eye machine the first three layers, representing the retina, consist of an outer layer of photodiodes simulating the bird's cones. These, as in the eye itself, convert light images into electrochemical potentials which feed the intermediate layer of bipolar cells, which in turn feed to a third layer of ganglion cells of the retina, then to the artificial optic nerve and the artificial brain. The actual electronic circuitry employed by Douglas is too involved to describe here, yet one can imagine the frustration felt by bionics people when R. J. Herrnstein of Harvard and D. H. Loveland of the General Atomics Corporation discovered that, far from being a mere detector of motions, the pigeon can be trained to be a sophisticated *people-detector*. In this case pigeons were taught by the usual food-award system to select photographs containing people and to reject photographs of the same background which did not contain people. The pigeons sometimes pecked when they should not, but this very significantly was only when the pictures contained, instead of people, objects which might be called "people objects," such as automobiles, boats and houses. It is quite obvious that in these crucial tests the pigeons had learned to conceptualize. They had, so to speak, learned to read. Ordinarily humans are said to "conceptualize" and animals to "discriminate." But "discriminating" between a picture of some trees and various pictures containing people by the trees in all manner of clothes, postures, sexes, ages and sizes, is something else again.. There is no movement involved—simply static images. By the bird, man has been conceptualized as a kind of complicated and various thing, man even in a skirt, man even in miniature and naked, man even in a topcoat and wearing a beard. This is a visual brain accomplishment comparable to the ability of a human being to pick out a friend's face in a crowd. It is impossible to teach a dog or a cat to recognize a picture of anything. This is not to criticize the intelligence of these good animals, but simply to emphasize the unexpected virtuosity of the eye-minded bird—even so humble and ridiculed a bird as the mooching pigeon.[10]

What we ordinarily think of in terms of bird vision is the gay and constant way in which mating birds recognize their own species. In such birds as gulls, for instance, several species that flock on the same beach are almost indistinguishable by an amateur. They differ only in eye-ring color. The female in choosing a mate invariably chooses one with the right eye-ring color, meaning the same as her own, the eye-ring color of the species. But how does she know what her eye-ring color is? Since she is not given to examining herself in the mirror of a stagnant beach pool, it must be assumed that she was "imprinted" on her parents and recognizes a potential mate only as one that is male and looks like her parents. Such a color-fixation is one of the reasons why birds so seldom hybridize and why species differentiation and evolution itself is so insistent among birds.

The extreme color consciousness of daytime birds is also reflected in the way some of them choose soil to live on that matches their plumage. Some birds even lay eggs colored to suit the soil. The widely scattered lapwing only on the Malabar Coast lays reddish eggs with dark brown specks to match the red laterite soil. Some birds have an almost frenzied fixation of certain colors. The satin bowerbirds of the South Pacific will steal anything that is blue. As a burglar he enters the complicated bower of a rival and tears down beakfuls of the walls and strews them around. If disturbed by the return of the owner he snatches up a beakful of blue feathers or blue glass as he flees from righteous wrath.

Mammals differ from all other vertebrates—from hagfish to eagles—in regard to what happens to the optic nerve fibers at the optic crossing (or chiasma). Everywhere except in mam-

[10] This kind of scanning and interpretative power could be most useful in missile warfare, as many military technologists have recognized. If, for example, you put a bird in the cockpit of an unmanned airplane or missile, conceivably he could be taught to recognize a city or a ship and, by pecking a button, could zero in as an avian kamikaze.

mals there is total cross-over, that is, all the nerve fibers from
the retinal ganglion layer of the right eye cross over to the
left side of the brain, and all the fibers from the left eye cross
over to the right side. In mammals only those fibers of the
retina nearest to the nose cross. Thus in man the fibers from the
right half of each retina reach the tectum of the right optic lobe.
Objects to the left of the field of vision (since they send light to
the left half of each retina) stimulate the visual centers in the
right optic lobe and vice versa. It is one of the many mysteries in
neurology as to why this partial cross-over was adopted in
mammals. That it must have something to do with binocular
vision is suggested by the fact that more and more fibers cross
over as binocular vision becomes more important to the animal.
Rabbits, for example, have only a small amount of overlap in
the fields of vision of the two eyes and a correspondingly
small number of fibers that cross over. However, there are
sharp-eyed birds such as the owl who do have binocular vision
and there are fishes with binocular vision, and in all these
animals the cross-over is still total. Perhaps we simply have to
admit that the mammal is a peculiar animal. For the most part
his early history concentrated upon a *smell*-brain, and the eyes
were only rough accessories for the nose. Until we get to the
primates, very few mammals are capable even of color vision.
The bull does not know red from blue.

In some mammals the eye has actually become a sort of
residual organ. The common and Western moles for example,
are all but blind. The eyelids have grown together over degenerate eyeballs and the creatures can only distinguish light
from darkness. In spite of popular opinion, not all bats have
poor eyesight. The semitropical bats of Trinidad use echo-
location in familiar territory, but when they migrate, after seven
hundred miles, they use visual landmarks and perhaps even sun,
moon or stars like certain birds. Even before we reach the eye
of the primate, we see some mammals operating on the ground
with exceptional vision. Deer may not be able to read a news-
paper or in fact make out the nature of a stationary object but
the slightest movement is detected at once. Their big reproach-

ful eyes are effective earlier in the morning and later in the evening than human eyes. Their relatives the antelope have a most interesting method of signaling an alert through a widely scattered herd. When aroused, twin white disks on the buttocks serve as heliographs. The reflex to the alarm causes a contraction of special muscles and multitudes of white hairs at the rear rise instantly. Simultaneously, as the rump signal is flashed, a strong musky scent is released from a set of twin glands located in the rump. Other antelope may see this warning a couple of miles away. They repeat with the buttocks flash and the warning is spread. Even antelope fawns a few hours old erect their brownish not-yet-white little rosettes. The large antelope jack rabbit of the Southwest also makes a rump signal. The white hairs bristle, reflecting more light. As the animal makes his zigzagging evasive run, the white flashes from hip to hip, nicely contrasting with his black tail.

Some members of the cat family have penetrating eyes, especially the lynx. In the daylight the pupils are mere slits and the yellow irises seem to cover the whole eyeball. Its light-absorbing tapetum (reflector in the back of the eyes which makes them luminous to a flashlight) gives it a considerable advantage over animals on which it preys. The name "lynx" in fact comes from a Greek term for "one who can see well in a dim light." The bobcat also hunts by sight rather than scent. Some rodents have remarkable sight, although this is not true of the common rat or mouse. The kangaroo rat has great black eyes, round as an owl's, that shine red at night.

Among large mammals the bighorn probably has the most remarkable distant vision. If he had wings, he would probably be as efficient a bird of prey as an eagle. Most bears have rather poor sight, but the polar bear is an exception. He pays little attention to sounds, probably because the polar sea is such a noisy place, with icebergs giving out their colossal grindings and ice floes cracking and crashing. Buffaloes have poor sight, which makes them seem stupider than they are. Their hearing and smell are good and they rely on wind scents. In spite of Kipling's famous story, an albino seal almost invariably has poor eyesight and seldom lives long enough to become a father, let alone a literary hero. The whale is something of an ocular cripple, not because his retina is especially poor but because his eyeball is fixed. He must move his whole body to shift his line of sight. Furthermore, the lens is set at just one focus. Everything beyond or in front is a blur. He sheds greasy tears, since aqueous tears would obviously do him no good under water. (Later in this chapter we shall have occasion to examine the tear-shedding process in other animals, including man.)

So much for a brief glance around from one observation tower. Now we must get down to business. One of the most important realizations of modern zoology is that among certain mammals, the same superbusy retinal apparatus that predigests visual information before signaling the brain (which we saw in action in the case of the frog and the pigeon) is also found in action in the rabbit and the ground squirrel. Clyde W. Oyster and Horace B. Barlow, both of the University of California (Berkeley), have found that the retinal ganglion cells (the third layer in the eye following the bipolar cells and the actual light-receptors, the cones or rods) perform an editing job on the messages that the rabbit's first-line cells of vision get from the outside world. Certain individual ganglion cells of the rabbit's eye signal the presence of a pattern in time and space that means something. They respond when the image moves across the retina in a particular direction and at a particular speed. When this kind of image is perceived, a remarkable automatic following device comes into play. The rabbit's eyes move precisely to reduce the rate of sweep of the image across the retina. This kind of servomechanism works without the knowledge of the brain. Clearly the corrective eye movements require error signals that indicate which direction the image is slipping over the retina, and the so-called "on-off" direction-selecting ganglion cells probably serve this function. If the rabbit's eye could be reproduced, with its muscular machines, and this automatic image-following ability, one would evidently have a radar that not only sees a moving object at a given rate and in a given direction, but which would also exactly follow the object,

enabling closer telescopic scrutiny and thus quicker identification. This goes the frog's eye and the pigeon's eye one better.
(It is a pity that most of our interest in the eyes of animals
seems to be inspired by the hope of military application.)

Charles R. Michael of Yale, in studies of the optic nerve of the
ground squirrel, found that this animal, which has only cones in
the retina (as fits in with its daytime activity), also responds
strongly to movement in one direction. A single fiber of the
optic nerve has in all animals what is now called a "receptive
field"; that is, a field consisting of all the cones in the pigment
layer of the retina that funnel into the optic nerve fiber. In the
squirrel such fibers respond vigorously to stimuli moving entirely
across the field centers in one direction only, not at all when the
direction of motion is reversed. (Some other fiber and its field
of cones takes on that job.) This curious directional property
is achieved, as most perceptive nervous events are achieved, by
an inhibition, which prevents the response to the reverse movement. Actually each field center is surrounded by a concentric
antagonistic region whose only job is to inhibit. Although this
is something like the inhibitions that we discussed in the compound eye to obtain contrast, it is primarily a time-in-motion
mechanism. It enables the ground squirrel, like the rabbit, to
obtain a super-keen picture of a moving object, perhaps a coyote.

When we get to an animal as advanced as a cat, we find ourselves out of the age of the automatic eye and into the age where
the brain insists on getting a complete, non-edited report from
the eye. Nervous elements which are uniquely excited by vision
and result in some patterned action are not found in the cat
outside the cerebral cortex. This results in a reduction of
fidelity, since in passing every visual sensation back to the brain
there is much channeling and convergence. Why and when did
this direct referral to the brain occur in evolution? It is probably
no coincidence that a cat, like a man, has complete binocular
vision, while a frog, a pigeon and a rabbit lack binocular vision.
Presumably when the vision of each eye overlaps to give the
stereoptic effect of a three-dimensional world, this effect can

only be realized back in the brain where the nerves of the two eyes deliver their separate messages. This tends to put the entire burden of sorting, inhibiting, exploring on the brain itself. It is a curious fact, quite recently discovered, that even if you surgically cut through the optical chiasma of a cat (where the separate optical nerves cross over) the cat still retains some binocular vision. It appears that there are certain cells in the visual cortex of one optic globe which can communicate with other corresponding cells of the other optic globe through the corpus callosum to maintain a sense of binocular eyesight. The optical sense of mammals has an amazing ability to regain its equilibrium. People who have lost one eye, for example, have no difficulty in continuing to see the world as three-dimensional. People who experimentally wear spectacles that make everything look upside down find, after a few days of nausea and stumbling, that they can adjust very well to an upside-down world. Indeed, in the first place, our eyes, without any spectacles, are so designed that, technically speaking, we not only see the world upside down but as a mirror image. It is the brain that straightens things out at a very early age.[11]

The exponents of the Lockean notion, so popular in the 1930s, that the human brain starts out as a blank slate and that we have to "learn to see" have had their arguments demolished by all recent experiments.

In his work on early form perception, Fantz found that, while freshly hatched chicks are born to distinguish a seed from a grain of sand, human babies and chimpanzee infants do not have to learn to look at things that are intrinsically interesting. Fantz's technique consisted of hanging various cards above the infants, and, through a peephole in the top of the closed crib, observing the image of the object mirrored in the subject's eyes. There was a definite preference in both chimpanzee and human infants

[11] As I have pointed out in my book *The Eternal Return*, studies by R. K. Luneburg have shown that we actually perceive the world in a non-Euclidean, hyperbolic geometry. The mind pretends that it sees a Euclidean world, because it is simpler for engineers to handle and, although it is a fairy story, it turns out to be a pragmatic fairy story. It may not be so useful for minds more advanced than ours.

for looking at complicated figures rather than simple ones, although the human babies were more quickly bored and tended to go to sleep. At all ages during the first six months, babies preferred to look at the schematic picture of a face rather than at scrambled patterns or two-colored flags. Solid forms are interesting from one month on and appear to give the baby a basis for perceiving depth. The general configuration of a face identifies a human being to an infant. At a later age a special person is recognized primarily by more precise perception of the facial pattern. Still later, subtle details of facial expression tell the child whether a person is happy or sad, pleased or displeased, friendly or unfriendly. When a baby looks at you, be assured he is sizing you up pretty accurately. In the chimpanzee this is the only way he will ever receive communication. The primate's inability to talk is to some extent compensated for by a tremendous range of facial expression.

We should note at this point that facial expression (as far as we know, since we do not spend much time going down Insect Row and scowling eyeball-to-eyeball at tough guys like female praying mantises) is confined mainly to vertebrates. We should call attention to some basic expressions among mammals. For instance, practically every mammal from mouse to monkey flattens its ears and narrows its eyes when startled by an alien growl or by some other sudden ungracious noise. This is a protective reflex serving to reduce the exposure of the sense · organs to insult. This ear-flattening expression is so natural that it spreads over other situations. Thus a male of some mammalian genera, preparing to approach a female to attempt copulation, likewise displays his lack of confidence (his basic fearfulness in a brutal universe where even females of his own kind may treacherously bite) by flattening his ears at the very start of approach.

Ear-flattening, originally a reflex act of protection ("Don't you *dare* bite my ears off!") becomes a communication device—a signal of intention rather than of defense. Consider all your own personal relations with horses and dogs. Do not all of them involve either the flattening or the pricking of the animal's ears?

In higher primates ear-flattening becomes less pronounced mainly because there is less control over the ears. What is retained (as emphasized by Richard J. Andrew of the University of Sussex) is a significant retraction of the scalp, which was a part of the over-all muscular movement in the primitive flattening of the ears. In macaques and baboons the scalp retraction is wildly exaggerated. (In our primate family we must admit a manlike tendency to temper tantrums and ham acting—behavior which would be incomprehensible to an ant or a fish and is probably incomprehensible to the angels.) Such monkeys go way out. Under emotion they automatically flatten a topknot of hair and there is a pull-up of folds of brightly colored skin from under the eyebrows, giving a look of deep clownish staring, almost a shaman wildness.

Where does the *frown* come from? The dog, the capuchin monkey, man and many other animals (again as observed by Andrew) typically lower the eyebrows in the frowning expression. What is the biological purpose? The fact that men frown when displeased or hostile does not explain anything. The frown may be partly protective or may help focus the eyes. In most mammals the frown is connected with a direct stare which indicates concentrated interest, perhaps aggressiveness, but very seldom does it show fear. A frowning animal is more likely an animal in a dangerous, fearless but businesslike mood.

What about the *grin?* At least two primitive origins seem likely. Drawing back the lips may be preliminary to biting or to *spitting*. The grin may be a signal of unease. A great many mammals from the opossum to the primates show this grinlike response when horribly startled. A braver man than I told me that in a long career of dockyard and barroom fights the most dangerous face he ever tried to defend himself against was a grinning one.

It seems to Andrew, however, that the grin must also be regarded from the human baby's point of view. Human beings find small changes in stimulation pleasant and *large* ones unpleasant. There is evidence that the higher vertebrates seek stimulation in the form of continually changing impact to the central nervous system. Babies show their first broad smiles on being tickled or by the peekaboo game (in which the main point is to startle, but not too much). The essence of all jokes throughout the world is a certain measure of surprise.

Advanced forms of the New World monkey and the Old World chimpanzee have a pronounced *pout*, as does the human child about to cry. In many primates the rounding of the lips, covering the teeth—which accompanies the sudden blowing of the breath—means "*Okay, you bastard,* here I come!" This same pout is familiar to us from annoyed presidents of corporations and even from Presidents of the United States.

Andrew believes that human speech may have evolved from apelike facial and tongue movements. Among baboons a common form of communication is *lip-smacking*, a display derived from movements of lips and tongue which they use in grooming one another. Lip-smacking is in this case a gesture of greeting and baboons use it more than the grin. With the lip-smacking they often grunt in a rather comfortable way. These are vowels and the nearest the baboons will come to vocal communication. (We shall discuss such matters in the next chapter.)

The development of visual displays of any kind depends on the extent of sociability of the animal. For example, the wolf—a highly social animal—shows an enormously greater range of facial expressions than the solitary bear. The most demonstrative species of baboons are those in troops on the plains. This is a hazardous profession. For these monkeys, mutual communication in one way or another is a military necessity. The leader is a George Patton and his lieutenants are ruthless in policing any fighting among the troops or among the females. It is significant that the forest-dwelling mandrill and the drill baboon make far less use of presidential frowns or pouts. Andrew concludes that living on the plains or savannas was essential in man's ancestry, since it probably not only promoted hunting and the use of tools but also the evolution of smiling, laughter and language itself.

Chimpanzees can communicate with each other as well as any

of us might do with someone whose language we did not know. In addition to what primatologists call "photic" communication with each other, some chimpanzees adopt "iconic signs" for use with humans. For example, the female Vicki (who was brought up by the Hayes man-and-wife team of primotologists) would bring a Kleenex to her "parents" to suggest taking a walk, evidently equating it with the diapers that were always taken with them on an airing.

The research team of Allen and Beatrice Gardner educated the infant female chimpanzee Washoe by a more direct method: they taught her the American Sign Language (ASL) used by the deaf of North America. Whereas Vicki, in spite of six years of anxious training by her human foster parents, learned only four sounds that approximated English words, Washoe learned to use a respectable variety of signals and concepts and is presumably still adding to her vocabulary. (Unfortunately when a chimp becomes physically mature—at about twelve years—at 120 pounds, it is stronger than a gigantically muscled man of 500 pounds. Since the Gardners taught Washoe by placing her hands in the appropriate positions for a signal, a slight degree of impatience on the part of a full-grown Washoe might result in the Gardners' having their arms torn out of their sockets.)

The sign language of the literate deaf is a combination of iconic signs (signs that imitate something), arbitrary signs and finger-spelling. Since finger-spelling assumes a whole background of human language ability, the Gardners did not try to teach this to Washoe.

As examples of ASL, the sign for "flower" is highly iconic, being made by holding all five fingertips together, and touching the fingers first to one nostril, then to the other. The sign for "always" is arbitrarily made by holding the hand in a fist, index finger extended, while rotating the arm at the elbow.

Young chimpanzees have a passion for being tickled, so when Washoe learned the sign for "more" she generally used it to mean "more tickling," but the "more" sign might also merely stand for something for which she had not learned the sign (a "whatchamacallit"). According to parents of deaf children being taught

the sign language, Washoe's inaccuracies in certain signs re-
sembled the "baby-talk" inaccuracies of their own infants.

In the case of "dog" and "cat," young chimpanzees are so
excitable that Washoe wasn't allowed to meet an actual dog or
cat face to face but could look at pictures of them and learn the
signs for them. The important point was that she could *transfer*
these signs from one modality to another. When she heard an
unseen dog barking she would make the signal for "dog." (This
is a more remarkable feat than it seems at first glance, since it
involves a deductive guessing process. How could Washoe be
sure it was not the unseen animal denoted by the sign for "cat"
that was not doing the barking?) Washoe at an early age was
learning (in fact, learning even faster than deaf children) to
generalize; for example, to associate the sign for "open" not only
with all doors in the house, but also with the refrigerator, with
cupboards, drawers, briefcases, boxes and jars. Eventually she
used this sign when she wanted water faucets turned on. It
is obvious that Washoe was on her way to the mastery of a
symbolic language. Chimpanzees, in other words, *can* acquire
language for which they are physically suited. Why then has
man prevailed? It is not simply the *ability* of man to communicate
symbolically that made him the lord of the planet, but some still
obscure incentive to *use* and to develop this ability.

Emotion can be conveyed by unlearned sign language. The
eyes as important organs for manifesting grief are used even by
geese, as Konrad Lorenz has shown. The lowering of tone in the
sympathetic nerve causes the eye to sink back deeply in its
socket and, at the same time, decreases the tension of the outer
facial muscles supporting the eye region from below. Both
factors contribute to the formation of a fold of loose skin below
the eye which as early as the ancient Greek masks of tragedy
had become the conventionalized expression of grief. Although
our repertoire of facial expressions has become somewhat limited
in comparison to that of the anthropoid apes, simultaneously as
our gift of language, including the gift of crying and sobbing,
increased, we respond still to grief and to laughter in faces that

we see around us and, perhaps most of all, to boredom. Yawning is universally infectious. Sometimes even our legs betray us. If you see a visitor in a chair at your house who cannot keep his legs still, his legs are giving the message "I want to go home." The once-popular idea that as babies we learn how to see by coordinating our eyesight with our sense of touch has been completely refuted by Irvin Rock of Yeshiva University and Charles S. Harris of the Bell Telephone Laboratories in experiments with both babies and kittens. The sense of vision is not only predominant over the sense of touch but vision educates touch. Babies and the young of most mammals have good depth perception before they could learn it any way but by seeing. When adults look through a reducing lens and touch an object at the same time, they are not aware of any conflicting sensory information. Their hands seem to be touching a small object. In one test a square object was made to appear through spectacles as a rectangle and was touched. So dominant was the sense of vision that most subjects said the square actually felt the way it looked. If they closed their eyes, they often thought, however, that they felt it changing shape from a rectangle to a square. After a sufficient time for the two senses to disagree about something, there is invariably a change in the sense of touch itself. The organism will insist that the touch be transformed into new touch perceptions that agree with the visual message. As a practical matter this enormous primacy of vision is one of the reasons why most astronautical engineers are urgently concerned with getting some better way of making actions mesh with eyesight. The optic brain of man is infinitely better than any imaginable physical device but the human hands as control-actuating devices are pitiful. In a tracking telescope the eye can quickly pick out and follow a target, but in high-speed situations even well-trained hands are relatively slow and fumbling.

The unexpected resolving power of the unhampered human eye was first fully realized when Gordon Cooper on Mercury 9 reported seeing roads, vehicles, buildings and smoke from huts in the Himalayas, while Ed White in Gemini 4 saw street lights and the smoke from trains, from 100 miles up. That all this was not an exuberant illusion was proved later in a series of Gemini flights with special targets laid out on the ground. How could the human eye see so far and so well? One could be romantic and guess that the animal man had at last attained his true environment—the place in space and time that three billion years of evolution had been leading up to. I think, however, that in order to explain this final splendor of vision we must now go back and review some basic facts of man's optic system.

The cornea on the outside and the lens are concerned with refraction of light so that the image falls on the retinal receptors.[12] The cornea is curved in a convex bow so that the light waves are already partly refracted before they pass through the lens. After the cornea, the light passes through the aqueous humor, a clear watery fluid that lies between the cornea and the lens. This is replaced periodically by blood-plasma filtrate drawn off special canals near the ciliary muscles and the iris and is reabsorbed back into the venous system, much as is the spinal fluid. After the aqueous humor, the light enters the pupil opening in the iris (a sort of automatic curtain); then the rays are bent twice, once by the front of the lens (or vitreous humor) and again bent by the back face. Having passed the lens, the light does not immediately encounter the retina but successively crosses the accumulating fibers of the optic nerve, the ganglion cells and the bipolar cells before striking the light-sensitive transducers, the rods and cones. The lens inverts the image which falls upon the retina so that, as we have noted, the image on the retina is not only a mirror image of the real object but is upside down as well.[13]

[12] In eye transplantations it is only the cornea that can be replaced. The mistaken impression that the whole eyeball is replaceable by an eye from an eye bank has been a frequent cause of grievous disappointment.

[13] We do not know for what reason all vertebrates have inverted retinas of this type. Embryologically, however, the retina is an extension of the brain. With its four-cell layers it looks like a small cerebral cortex and, like the cortex, has independent synapses between the neural elements. In embryonic development the optic vesicle pushes out from the brain,

The vitreous humor in the lens is heavier, more gelatinous than the aqueous humor and remains in place permanently without replacement. When the ciliary muscle contracts, the lens assumes its most rounded shape for looking at close objects. When this muscle system relaxes, the lens flattens for accommodation to distant objects. This reflex reaches full development several months after birth. There is a brain mystery involved here. The reflex of accommodation is triggered by visual impulses reaching the optical area in the occipital cortex, saying in effect that the retinal image is not clear. The cortex, having said "Roger," sends a message to the motor centers which in turn instruct the ciliary muscle to contract—or relax, but how this message is coded is not known. (Our whole body is a silent rustle of codes, but as far as our technical understanding is concerned they might as well be in ancient Mayan.) Recently it has been made plain that the lens actually keeps growing at a small rate until we die, which means piling layer upon layer of cells, like the skins of a transparent onion. Accommodation does not increase at the same time so the lens gets compressed and its focusing power diminishes. The lenses of rabbits, horses and rats stop growing at about eighteen months. The growth regulator is a protein fraction called "chalone." Man's eyes have chalone but less than those of other mammals. R. A. Veale of London's Institute of Ophthamology has proposed that we stimulate the production of chalone or provide it artificially to delay the aging process. The mechanism of the pupil's contraction or dilation, like that for accommodation, is triggered by reflex reactions to the visual input, too much or too little light. This reflex is known to be active at or even before birth, since otherwise a baby's eyes could be irreversibly damaged by exposing him to bright sunlight. Pigment around the radial or circular muscles of the iris give the eye its color of blue, green or brown. It is not surprising that most individuals in most species of mammals, including man,

---

then folds back upon itself to form the optic cup. This double folding is the *anatomical* reason why the bipolar and ganglion cells are between the light source and the rods and cones. But that does not tell us why all vertebrate eyes should be designed this way.

have brown eyes, since this pigment gives the eye the most protection, especially in the burning suns of the tropics.

The retina has about 10 million cones and about 120 million rods but since the number of optic fibers in each optic nerve is about 1 million, there is obviously a good deal of channeling or funneling, leading us to the previously mentioned concept of receptor fields. Several rods or cones funnel their fibers into single bipolar and ganglion cells. The axons or fibers of the ganglion cells form the optic nerve. The point, towards the nose, of each eye where the optic nerve leaves toward the brain becomes a blind spot. Now an exceedingly important exception must be pointed out with regard to the funneling of rods or cones. In the fovea, the central spot of best sight, which contains only cones, each cone connects with a separate fiber of the optic nerve. Here also the bipolar and ganglion cells are drawn aside at oblique angles so that the cones are more directly exposed to light and the innate disadvantage of the inverted retina is obviated. It is believed by many neurologists that the fovea is the sensory basis of human attention and concentration. In mammals, only the later primates have foveas and only the primates, perhaps only the anthropoids, have color vision. What is the significance of this and what is the basis of color vision?

Color vision is a property of the cones. Areas of the retina where rods predominate, as they do around the outer edges of the eye, are highly sensitive in dim light but lack color sensitivity. In the early 1800s an English physicist, Thomas Young, proposed that ability to see color is due to three different pigments in the cones. By mixing red, green and blue light, white light is seen. Consequently special pigments sensitive to three wave lengths would seem to offer a plausible basis for color vision. A pigment that absorbs the red and one absorbing the green have been known for some time. It was not until 1964, over a century and a half after Young's suggestion, that the existence of two pigments which absorb the blue region was demonstrated. This was done by using a microspectrometer capable of measuring the absorption of light passing through a single cone cell. The generally accepted assumption now is that there are three types of cones and our ability to distinguish colors depends on the proportions of different cones stimulated.[14] Even though there are over ten times as many rods as cones in the human retina, the rods do not interfere with color vision, probably because the rods do not function in bright light. In color blindness the light waves of red wave length stimulate not only the cones sensitive to red but those sensitive to green and green light in the same manner stimulates normally "red" and "green" cones. The color-blind still see blue, yellow and violet as they are, but red and green appear as various shades of yellowish gray.

Let us now follow the path light takes to the brain. As we have mentioned, the process begins with the responses of some 130 million light-sensitive receptor cells (rods and cones) in each retina. From tiny differences in the two retinal images there results a three-dimensional picture. From the retina of each eye, visual messages, having been funneled through bipolar and ganglion cells, travel along the optic nerve which consists of about 1 million fibers. At the junction known as the "chiasma" about one-half of the nerves cross over into the opposite hemispheres of the brain. The first way station in the brain is a pair of cell populations called the "lateral geniculate bodies" in the thalamus. We can think of the pathway to the sense of vision as involving six kinds of nerve cells (three in the retina, one in the geniculate body and two in the cortex).

The retinal ganglion cells fire at a fairly steady rate even in the absence of stimulation. The resting discharges of these cells

14 This is, as I have said, the "generally accepted" theory of color vision. In 1959, however, Edwin Land, the genius who invented the Polaroid camera, reported some experiments that seemed to show that it is not necessary to mix blue, green and red to produce all the hues in the spectrum. The retina, according to Land's work, need not have a specific receptor for each primary color and colors in images arise not from a choice of wave length but from an interplay of wave lengths over the entire scene. This subtle concept immediately enraged the professional psychologists who claimed that Land had stumbled upon an unusual instance of simultaneous color contrast, but how much of such objection proceeded from the fact that Land had been able to make $100 million by capitalizing on his knowledge of optics is still a question.

are intensified or diminished by light in a small and more or less circular part of the retina. That region is the cell's receptor field. A particular ganglion cell's firing rate may be *decreased* by light, thus enforcing the contrast or contour effect, which has been discussed in connection with compound eyes. Lighting up the whole retina diffusely does not affect any given ganglion cell nearly as much as a small circular spot of light covering precisely the center of this cell's receptive field. In the geniculate bodies of the mid-brain this contrast is even more specialized. It has the function of increasing the disparity (already present in the retinal ganglion cells) between responses to a small centered spot and to diffuse light. These messages of contrast are then passed on to the stupendous complexity of the visual cortex. Some idea of what happens there has recently been obtained by David Hubel in the case of the cat's brain. There are no cortical cells with concentric receptive fields, but instead there are many different cell types with fields markedly different than anything seen in the retinal and geniculate cells. Roughly they can be grouped into "simple" and "complex" functions. The simple cells respond to line stimuli and edges. They will respond only if the line is in a particular direction and will not respond if it is moving. The complex cells will also respond only to lines in a given orientation but will continue to fire if the line moves. It is evident that each complex cell is in fact responding to a number of simple cells. The number of such cells involved when the eye observes a slowly turning propeller must be unimaginably huge.

We still have only the vaguest idea of what the complex cells do with *their* responses. Each cell in the visual cortex is connected by obscure and elaborate networks with the rest of the cortex. Exploring the visual cortex with a microelectrode one finds it subdivided like a beehive with tiny columns or segments, each of which extends from the surface down to the white matter lower in the brain. Such a column is defined by the fact that the hundreds of thousands of cells in it all have the same receptive field orientation. The cells in a particular column tend to differ, some being simple, some complex, some respond to slits, others prefer dark bars or edges. A column may thus be looked upon as an independently functioning unit of the visual cortex, in which simple cells receive connections from lateral geniculate cells and send projections to complex cells. In sum, the visual cortex rearranges the input from the lateral geniculate body in such a way that makes lines and contours the most important stimuli. Although the tagging of such functions represents progress in neurophysiology, it is a long way from telling us why we appreciate the contours of Miss Universe or in fact how we can see railroad smoke from 100 miles in the air.

To come closer to the mechanics of the eye's precision, we need to focus attention on the extraordinary involuntary movements of the eye. Roy M. Pritchard of McGill University has studied so-called "stabilized images" on the retina by attaching the visual target to the eyeball itself by means of a tight-fitting contact lens on which is mounted a tiny, self-contained optical projector. This is a most abnormal condition for an eye. Normally the eye is constantly in motion. Small involuntary movements persist even when the eye is apparently "fixed" on a stationary object. Try the experiment of staring somebody down "eyeball to eyeball." One movement of the eyeball makes the image drift slowly away from the center of the fovea. The drift ends in a sudden flick that brings the image back toward the center of the fovea. Superimposed on this drift motion is a constant tiny tremor with frequencies up to 150 cycles per second and an amplitude of about one half the diameter of a single cone. All three of these involuntary movements are involved in reading or looking at the world.

Now one finds, when using Pritchard's image stabilizer, that the image begins to fade and disappears bit by bit, leaving a gray field of light that may later darken to intense black; then after a while the image regenerates and becomes visible in whole or in part. Simple images such as a straight line vanish quickly. More complex images, such as the profile of a face, take longer to fade and may disappear in a gradual and selective manner, the most interesting or meaningful feature being the last to go. The disappearance shows a certain esthetic property. If an amoeba form with one swollen protuberance is the image, the protuberance is the first to go, thus giving a more rounded and acceptable pattern. Color disappears very rapidly. In a field composed of the three primary colors, red, green and blue, all disappear to leave a colorless field of three degrees of brightness. This seems to mean that the perception of hue is maintained by continuous changes in luminosity of light rays falling on a receptive field of cones. The *movements* of the edges of a patch of color across the retina, produced by normal eye movements, therefore seem to be necessary for continuous perception of color. Thus, in order to see well and in color, the eye must be able to dance.

Perhaps in a state of zero gravity, the eyes of an astronaut are in a condition that is the exact opposite of those of the subjects whose retinas were compelled by Pritchard's device to keep confronting the same image and to see it fade and reappear and fade again. Perhaps the eyes of astronauts work so superbly just because the eye can keep effortlessly scanning and rescanning. The weightless eyeball may simply move more easily in the socket. We must keep remembering also that the eyes of advanced primates were first made for a life in the trees, where gravity was indeed an important opponent and the sense of balance was strongly linked with sight. It is not easy to stand upright without swaying if the eyes are closed, especially on a waving branch. Stimulation of the inner ear and some disorders of this organ, where the sense of balance is located, can make the eyes flick aimlessly back and forth. In the weightless condition, the normal interaction between the inner ear and the eye is disrupted. The eye is set free from the inner ear. There are grave reservations about some of the effects of weightlessness in space, but surely this enhancement of the eye is a sparkling incentive. If we can see so well up there, might we not start to think better up there?

In a rather pitiful sense, since the australopithecines came out of the trees and more cogently since ancient man became a farmer rather than a hunter, it became sometimes an advantage to be nearsighted. Almost all the higher rates of nearsightedness are found among populations which have had agricultural or pastoral economics for at least several thousand years. Myopia was an advantage even in more primitive communities for those possessing it by giving them the safer jobs, such as shaping arrow points. The Chinese and Japanese are more commonly nearsighted than the Anglo-Saxon, while optical errors are as frequent among Arabs living in the desert as among members of industrial communities in Europe. Dark-eyed people have higher resolving power under intense glare than the blue-eyed, since the pigmentation of the retina is partly an anti-glare mechanism. The survival of hunters depends so much on ability to spot game at great distances that in the hunting stage dark-eyed people have always had an advantage in desert lands.

Even the most normal human eye has peculiarities, many of them connected apparently with the intense development of the fovea. Especially at night or in dimly lighted places, the population of rods are alert to movements that the densely packed cones of the eye center cannot see. One glimpses a stealthy movement out of the corner of the eye but when one focuses the fovea, the sly spirit has gone. This is why people see ghosts in dimly lighted places. Even daytime seeing, under conditions of more than adequate illumination, has its moments of mirage. Sometimes looking at the bright sky one sees semi-transparent *muscae volitantes*, or "curlicues," which are the shadow of substances contained in the vitreous humor of the eyeball, projected upon the retina. Exhaustion and alcohol can break down the co-ordination of the reflexes of the two eyes, so that we see two pink elephants instead of one. When the shifting of the gaze is willed but prevented by a local drug paralysis of eye muscles, the surroundings seem to move and in a direction equal and opposite to the one occurring upon manually moving the passive eyeball. Alcohol, drugs and exhaustion are perhaps not as effective in distorting the vision as pure boredom. When you place people in an experimental blank cubicle, with nothing to look at, they begin after a few days to have hallucinations. The starved visual cortex begins to manufacture figures—marching eyeglasses, floating skiffs, ants carrying banners, etc. As in dreaming, the cortex, through deprivation, has to put on its own show, although in this case the eyes are open.

There has recently been a revival of practical interest in these false images (the "prisoner's cinema") which are scientifically called "phosphenes." They may be part of the process of brain-washing, in which suspected spies or political prisoners are left for a long time in solitary confinement with nothing to do but stare at a featureless wall or at the darkness. Phosphenes may actually be the ghosts that many people used to swear they saw especially in the rural South before radio and television gave them something to occupy their minds with after supper.

One must distinguish, however, phosphenes or phantoms seen in lonely revery and those that can be mechanically evoked. Blindfolded pilots on take-off in a rocket will automatically see phosphenes at an acceleration of about three and a half Gs (gravitation measure). On the other hand, as the pilots of the future pass their lonely vigils on a months-long trip to a planet, such as Mars or Jupiter, the other kind of phosphenes— the phosphenes of desuetude—may take over and they could be dangerous to the extent of madness. In any such venture, either men of great inner resources—men capable like Cervantes of turning imprisonment into a period of intense creativity—should be selected for the long voyages or an appreciable part of the rocket's load should consist of books and entertainment or educational cassettes.

Children have a special ability, which falls off with adolescence, of evoking phosphenes quite easily. One woman mental patient, after rubbing her eyes with a towel, would see phosphenes superimposed on her normal vision for hours afterward. Mescaline, psilocybin and LSD evoke phosphenes of a polished and abstract quality. Dr. Gerald Oster of the Mount Sinai School of Medicine of New York (who is perhaps the best authority we have on phosphenes) reports that six months after taking a small dose of LSD in an experiment he was still seeing magnificent phosphenes at bedtime.

The electrical induction of phosphenes was discovered in the late eighteenth century when it was considered a fun thing at a party to sit around with joined hands in a circle and receive a shared shock from an electrostatic generator. Benjamin Franklin (that unbelievable combination of swinger and scientist) was the first to observe that along with the shock came a flash of light that could be seen with the eyes closed.

Max Knoll of Munich, who shared in the development of the electron microscope, studied phosphene generation in a systematic way. He found that electric pulses in the same frequency range as normal brain waves (five to about forty cycles per second) produced the most elegant phosphenes. As Knoll varied the frequency of applied pulses, the patterns changed. Knoll claimed to identify fifteen distinct classes of these optical illusions, depending on frequency of the electric current. This frequency effect suggests some kind of resonance phenomenon, with different groups of nerve cells acting together when driven electrically at a certain rate. Knoll and his group found that electrically induced phosphenes were gaudier when the subjects had been given previously a very small dose of LSD.

Oster and Mordecai Schlank discovered a weird thing: Above a certain frequency of current (about forty cycles per second) the electrically induced phosphenes suddenly vanish. It is as if a fairy world had been annihilated with the wave of a wand. One has a feeling of being left alone in deep space.

Wilder Penfield and his associates at the Montreal Neurological Institute applied alternating current to closely spaced electrodes over various surfaces of the brain. Stimulating the visual cortex at the rear of the brain merely interrupts the patient's normal vision, making him see what appears to be a raining and spotty TV picture. When the electrodes are moved to the nearby visual association area, the patient sees phosphenes of geometric design. When the electrodes are moved farther forward the patient may enter upon a nostalgic visit into his past—he may report a visual scene long forgotten, a sort of Citizen Kane's "Rosebud." People born blind see no phosphenes but people blinded accidentally or by disease can see them and in fact eagerly enjoy them.

One feature of the eye that until recently had been regarded simply as a window that could be changed in size by reflex action—the pupil—now is found to undergo very complicated psychological behavior. It was not until the 1960s that the pupil's *emotionality* was fully realized by psychologists. With changing light the pupil contracts and enlarges by reflex as a result of innervation by the parasympathetic nervous system. However, the pupil is also innervated by the sympathetic system—a rare situation. As a result the pupil responds not only to light but to emotion and even to concentration. It enlarges with interest and contracts with disgust or boredom. Eckhard Hess of the University of Chicago has ingeniously used this principle to discover facts that sometimes prove a trifle embarrassing.

Magicians and other tricksters have known this all along. It is part of the secret of the trade. Magicians doing card tricks can identify the card a person is thinking about by watching his pupils dilate when the card is turned up. Professional gamblers take advantage of this behavior. In a modern game of high-stakes poker one can identify the real pros because they will wear polarized colored glasses to hide their own pupils, but thus equipped they can still study the pupils of the sucker in the crowd. They know when he has filled an inside straight. Those sharpest of sharpies, Chinese jade dealers, watch a buyer's pupils to know when he is impressed by a specimen and is likely to pay a high price.

Men's pupils dilate, of course, when they are shown a picture of a nude female. Although she would indignantly disavow any interest in a male pin-up, Hess found that a woman's pupils would give her away. Her pupils sharply contracted on the other hand when shown a picture of a shark or of a crippled baby. The pupil response is a devastating puncturer of pretense and Hess's technique may be the best debunking weapon yet discovered. For example, constriction or negative response is shown almost invariably to modern paintings, particularly abstract ones, even by those who buy them (or talk about "relating" to them) and indeed even by those who *paint* them. However, one never detects a pupil constriction, even in the case of the most adamant and babbling modernist, to Andrew Wyeth's *Christina's World*.

Horror pictures (with dead and mangled bodies or vampires in action) cause dilation (horrified interest) followed by constriction (disgust).

Hess has demonstrated a fact of sexual attraction that was known by women in the Middle Ages but apparently forgotten by the average modern man. He showed a series of pictures to a group of twenty men. In the series were two pictures of the same comely young woman, except that in one picture her pupils had been retouched to make them look abnormally large and in the other extra small. As shown by their own pupil responses, the men were attracted twice as strongly to the picture with the large pupils. Upon review, most of the men claimed the pictures were identical. Some admitted that one picture was "more feminine," "softer" or "prettier" (indefinably) than the other. None noticed that the one simply had larger pupils than the other and in fact had to be shown the difference.

Women realized this fact of nature and exploited it shamelessly after the discovery of belladonna (which means "beautiful woman" in Italian). Perhaps the attractiveness of large pupils is that they denote interest in the man the woman is with. It may be more subtle. A movie expert once told me that a large part of Elizabeth Taylor's goddesshood depended on the fact that she not only showed large pupils but never blinked.

Hess has shown that the pupil response will correlate exactly with verbally expressed food preferences. However, in politics the technique is incomparably more precise than a Gallup Poll and in fact the pupil response indicates that a good many people in the solitude of the voting cubicle do not vote the way they talk.

The technique is capable of showing up even more curious aspects of political science. During the Johnson-Goldwater presidential campaign of 1964 some extremely heavy anti-Gold-water material, which one of Hess's assistants found very easy to write, had unexpected effects on an audience. It not only caused the expected decrease in pupillary response to a picture of Gold-water but also caused a large drop in response to a picture of Johnson and even one of Eisenhower. Only Kennedy (evidently because of martyrdom) retained the same status as before. What the pupils were reacting to was what might be called "politics in general." The lesson to be drawn perhaps is that a bitter and vindictive campaign speech lowers the status of *all* politi-cians, not simply the status of the speaker's opponent. Sociologists may eventually, by means of the dead giveaway of the pupil re-sponse, be able to accept the fact that people often regard a politician not as a specially favored citizen (*as one of them*) but as a representative of a sort of psychic underworld.

It is clear that the pupil is an unexpectedly eloquent organ. But with it we are merely on the outward skin of the complex process of sight and recognition. What we see may or may not affect our emotions or even our consciousness as a tactical animal. One of the most astonishing things discovered in recent years about human sight is that, even though we don't realize or utilize the fact, *practically everything we see is indelibly and infallibly recorded in the brain*. There is a great mystery here. Since the underlined statement seems to contradict practi-cal experience (the notorious unreliability of visual witnesses to a crime, the failure to remember things we have read), we must dig a little deeper. Among scientists that have studied visual memory is Ralph Norman Hafer of the University of Roches-ter. He and his colleagues make use of tachistoscopes—devices that can display a series of images in rapid succession. Other tools are slide projectors and screens, instruments for following eye movements, instruments for measuring the time needed for response to stimulation and various kinds of pictorial and linguistic apparatus.

One of the first conclusions that comes out of such work is that the memory for pictorial material is distinct from the *linguistic memory*. This seems a simple thing to say but it is hard to appreciate. Even though your brain has total and exact recall for *scenes* or even *symbols* (words in a book, for example), this does not mean you can answer the question, *What was the first thing you saw after you were born?* The reason you cannot answer this question is that it involves language and therefore linguistic memory as well as visual memory. Shortly after your birth you did not know how to *describe in words* what you saw. Although the scene is still in your brain and could possibly be excavated by a twenty-second-century technique, there is no way known at present to get it out linguistically. Because of the immense recent bias in the human brain toward language, we have forgotten how to remember sights (including words on paper) because we do not use words as sights but as ideas.

The true visual memory (what might be called the "Rosebud" memory) is much older than the linguistic memory but has been hopelessly contaminated by the latter. This is a great pity, but we are probably not alone. Previously I have pointed out that in lower animals, such as insects and frogs, and even in animals higher on the scale, such as rabbits and pigeons, the retina itself decides what shall be truly *seen*. When we go farther up the ladder, to cats and monkeys, for example, there is probably total visual recall, but the total visual memory is not used, this time not because it is confused with linguistics but because the animal does not need all that information in his business. A cat may on his excursions come across, let us say, a diamond ring. Even if the ring retains a faint odor of humanity, it is otherwise completely meaningless to the cat. It is not edible, it is not threatening, it is not even alive. The sparkle of the ring makes a visual impression but the cat will make no use of it. Nevertheless (and philosophically this is an important point) *the cat's memory of the diamond ring endures.* It is as real a thing in the world as the ring itself.[15]

Hafer and his group believe (and I agree) that the human capacity of memory for pictures may be unlimited. Almost

[15] One of the most pathetic photographs I have seen is that of a circle of cows facing the remains of a fallen earth-orbiting rocket in Arkansas.

everyone has had the experience of recognizing a face he saw only briefly years before. Together with Lionel Standing, Hafer carried out experiments showing that people can recognize at least 2,400 pictures they had seen for only a short period of time. The high scores in recall were maintained even when the pictures were shown as their mirror images. Hafer and Standing suggest that the results would have been the same with 250,000 pictures. But when the images are formed unassociated with language, it is impossible to record these remembered images in the form of words that can be communicated to another person. However, by use of the device of free association (thinking visually and linguistically about similar images), it is sometimes possible laboriously to extract more and more visual memory—to make the subject, in other words, a better witness. Needless to say, people would be better witnesses in the forensic sense if they tagged visual memories with words. For instance, you are walking through the park. A man suddenly confronts you. As you are handing over your pocketbook, you should be verbalizing your visual impressions: *weak jaw, pimple on nose, eyes gray, unshaven but brown hair not especially long, dirty blue scarf, about my height but maybe twenty pounds lighter, holds what looks like .38 revolver in left hand while removing cash from my pocketbook with his right,* and so on. The fact is that, although armed robbery has become all too commonplace, the victim is usually in such a state of shock and beflusterment that he cannot for the life of him give anything close to an accurate description of the robber. It is accepted police doctrine that so-called "eye-witness" accounts by inexperienced observers are worthless and may be actually misleading. (It is common these days even to mistake the sex of the criminal.)

Words themselves are remembered as ideas, not as a literal collection of words. A road sign is not remembered as a brightly colored object with an arrow or a warning but as a message. This particular (linguistic) memory process accounts for the ease with which a reader may overlook spelling errors in a printed text.

Reading itself is a task of viewing a rapid succession of brief visual exposures containing large amounts of information. Given the same innate intelligence, what makes the difference between the slow and the fast reader? The slow reader fixes his eye on each word for about one quarter of a second. A fast reader also fixes his eyes for about the same amount of time. (This time, in fact, seems to be a constant of nature—the time for iconic, or visual, storage). The fast reader attains his speed by reducing the number of fixations; that is, he looks at and processes several words instead of one word during each fixation. Both kinds of readers need from thirty to fifty milliseconds to shift their eyes from one fixation point to the next.

Now for temporary purposes each word or group of words has to be erased as an image; it has to get out of the way so that new images can be formed as reading progresses. The linguistic memory has to recall them later in order that what is read makes sense. However, there is evidence that these images are not only linguistically stored for a respectable length of time, but also visually stored (unknown, so to speak, to the reader) for a lifetime.

Some very exceptional and gifted people are able to use these indefinitely stored images. They are said to have a "photographic memory" or to possess "eidetic" imagery. The remarkable, almost alarming feature of an eidetic image is that it remains fixed. The possessor of such a memory inspects the image in his mind in detail by actually *moving his eyes* as if he were reading. Quite recently C. P. Stromeyer of MIT and J. Protka of Harvard described an individual with this kind of memory. The memory belongs luckily to a gracious and highly intelligent young female MIT faculty member. Thus we shall hope to have a chance to learn at first hand more about the nature of the ancient and primary optical memory that doubtless we have neglected to our detriment in imagining that we could create a workable Platonic world of pure linguistics.

Man is the only animal that sheds emotional tears. We do not know why. The tear duct system is quite complex and the most obvious purpose is to keep the cornea transparent, clean and lubricated. *Reflex* tears are caused by the excitation of sensory receptors in the surface membranes of the eye and nose (the conjunctiva and mucous membrane). These tears are shed by perhaps all terrestrial vertebrates except snakes. Even snakes give out the tears known as "continuous" to form a liquid film on the surface of the eye. Invertebrates, whose eyes have no movable parts, have no lacrimal system, nor do aquatic animals, for whom water plays the part of tears. Whales and seals are exceptions, possibly because they spend so much time using their eyes in the air, but their tears are oily. A fourth kind of tearing is caused by pilocarpine and some war gases which do not, curiously enough, act on the eye or nose but reach the tear glands through the bloodstream. The tear gases, now so universal in our urban civilization, like peeled onions, induce reflex tearing by directly irritating the nose and eye. Tears probably developed for the purpose of moistening not only the eye but also the nose and mouth. There is a pronounced similarity between the lacrimal and the salivary glands. (In Sjögren's disease both gland systems dry up at the same time.) Everyone is familiar with the fact that hot chili or a bolt of unaccustomed brandy brings an outpouring of tears from both eyes and nose.

The film of tears that continuously bathes the human cornea consists of a deep mucous layer, an intermediate watery layer and a superficial oil layer. Each layer is secreted by a different group of glands. The chemical composition of tears is somewhat similar to that of blood serum in salt content, but the amount of sugar and protein in tears is much lower. However, the tears of mongoloid idiots and of victims of cystic fibrosis run high in protein. It is agreed now that the parasympathetic nerves are responsible for reflex and emotional tearing, but the precise mechanism of how the glands secrete the liquid is not known.

It is difficult to imagine how the basic plan of the human eye could be improved greatly for the purposes of terrestrial man, but in another book we shall present some ideas on eyes designed for superman. In the meantime, progress has been made in eye surgery by the use of laser beams. Perhaps the greatest achievements in optics, however, have been along the line of making photographic reproduction more closely simulate the subtle contrast and contour shadings that the eye introduces into the images it presents to the mind. How this can be done by computer adjustment of raw photographs of the moon and of Mars has been demonstrated by the Jet Propulsion Laboratory at the California Institute of Technology. The Japanese are developing a TV camera to match the selectivity of the eye. As we have noted, the retina perceives color and detail best in the center of the retina (fovea), but detects *movements* best toward the edge of vision—to about sixty degrees up, down and to each side. When the peripheral activity is noted a feed-back mechanism instantly brings the movement to the center of vision. In their experiments, the Japanese project the viewing point, represented by a white dot, onto a screen carrying a picture of the eye's field of vision. The viewing point jumps about, never focusing on one spot for over two tenths of a second. In scanning a letter of the alphabet the eye does not cover the whole area as a TV camera would. The eyes saves time by seeking out contrast and transition points (thus in the letter "K" only the points of intersection of three lines). From these few selected signals the brain "recognizes" the letter—a feat still beyond the abilities of computers. In any given scene, the eye instantly focuses on anything that moves. A TV camera with the same ocular sprightliness would greatly improve the TV coverage of live events, sports, etc. TV would automatically anticipate the behavior of the viewer's eyeball. What effect this might have on Marshall McLuhan's notion of television as a viewer-participating medium (precisely because the eye has to do so much work to amplify and to build contrast into an essentially coarse reproduction) remains an interesting question. Perhaps TV scenes of violence may then become so vivid and identification so intense that we may raise a new generation of assassins and cutthroats.

We cannot leave the subject of sight without trying to explain a new and very difficult optical technology of much greater importance than the "foveal television camera" just described.

This is holography. Those who have seen the performance of holograms are rendered speechless. Their eery loveliness and their possibilities for drama and horror are nearly unendurable for the sensitive, eye-minded esthete. All agree who have glimpsed them that holograms are the unescapable optical medium for the artists and the pictorial scientists of the future, but the viewer must prepare himself for the shock of seeing, for example, a full-sized tiger not only burning bright but stalking three-dimensionally toward one in the living room or library . . . Here he comes! His tawny head has blanked out the coffee table . . . Help!

How is such an instant muscular phantom produced?

The hologram is one of a great many by-products of the laser and I am not required to go into the complexities of this instrument, except to say that a laser gives out light waves that are *coherent*. Unlike ordinary light, the waves from a laser source are identical in length and march in step.

In taking a hologram the object to be recorded (say, a tiger) is placed on a solid platform and flooded with light from a laser. The light reflected by the object falls on a photographic plate. The plate is simultaneously flooded by a second set of laser rays, called the "reference beam," that is reflected by a mirror. The reference waves travel on a path that bypasses the object. After exposure (and the tiger has been given his raw porterhouse steak) the plate is developed. It is now a hologram.

No lens has been used to form an image and no image therefore appears on the completed plate. Instead the emulsion records an abstract pattern of fine lines and whorls. It looks like a big thumbprint. If rays of colored light are now directed through the hologram along the previous path of the reference beam, a new set of rays emerges from the back of the hologram. The new waves are in every respect identical with those that were reflected by the object on the platform. In other words, there is your tiger burning bright! The image in free space is more realistic than any image ever projected. It *is* the tiger.

People looking at such holograms may, unless carefully warned, have heart attacks. One has a sense of complete three-dimensionality with full perspective and all the effects of parallax. For example, background details that may be hidden behind, say, the tiger's foot in the foreground can be brought into view simply by moving one's head to one side or the other. In a similar way, one's eyes must be refocused when attention is shifted from the foreground to the background—from the tiger's eyes to his tail.

The laser is not an imitation of nature. It never occurs, as far as we know, in nature. Evolution never thought of holograms. But IBM has gone back to one of evolution's trickiest successes in developing a technique for producing holograms from photographs taken of scenes illuminated with ordinary incoherent light rather than with laser beams. The key is the use of the "fly's-eye" lens, composed of hundreds of individual optical facets. This peculiar lens samples and records intensity, curvature and direction of light waves coming from every illuminated point in the field of view of the camera. Correspondingly, this produces hundreds of individual exposures on the film, each showing the scene at a different angle. (Such image storage is related to that described above in a hologram by reflected laser light interfering with a reference laser beam.) One then makes a conventional hologram from the multi-imaged picture by passing a laser beam through the film and through another multi-faceted lens while simultaneously causing interference of this beam with a reference laser.

The advantage of this approach is that the lasers (which are rather uncomfortable and complicated engines to work with) are used only in processing the film. The camera owner or the "producer" uses only the camera with the "fly's-eye" lens.

By a combination of man's and evolution's inventiveness, one hopefully arrives literally at a new dimension in visual reproduction.

CHAPTER 2

To Hear and Be Heard

THE SENSE of hearing was originally a sense of gravity. We are dimly aware of this close connection between hearing and equilibrium, or balance, because of the structure of our own hearing system, in which the part of this outrageously elaborate apparatus intended for telling us whether, when blind, we are standing up straight or lying in the gutter is on terms of anatomical intimacy with the part that hears the voice of God or of the policeman. Evolution seems to have been hesitant about giving a sense of hearing to its earliest creatures. It is doubtless true that life evolved in the water and that water not only conducts sound much faster than does air[1] but sound is also retained very precisely *within* the water, yet one can see the grounds for evolution's hesitancy. What good is hearing to a very small animal whose prey and whose predators are within smelling or feeling distance? The jellyfish is amply supplied with statocysts (organs of balance) but cannot hear, nor can any of the

[1] The velocity of sound under normal conditions of temperature and pressure is 1,087 feet per second in air, while in water it is approximately four-and-a-half-times as fast and is reflected back into the water from the surface so efficiently that only about one tenth of one per cent of water noises ever get out into the air. The film separating water from air is one of the most potent sound-deadeners that we know of, and it works both ways.

great phylum of mollusks. Some gastropods (snails, etc.) do have organs that sense ground vibrations, but this seems to be a highly elaborated touch system. Such otocysts enable the mollusk mainly to determine the direction of the force of gravity. They are located in the foot and consist of membranous pouches in which float sandlike grains. As the mollusk moves, the tendency of this small grain to fall on the particular sensory hair that the animal's movement happens to bring into line with the force of gravity enables him to keep his equilibrium. But in some snails there is a pair of otocysts or ear sacs that contain from one to over a hundred otolites (ear stones) and nerves that transmit impulses to the hindquarters for action. These have sometimes been called "ears" by malacologists, who want the mollusks to look good, but there is no evidence of an eardrum, or tympanum, that can distinguish sound. Probably such snails hear vibrations only in the sense that a deaf man can feel an earthquake.

However, we must be prudent about such distinctions. In spite of the fact that no one has been able to find a true ear in the enormous class of crustaceans, they possess such a complicated repertoire of sound-*producing* organs that it seems incredible that sound would not have some more significance for them. A coral reef is noisy with the loud "pops" of "pistol crabs" (alpheid shrimps). The popping is made by a movable finger provided with a little plug that fits snugly in a tubular pocket in the opposed fixed finger. (One can make the same noise by jerking a finger out of a small-necked bottle.) In fact nearly all land crabs act as if they can hear, and the underwater noises of lobsters seem to have biological meaning. Perhaps we have been looking too scrupulously for the tautly tuned drums of hearing that are used by insects and vertebrates. A slender free hair, adapted primarily for touching, can act as at least a rough detector of sound, even if it is waving freely in the water or air, because, if it is fine enough, it will move with the cyclical air (or water) displacement that sound consists of. This is certainly not a very good kind of an ear, but it may be adjusted to a few sounds that mean life or death to a crustacean. There is evidence that the larvae of barnacles can be warned off by steady, loud humming sounds, and this has been proposed as a way of protecting ship's bottoms. (We must remember that the barnacle is a crustacean, not a mollusk.)

In the last chapter we concluded that evolution's way of putting down the otherwise intelligent dibranch mollusks (octopus and squid) was to deny them a sense of hearing. This seems to be an especially dirty trick, since the water is the place for a fairly large animal to hear things, and, as we shall see later, mammals that have made the decision to return to the ocean from the land (such as the seals, whales and porpoises) have developed incredibly good ears and even "sonar" (or echo-location) abilities. When the arthropods came out of the water and became insects, curiously enough many of them became extremely ear-minded. Perhaps we can see a reason for this that depends on a little elementary geometry.

One of the reasons for hearing in a very small animal, such as an insect, is to locate something (a mate, enemy or prey). But *directional* hearing is dependent upon a difference between either the time of arrival or of the pattern of the sound wave that arrives at two distinct points on the animal's body. It is no use to have only *one* ear, because this won't do the job of getting an auditory fix on the source of sound. In water, sound is so fast that it would take an extremely delicate brain mechanism to make the differentiation between the sound heard in one ear and another, especially since the width or length of the animal might be less that a wave length of sound. I believe this is the reason why evolution waited for small animals living in air before it decided that a sophisticated ear was worth trying to develop.

We see this development taking many directions. The so-called "chordotonal" organs are scattered singly or in groups throughout the body and appendages of insects. Some highly advanced groups form hearing organs that work by the sensing of the vibration of tympani, or little drums. Other rather mysterious and versatile devices (Johnston's organs) at the base of the antennae can detect sound, wind direction, flight speed, direction of gravity or (in aquatic forms) the velocity of water flow. Another similar group (subgenual organs) in the leg act as sensitive detectors of vibrations on the surface of the ground or substrate.[2] In general, insects are tone-deaf. Their eardrums and some fine-hair sound receptors are designed mainly to hear repetition rate and other patterns of sound intensity (rather than pitch), although their sensitivities to *certain* frequencies may sometimes get them into trouble. A flesh fly, for example, is bored by a firecracker, but the sound of a rubber cork being turned in a bottle will drive it into a nervous fit.

The enormous degree to which insect receptors can be specialized for extreme sensitivity to a given *range* of sound frequencies is shown in three families of night-flying moths that have had to develop a defense against the bat. (Because the eyes of these moths shine at night when light strikes them, they are also called "owlets.") The bats are able to detect prey quite precisely by echo-location; that is, they send out ultrasonic signals (that are of too high a frequency for us to perceive), and from the echoes of these sonar beams are able not only to locate the object but to tell what it is. The night-flying moths are still here, even in bat country, so their various defenses against this diabolic hunting scheme must have been successful enough to bring about an offense-defense stand-off. First of all, moths have soft, sound-absorbing wings to make the echo-location as tough as possible. But they have also developed an absolutely incredible sensitivity to the bat's ultrasonic signals by the use of only four nerve cells. That this would be accomplished with such an extreme economy of design is enough to make an acoustical engineer drown his blueprints in a cask of beer. Compare, for example, the effec-

[2] In the spiders, the lyriform organs in the legs are of this type, but some can also hear air-borne sounds after a fashion by raising the leg off the strands of the web. The web-building spiders are extremely sensitive to vibrations of the strands, either by prey or by a courting male. Some predacious spiders take advantage of this sensitivity by imitating the frenzied tugs of a trapped insect and, when the half-blind web-owner rushes out to retrieve her supposed prey, she is herself devoured.

tiveness per pound or per anything of the radar warning device of state highway police with instruments equivalent to those of the noctuid moth. The moth's ears are located on the rear part of the thorax and directed outward and backward into the constriction that separates the thorax from the abdomen. Each ear is a small cavity and inside it is a transparent eardrum behind which is an air sac. A fine strand containing the sensory apparatus extends across the air sac from the center of the eardrum to a skeletal support. Two acoustic cells (known as A-fibers) are located in this strand. The two A-fibers join a large non-acoustic (B) cell and continue as tympanic nerves into the brain. By listening in electronically at the two A-fibers, Kenneth D. Roeder and his associates have been able to find out what happens when a moth hears a bat.

A bat actually sends out a frequency-modulated beam of ultrasound. Their cries start out at 70,000 cycles per second and end, a millisecond or so later, at about 35,000 cycles per second. But the moth pays no attention to this FM effect because he is tone-deaf. The reception of the first pulse (and the bat repeats his pulses from 10 to 100 times a second) causes an action potential to travel in the moth's A-fibers to the brain in less than 2 milliseconds. What he does then depends on whether he has located the bat at a fair distance or close upon him. It should be noted that actually the absolute sensitivity of the moth's eardrum is not very high. To get a response from an A-fiber cell requires ultrasound about 100 times as intense as the sound that human ears can hear. But there are not many ultrasonic pulses in the night of the same pulse rate as a bat's, so the moth can detect the bat at distances of over 100 feet, but most importantly he can detect the loudness and the pulse rate and can tell, from the difference in sound in the two ears, where the bat is. From loudness and direction the moth decides what to do. If the bat is far away, the moth under "early warning" alert will turn about and fly at top speed away from the sound source. Even though the bat can fly faster, this is a good tactic because the moth can hear farther and he may not have been detected by his mammalian predator. If the bat were close, this maneuver would be futile, so the "red alert" dictates either going into an evasive loop or, best of all, folding his wings and dropping instantly to the ground. That such fluid and complicated tactics can result from the activity of two pairs of nerve cells is fantastic, but certain moths of the arctiid family (including those whose caterpillars are known as "wooly bears") have gone beyond this into the realm of what would once be regarded as science fiction. They have developed sonar countermeasures. From the "hip" joints of the third pair of legs they are able to send out clicks by a mechanism somewhat similar to the way a child's spring-steel toy makes a noise when you press the spring with the thumb. Only this comes out as pulses of ultrasonic sound in a frequency range which the bats can hear. They don't like it and veer away. Even though a bat can hear other bats making somewhat similar noises, he detects an alien menace and decides he's had it for the night—at least in that area where moths behave like bats. That these arctiid moths have got it made seems evident from their much higher rate of survival than their less gifted cousins in bat country. Entomologists believe that this is a relatively new invention and, in the deadly chess game of offense and defense between bats and moths, one could predict that some bats sooner or later will develop an immunity to the frightening effect of a moth that sounds like a bat.[3] But we have to await evolution's leisurely pace, and who knows what catastrophes of pollution or air chemistry evolution's Bad Boy—man—may provide in the meantime to wipe out arctiid moths and flying mammals alike?

Although not so technically prodigious, the sound and the hearing of the cricket have been perkily interesting to man throughout historical times. Male crickets sing to prospective mates with a sort of amiable creak which is produced by rubbing a scraper on the left wing against a file on the right—a

[3] As far as I have been able to ascertain, this is the first and only case in which an animal of one phylum has been able to establish communication (even though it is one of doubtful cordiality) with an animal of another phylum in a language both can understand.

built-in fiddle. The love song seems on the face of it the height of futility since in most species the female is deaf. Investigating this absurd situation further, entomologists found that while the cricket is fiddling, a small cup between his wings fills with a fluid called "seducin." That this is the real source of his male attractiveness becomes apparent when the female crawls up on her sweetheart's back to drink and is quickly impregnated. It would seem that the cricket's song may be of a territorial nature—an admonition to other males— and, indeed, in the Mediterranean world people have found amusement in the sexual battles of crickets. Every cricket has his own hole, which is home to him, and he sits in front of it fiddling. When two male crickets whose territories overlap chance to meet one another while seeking food or mates, they try to fiddle each other down and finally leap at one another, biting. Showmen at Italian county fairs put two male crickets into a narrow cage, which the loser cannot escape. Fighting crickets have been reared since the tenth century in China for the amusement of the well-born, much as fighting fish were raised in Siam. In a quite different context the song of the cricket has made its way in a symbolic sense into modern industry. The frequency with which a cricket broadcasts is proportional to the ambient temperature. So-called "mechanical crickets" are used in the fluidized catalyst beds that serve to convert heavy oil to high-octane gasoline, signaling a servo-mechanism that keeps the temperature just right.

The grasshopper (or biblical locust) hears and makes himself heard at higher frequencies than the cricket. At reasonable loudnesses, the cricket's upper limit is 10,000 cycles per second, while the grasshopper can hear up to 45,000 per second. The thresholds are such that a large grasshopper can be heard by another at a distance of about forty-five yards and at swarming time locusts can hear the flight noise of a passing swarm. As in the moths, hearing does not seem to involve tone or pitch discrimination, as long as the sound is within a certain tone range. This is shown by electrical recording of the nerve fiber responses to pulses of sound, which are the same regardless of change of pitch. The behavioral response (what the insect does when he hears) depends on how loud the sound is but not its tone. An insect's tympanal ear shows the typical inhibiting or contrasting capability that we have observed in his compound eye. A constant sound gives only a nervous "on" response and the background noise is then quickly inhibited. In other words, the insect when alerted is able to concentrate on only what he wants—or needs—to hear. In grasshoppers the eardrums can easily be seen on the sides of the first segment above the hind legs. Unlike crickets, grasshoppers fiddle with their thigh bones. The grasshopper stands on his "hands" and lifts his back legs until the femurs rub against a line of small stiff pegs on the wing. This produces the meadow song that sounds to us like a boy trying to start up a miniature automobile with a dying battery. The grasshopper makes an entirely different sort of noise when he jumps, snapping his two big top wings against the smaller inside ones and making a lively crackle as he takes off.

The katydid is a more subtle musician, since he can not only be made to change his characteristic rhythm, but he also has an extraordinary amplifying system—he is a sort of winged loud-speaker. He makes his sound by lifting his wings and running the edge of one over some two hundred sawlike ridges on the other. At the base of the wings are miniaturized amplifiers less than one-eighth inch diameter, made of that universal insect plastic, chitin. These are membranes thinner than paper and can amplify sufficiently to be heard a mile. The U. S. Navy has used some of the principles of this amplifying system. In the Harvard laboratory of George W. Pierce, katydids were taught to change their normal two-beat rhythm. By imitating a mechanical katydid, they were conned into shifting to a three-beat and a four-beat rhythm, but above this they lost count and when the teacher got to a seven-beat rhythm, they went into a sulk and stopped singing. (This sulkiness is a constant stymie for every ethologist trying to teach an animal or even a child.)

The cicada, when the summer is hot and sticky, is about

the noisiest animal around. In general principle one could duplicate his noise by snapping the bottom of an empty beer can with the thumb, but one would need to have a thousand beer cans and thumbs and the snapping would have to be accomplished much faster than is done by a sweaty man at an August baseball game. The cicada has drumheads vibrated by formidable muscles and an amplifying system that is more like a bull horn than the katydid's ladylike megaphones. The sound organs are small pits on either side of the belly just under the wings. Two large plates, which can be raised and lowered to control volume, fit over them. The drumheads are in these cavities, together with the amplifier—a folded membrane, or "mirror," and a tube that lets in air to be vibrated. Under control of the muscles the little drumheads shudder slowly at first and shake up the air in the cavity. Immediately the trembling air expands within the folded membranes, then bounces off the mirror for more intense magnification. The plates open and that terrific metallic din emerges to intensify summer headaches and to remind one that August is indeed a month of noise and of guns. The cicada may deserve his short time of noisy courtship because to enjoy these brief summer weeks he has endured from one to seventeen years in the soil and has left many molted exoskeletons there.

In the case of mosquitoes and the like, the noise is produced by special vibrating blades in the base of the wing, but there are three basic sounds. One is of irritation, as when the mosquito has failed to get a productive bite at you. Another is a cry for help. Another, used by the males, when amplified in the laboratory resembles a wolf whistle. And that is precisely its function. If the passing female utters a certain cooing noise, it's a date. Acoustic engineers have been amazed at the selectivity of this process, since the communication between male and female mosquito may take place across considerable distances and in the middle of a noisy city. Apparently the wave form is distinctive and once heard, the inhibitory processes go into effect so that that's *all* that is heard, at least until boy and girl mosquito have located each other and introduced themselves.

H. C. Bennett-Clark and A. W. Ewing of the University of Edinburgh have devoted a good deal of unromantic attention to the love communication between opposite sexes of that exhaustively studied genus *Drosophila*, the fruit fly. We have used and abused this animal so extensively as a laboratory robot that it is refreshing to find somebody interested in its natural life outside the range of the X-rays used for studying mutations. As in mosquitoes, the fruit fly's love song is expressed by the wings. The call of love is usually a wing vibration, but some flies are peculiar in that the *posture* of the male's wings may be more important than the noise. In fact, one species *D. obscura* sings no song at all and courts only by means of a wing display. In this species, the female must have very sharp vision, since without the wolf whistle or the lute of the troubador, she can only respond by thinking, "I like the *looks* of that guy."

This way of flirting requires a small insect city. The girls cannot see over much distance, while in the case of certain moths we find a *chemical* response between the sexes of thousands of feet apart.

The chief technique of love calls, however, in this tremendous genus of insects is a telephonic one.[4] Typically the male blows his horn (by specific vibrations of his wings). The female can pick up this lascivious invitation through her arista organ—a feathery projection of the antennae. If she is an unreceptive female, a member of Woman's Lib, too young, already mated or of a different species, she produces a countersong of a squawky quality that sounds curiously like that of a Marseilles fishwife or like the imagined voice of some sort of Dickens' character (most all of at least the older women characters in Dickens apparently squawked). In some species the frequency

[4] It is one of the great mysteries of biology that in the lower animals a *sound quality* should result in the purity of species. It is as if an American boy and a Japanese girl could not indulge in sexual intercourse because they could not (at least initially) speak a common language.

of the squawk is 300 cycles per second, and for reasons we do not understand, this buzz not only discourages the courting male but causes him to turn and retreat in panic. We thus see in certain species of *Drosophila* a completely liberated kind of female. (But why do liberated females always converse in squawks?)

If the female has abandoned her Lysistrata mood and is inclined to add to the number of the species, she is quite music-conscious. In some species the female responds only to a veritable din of male wing sounds, in certain cases about 115 decibels, which is roughly equivalent to the climax of Tchaikovsky's "1812 Overture."

Some closely related species can hardly be told apart simply by looking at them, but their love songs are as different as "Hey Jude" and Mozart. Thus hybridism is discouraged by musical style. On the other hand, two closely related species of fruit fly have an almost identical song (curiously similar to "Yes Sir, That's My Baby!"). Hybridization on this ancient jazz theme might be possible, except that one species is confined to North America and the other to the Southern hemisphere.

What is evolution trying to do here? Why this huge number of species of a fundamentally similar fly? Note especially that the species are often identifiable as separate *only* by their love songs. This does not seem like good taxonomy, because in man it would make separate species of acid-rock hounds and lovers of Beethoven. The crucial point, however, is that practically all of the fruit fly species are mutually infertile. The rock lovers and the symphony-concert esthetes are not mutually infertile. Putting it in another way, one would expect that, despite this communication gap, there would have been just one great species of fruit fly, like that of man who is specifically fertile but speaks in a babble of tongues. The point is worth emphasizing.

The fruit fly uses his song or wing gesture to express only sexual provocation. This is not a symbol but an identification. ("I am a fruit fly of the type *Drosophila pseudoobscura.*

If you are a female of the same species, let's make a date.")
Furthermore, the male fly may be addressing this message to
his sister. Because of the human invention of symbolic communication, in which one can *translate ideas* from English into
Bantu by means of signs or even facial expressions and because,
further, of the almost universal human abhorrence of inbreeding,
we remain one big species, while the fruit flies observe anti-
hybridization and maintain at least 2,000 species (1,000 in Hawaii
alone) by varying their love songs. It is actually a misnomer
to call these noises "love songs," since they represent pure
signals, denoting not a tender state of mind but a specific
condition of the glands. One might better call them "gland
songs."[5]

Although insects do not communicate by frequency modula-
tion, it is interesting that the single frequencies, or narrow
bands, that they use are nevertheless often close to pure tones.
Musicians have noted, for example, that the housefly buzzes
at a nearly pure F natural in the middle octave, vibrating its
wings 21,120 times per minute. However, if the weather turns
unseasonably cool it may go to F-flat.

The sound and hearing of termites and ants are in dispute,
but they seem to have some kind of vocal alarm system. A
colony of termites will go quietly about its business of swarming
for several hours, but if a worker or soldier becomes disturbed,
for some obscure reason some kind of panic bell seems to
be rung, whereupon the entire military guard withdraws and
the swarming stops until the all-clear is sounded. If an ant
colony is invaded by some gross beast, such as a mouse, an
undoubted stridulation (a faint squeaking) sets in and the intruder is encouraged to leave before the sharp jaws of the
soldiers. The source of this stridulation has been located in some
ants of the subfamily *Myrmicinae*. The gaster, or back part of
the abdomen, rubs against a scraper of the nearest segment. As is
the case with spiders and crustaceans, these ants (especially the

[5] Unfortunately I must admit here an oversimplification. A good deal of
modern gut music, consisting of highly amplified guitars, drums and
hoarse shrieks, might also be classified as "gland songs."

Western Hemisphere species) are much more sensitive to vibrations in the ground than in the air. No frequency of over 15,000 cycles per second can be detected by an ant, which is natural since sounds of higher frequencies in the earth disintegrate by losing energy and thus would not be heard far enough to be of any use. The chirp patterns of the ant can be modified into pulses and pauses between pulses and hence may constitute an ant language.

The cries of some insects have been scrutinized with research thoroughness for ulterior motives. For example, bedbugs let out a little yowl of excitement when they sense the nearness of human flesh. Scientists at the U. S. Army's Limited War Laboratory in Aberdeen, Maryland, have been working to perfect a sound-amplification system that will make these cries audible and thus develop a system for detecting a lurking enemy —presumably one whose habits or body condition attract such insects.

Some of the sounds that insects make are mere by-products of their work and they may not hear them themselves, although in many cases they are direfully audible to human beings. Such is the case of deathwatch beetles that tunnel through wood. They make tapping sounds with their heads which can often be heard in old log cabins. By our ancestors the tapping of these insects could be heard at night when all else was quiet and the spirits of dead pioneers were about. Since this beetle is remarkably long-lived and of infinite patience, he may tap in some wall or in some old wooden desk for a score of years.

The experiments of Harald Esch of the University of Notre Dame and the parallel ones of Adrian M. Wenner on the sound language of bees have been fully as fascinating as the original discovery of the wagging dance by Karl von Frisch. Esch joined Von Frisch's group in Munich in 1960 and his first research deed was to build an artificial bee that could mimic exactly the dance of a live forager bee returning to the hive with full belly and glad tidings. The real bees showed the dummy considerable respect and showed great interest in her dance, but did not leave the hive. Some element of the message

was missing. Since Hans Antrum of Germany had proved
many years ago that a bee can detect sound through its legs
(can in fact detect vibrations of the honeycomb with an amplitude as small as thirteen millionths of a millimeter), Esch
concluded that his dummy bee needed sound effects. He noted
as many as 15,000 returns on the part of "silent dancers"
who forgot or were unable to get the sound part of the message
across. Esch's first artificial bee with a loud-speaker was ex-
ecuted by the real bees as a spy, however, because Esch forgot
to take account of the time necessary for audience response.
The reporting bee is supposed to pause while the listening
or antenna-thrusting workers utter beeps which mean, in effect,
"We dig you," and then a short time for smelling the nectar.
On the other hand, the sound without the dance wouldn't
convey the information either.

It appears that the evolution of the dancing-talking bee has
reached culmination only within the family Apidae. Going down
the evolutionary ladder, the bumblebee, a stupid animal, does
not know of any way to communicate. In the genus *Trigona*,
the foragers make scent trails and can guide a party of com-
panion-workers back to the nectar. The genus *Malipone* makes
various sound signals to tell how far the food site is, while
in the gifted genus *Apis* both the distance and direction are
given. The stingless bees of Brazil don't dance but do communicate with sound and give out samples of goodies. They
make a series of short dashes to show that the food source
is nearby and a series of drawn-out passes to indicate a distance
of up to several hundred yards.

Esch gives a plausible explanation of how such behavior
might have come about. Even so primitive an insect as a
moth, alighting from flight, rocks back and forth rhythmically
on its feet, the duration of rocking being a measure of the
length of flight. This is a response to a basic physiological
need, and in the highly developed social bee, the wagging
walk could have started out as a similar physical reflex that
later achieved symbolic significance. At the primitive level the
problem of direction is solved by the forager's simply leading

the group to the food, as the ant scout does. Occasionally on a hot sunny day even the sophisticated honeybee forager will revert to semidirect rather than symbolic guidance. She will perform her wagging dance on a horizontal surface in front of the hive, pointing her run in the *actual* direction of the food and buzzing her wings as if to take off in that direction. Esch found that by changing the hive conditions so that the honeybee could no longer resort to symbolic language (for example, by laying the hive horizontal so there were no longer any vertical surfaces on which the foragers could dance) the advanced bees would take one step down in evolution and, like the stingless Brazilian bees, simply indicate the distance by sound and neglect the direction.

Wenner in California identified the sound of distance as a low frequency of 250 cycles per second. The bee emits a train of sounds during each straight run of the wagging dance, the average length of the sound train during a given dance and also the average number of pulses in a train being a direct measure of the distance the bee has traveled from the food source. There seems also to be a message in the rate of pulses indicating the strength of sugar concentration in the food (*Apis* cannot be bothered to hand out samples).

In addition to the food-source song and dance, bees in a hive make a lot of other distinct sounds, some of them peculiar to female autocracy. The characteristic hot weather hum of a beehive is produced by worker bees acting as ventilators. They stand on the comb and create currents of air by beating their wings—a sort of attic fan system. Their sound has a basic frequency of 250 cycles per second but is rich in overtones and is enhanced by the resonant vibration of that part of the comb structure on which the ventilator bee stands. The worker bees are exceedingly home-conscious. When an intruder, such as an ant, approaches, guardian bees rock forward on their legs like watch dogs and issue short bursts of sound every two or three seconds for ten minutes or more. Whether this bee-barking is heard by the ant probably depends on whether it is walking on the same comb structure as the one the bees are standing on. When the hive is jarred, as by a sharp wind or a careless bird, the collective reaction of hundreds of guarding bees is heard as a shrill, loud buzz. This is followed by a piping of workers throughout the hive—faint beeps at half-second intervals, a complex sound with a fundamental frequency of 500 cycles per second. This seems to be a message, something like "Cool it, girls!" because when a recording of this piper's song is played, it will quiet down any disturbed hive.

Her majesty the queen, on assuming the throne as a virgin, begins a song which is called "tooting." In order to explain this, we must understand something of the cruelty and despera-tion surrounding apian sovereignty. A hive cannot tolerate more than one queen at a time, yet in queenless hives several queen-bearing cells develop simultaneously in a comb, one always maturing first. Once the first-hatched is strong enough to walk, she visits the other queen cells, tears them open and stings the potential rivals to death. (Unlike the workers, she can use her dagger without damaging herself.) Quite often, however, the worker bees don't allow her to kill *all* of her unhatched rivals. They bar the bloody virgin from some of the cells. Incensed at this, she begins to toot, night and day, for a week or more. She is crying, "I am your one and only queen. Let me at those pretender wenches!" The surviving rivals are glued back in their cells as soon as they start to escape and they start to pipe in a lower tone and in a different pulse pattern than the free queen. This has been called "quacking" and probably means something like "Let me out. Let me fight her." In their own time the workers do just this, but they release only one rival queen at a time, who then does battle with the reigning mistress of the hive until one is killed. This deadly elimination tournament generally continues until only one queen is left in the hive. The surviving virgin then flies away with several drones and returns later to begin her prodigious life as a mother.

The communication involved in all this, although of a phatic (emotional) nature, is important to the workers, since the tooting announces a live queen and the quacking response signals the

liveliness and eagerness to challenge on the part of the caged
queens. Wenner has found that if the queen's tooting is recorded
and played back in another hive containing free and caged
queens, the caged queens will immediately set up their quacking
challenge. A wise hive (we refer to an instinctive community
wisdom among the workers) will sometimes keep a caged queen
in reserve for even an egg-laying queen will be seized with a
strange restlessness that will infect some of the worker bees
(perhaps a younger generation tired of the Establishment) and
she will take off with these leftists in a swarm, leaving the
decimated hive queenless and forlorn.

As to the mechanics of bee sounds, there have been many
theories. The first, very attractive one was that the bee ejects
air through its spiracles (surrounding the lungs), manipulating
these as a sort of bagpipe. This doesn't hold up, however, since
the frequency stays the same if the experimenter substitutes
helium for nitrogen in the air of the hive. (The frequency of a
sound varies with the density of the medium. An astronaut
talking in an oxygen-helium atmosphere sounds like Donald
Duck.) The tentatively accepted idea is that the source of sound
is at the hard little platelets at the base of the wings. If one
clips a bee's wings, the frequency of her sound is increased
and the loudness is muffled in proportion to the amount of
wing removed. Bees do not hear through the air but, like
spiders and ants, mainly through some sensory apparatus in
their legs below the knees. The queen responds only when
a sound is transmitted via vibrators attached to the hive structure.
It appears, however, that bees may hear with their antennae
when the sound is close enough for direct contact. Thus the
numerical sound message during a wagging dance may, in the
general din of the hive, be perceived much as the late Helen
Keller used to "hear" human speech by placing her sensitive
hand on the speaker's throat.[6]

[6] Sad to relate, Adrian Wenner and his co-workers have quite recently
concluded that bees do not have a food-source language, visual or auditory, and that recruitment is done by direct imitation or by odor.
Esch and Von Frisch, although admitting that much of the foraging is

For a long time it was believed that fishes had no sense of hearing because if one went up to an aquarium and shot a gun off in the air, the fishes would not even bat an eye. The fact is that a fish cannot hear air-borne sounds but can hear very well in the water and, although not endowed with a specific noise-making gadget with amplifier like a katydid, is in practically all cases able to state his case in one way or another. If you submerge a hydrophone (an underwater microphone) in a fish-populated area you will hear all manner of grunts, rattles, snaps and honks, and sometimes with particular species in a vocalizing disposition there is a rather comforting barnyard racket. Since the fish was the first vertebrate, his hearing apparatus is of family interest to us, although anatomically we derive our ear structure from a gill arch that was no longer necessary out of the water and which the fish did not of course use in connection with hearing. Embryologically the mammal's eardrum is derived from tissues which became a gill slit in a fish, while the stapes of the mammal (the bone that transmits the vibration of the eardrum to the inner ear) is an embryological parallel to the hyomandibular bone of the fish by which the jaw is articulated to the skull.

The fish in the earliest evolutionary state probably developed the ear as a balancing organ. Sharks have large semicircular canals and sound waves pass directly through the head to the lower part of the inner ear. There is nothing corresponding to the human external ear (the pinna) and our very elaborate middle ear. Most fishes, however, hear virtually with their whole bodies. For low frequency sounds, in the same band width, for example, as the underwater vibrations of a submarine engine, the fish has a system of pores that extend through the skin and scales and are visible as slight surface bumps. On the head, these pores with attached tubes are called "cephalic,"

---

carried out in this prosaic way, maintain that bees *do* resort to symbolic communication when they are in the mood. To one exposed to the distressing repercussions of this controversy, it would seem that Esch with his greater experience with the pattern of evolution of bee-talk has an edge in the debate.

while this system along the side of the body is known as the "lateral line." All the cephalic and lateral-line systems are supplied with tiny organs, responsive to changes in water pressure. Each little surface organ has a nerve fiber that goes to the brain. In some cases "body-hearing" may be enhanced by a special device. For example, fresh-water carp and catfish, who have particularly acute hearing, have thin air bladders connected to the inner ear by a chain of small bones.

The kind of sounds that fishes (and other aquatic animals) make has become of military importance, since the Navy does not want its underwater submarine detectors confused by the noises of fishes and porpoises or even by the snapping and crackling of shrimps. Thus, under Navy support, phonographic records have been made of fish sounds over the world of oceans. There are quite a number of ways that fishes produce sound. One is by grunting by the expulsion of air through the duct leading to the air bladder and usually connecting with the mouth, although one of the Asian loaches is so uncouth as to expel the air through its anus. Certain sculpins use stridulation or frictional noise, like insects. When they vibrate their gill covers against the sides of their head, a humming sound is heard which may or may not mean something more significant than "Here is a sculpin." Horse mackerel, ocean sunfishes and certain triggerfishes use their pharyngeal teeth, which lie far back in their throats, for making a rapid gnashing sound. On the other hand, the grunt (a typical shore fish) uses the same teeth to give a loud rasping croak. The sea robin grunts but by a different method, using special muscles in the air bladder. The toadfish with the air bladder scheme actually achieves a low-pitched blast like the whistle of a miniature ocean liner. Some triggerfishes have taut membranes just behind the pectoral fins and above the air bladder. When they move their fins rapidly back and forth the fin rays act as drumsticks and the membranes vibrate, acting as resonators for the underlying air bladder, precisely like the skin of a drum. In open water the croaker makes more noise than any other fish by the action of special muscles on the air bladder. With certain South

American catfishes the air bladder is divided into many sections. The first four vertebrae are modified into an elastic spring and, like a bony cap, one end of the spring fits onto the end of the air bladder nearest the head, the other to strong muscles reaching to the rear of the skull. These fishes are able to speak a complicated code by vibrating the springs and muscles, the air bladder resounding and the partitions acting as amplifiers. What they have to say is obscure to us, but, to justify such an elaborate system, it must be important to another South American catfish. One of these genera, *Galeichthys*, must constitute a race of orators since, in addition to the rythmic drumming of the air bladder, they can make a sort of mewing sound by stridulation. This fish has a movable pectoral fin spine that locks in the forward position when the fish rotates it counterclockwise in an angry or defensive mood. This locking process is quiet, but the clockwise unlocking gives out a creaky mew, like a hoarse cat, and apparently signals, "I have won the fight."

Since the systematic study of fish sounds is only recent in ichthyology, the sounds and the behavior associated with them have been studied only in the case of small species suitable for observation in an aquarium. In many small fishes, it is difficult to determine exactly how they vocalize, but as a rough rule it is usually assumed that a low-frequency sound (say, 300–500 cycles per second) is made by use of the swim bladder while sound above 3,500 cycles per second are produced by some sort of frictional process (stridulation). In the cichlid family cry, "Br-r-r-" (low frequency), warning is connected with aggression, the frequency increasing as the size of the fish decreases. Usually the male has a deeper voice than the female. When she is guarding her eggs or recently hatched young, she will give her tiny growl just before attacking an intruder. She will give the same sound during the courtship period while she is aggressively holding her ground against the male as he tries to bite or ram her. In some species the male produces the "Br-r-r-" noise during courtship and also when his mate is returned to the tank, but he makes a curious thumping noise during the early stages of fighting a male of the same species.

Unlike *Galeichthys,* the victory ceremony of following the loser and ramming him is conducted in silence.

Perhaps the most important objective of a fish small enough to be a prey for a bigger fish is to make no sound at all. Fishes accomplish their swimming with a lack of hydraulic noise unbelievable to a hydraulic engineer and we have never come close to devising any mechanisms that can travel through water so quietly. As we shall see in Chapter 5, this ability is innate in a *living* marine organism and perhaps may never be duplicated artificially. We come closer to it with our own bodies, yet even the graceful turnings of an experienced scuba diver sound like a threshing machine to a distant shark. The shark can pinpoint the source of low-frequency sounds at distances of over 200 yards, apparently with the help of the lateral-line cells along his sides. Although the prey fishes normally do not make enough sound for the shark to detect, if they get into a fight among themselves or if they struggle in the clutches of some lesser predator, low-frequency sound is propagated in bursts, the frequency being involved well within the shark's audible range of 7 to 400 cycles per second. The same pulses also attract other fierce fishes such as barracuda, jacks and groupers. Neither the shark nor these other predators are attracted by pulses of high frequency, such as the whistles of a porpoise or the shrill singing of a white whale.

As evolution gave the signal for vertebrate animal life to come out of the sea, some changes had to be made, for the air is not only a slower sound medium, but also tricky on account of the wide variety of wind noises and the stridulations of the vast alien phylum of insects, which, however, have to be perceived because the insects are good to eat. The wide spectrum of air noises brought to the fore the application of the principle of inhibition and contrast, exactly parallel with the similar capability of the eye.

One anatomical peculiarity that we see in all air-breathing vertebrates from frog to man is that the air to be breathed has to cross the route of the food to be eaten. The glottis, a slitlike opening on the floor of the mouth back near the esophagus, leads into a boxlike cavity, the larynx, which in turn opens into the lungs. Cartilaginous rods support the larynx and from its *sides* hang a pair of horizontal membranes, the vocal cords. This is the way vertebrates began to use the sound-carrying properties of air. If you have something to make a noise with, you should also have a tympanum or eardrum to pick up these vibrations (although in many reptiles the ear is regarded as dispensable). In frogs and toads this tympanum is flush with the surface of the head and is stretched across the old first gill slit, the spiracle in sharks. The gill slit itself now becomes the Eustachian tube.

The various peepings and croakings of frogs are mainly male sexual calls (practically all female frogs are mute), but there is a tribal reason for them too. Although a lake or a pond may be too small for us to have much fun in, it is a big place for a frog. The chorus of calls serves to keep everybody in the community together. Species like *Rana sylvatica*, the wood frog that wanders vaguely around far from the water, might find it hard to find his way back home if it were not for the passionate croaks of his male companions from the pond. Different species of frogs respond preferentially to the mating calls of the species and actually probably do not even hear the croaks of frogs of a different species. Thus at this level of evolution a precoded and preprogrammed system is tuned to process only biologically useful communication. Thus as the frog only sees what it wants to see, it also hears only what it wants to hear.

The ears of reptiles are intermediate between those of the fish and those of the mammals. The inner ear shows the least change. The three semicircular canals are there, but a new structure, the lagena (flask), has appeared and in birds and mammals will be the cochlea (shell). In reptiles it is scarcely more than a small knob containing the nervous organ of hearing. In reptiles as in amphibians, the middle ear still contains a single bone, the columella, which transmits vibrations from the eardrum to the inner ear. (In the mammal two other bones at the hind end of the jaws join up with this columella, now called a "stapes" to add a rather exasperating degree of complication to the ear structure.)

Crocodilians and some lizards are the only living reptiles who actually detect air-borne sounds. Turtles have no sense of hearing. The snake has no exterior ear or eardrum, but the inner ear is developed and he probably hears sounds carried through the ground fairly well, just as do ants. Since all the snakes are deaf to air-borne sound, the absurd superstition about snake charmers is at once exploded. Indian snake charmers do not charm cobras with music but with the sway of their bodies from side to side. The highly sensitive animal is simply being induced to imitate a sort of dance motion. Although snakes are in our sense deaf, some of them can make noises which they probably don't hear but which may serve to terrify an enemy or prey. Thus the rattlesnake and the famous, vicious saw-scaled viper which has a habit of making a noise like violently boiling water. This comes from scales being rubbed together when the animal inflates and makes a figure eight. The dasypeltinian subfamily of egg-eating snakes make a bluffing sound by the same method. Birds are supposed to be scared by this and usually are.

Lizards at one extreme have no more air-vibration sensitivity than the snakes but most of them have some sign of an external ear. The gecko makes a call that sounds exactly like his name, and all members of his family can at least squeak. It is assumed to be a love call. The crocodilians are noisy. The alligator even makes its first sound while still in the egg—an "Umph." The adults when frightened give out a curiously sissified quavering hiss. But during the mating season the bulls bellow or roar and some of them bay like hounds.

The average bird's inner ear resembles that of the crocodile, which is not surprising in view of the reptilian origin of birds. What a bird hears does not include as wide a range of frequencies as a mammal can distinguish, but the bird is more aware of slight differences in loudness. However, he can hear and respond about ten times as rapidly as man to rapid fluctuations in the song of his own kind or of insects. The perception of young birds that enables them to imitate bird songs is remarkably delicate and can only be appreciated by taking a sound spectrograph, which shows the reproduction of speedy intricacies of sound pattern that are inaudible to human ears. Although the bird does not hear as wide a range of frequencies, the range within which it operates is special and critical. For example, baby chicks are sensitive to the low clucks of the hen (400 cycles per second) while the hen is very aware of the high cheeping of the chicks (over 3,000 cycles per second).

The location and range-fixing of the sound source is as important for birds as for insects and these functions again are achieved by having ears at both sides of the head. Not only the time of arrival but the loudness and *phase* of the sound (that is, the instantaneous form of the wave) are used for the purpose of localization. Whenever possible, an animal uses all three of these cues. Difference in loudness at the two ears is the most efficient with high-frequency sounds, especially when the wave lengths are shorter than the width of the head and when the sound-shadowing effect of the head is considerable. Localization by phase is most effective when the wave lengths are *longer* than the distance between the ears. For localization by means of differences in time of arrival at the two ears, there must be transient frequencies and abrupt discontinuities, the timing of which can be compared at the two ears. It is no use for a bird (or for a man either) by this technique to locate where a long, steady factory whistle is coming from. The kind of signal a bird likes to hear is one that includes cues for all three methods of localization. It should be repetitive but with a wide range of frequencies, and luckily these are properties shared by most of the sounds all animals make.

In many bird species the ear openings on the two sides of the head differ slightly in size and location. Evidently this asymmetry is helpful in pinpointing the origin of faint sounds but in precisely just what fashion is not known. Coupled with these external structural advantages, such night birds as owls have very large eardrums and cochleae. The wide head helps.

The barn owl can locate mice by ear in complete darkness. In one experiment, mice moving through a pile of leaves in a black room were pounced upon and devoured in thirteen out of seventeen trials. If by special sound filters, you remove all the rustling noises above 8,500 cycles per second the owl will always miss the mouse. When all frequencies above 5,000 cycles per second are removed, the owl will not even budge from its perch.

Although the raw mechanism of the bird's hearing is not unusual in the animal kingdom, its way of making itself heard is unique. Evolution has provided for birds a special location for vocal cords in a boxlike syrinx, at the lower end of the trachea (much lower than the larynx of mammals) at the point where the two main bronchi of the lungs begin. The voice box contains a bar of cartilage called the "pessulus." Air passing through the syrinx from the lungs causes the pessulus to vibrate. In swans the trachea is very long and coiled within the breastbone, serving the same function as the coiled tube of a trumpet.

There is something mysterious about the passionate and subtle vocality of birds, as compared to the muteness or grunty vocabulary of their reptilian cousins in evolution. What good is it for a mockingbird to learn the songs of others or of a mynah to be able to imitate a wolf whistle so precisely that young women for yards around will start to smile primly and to pat their hair? Some bird sounds, of course, have obvious survival value. Precocial birds (that is, domestic fowl and others who need to be born ready, rather than helplessly opening their yaps in a nest) can actually be taught sounds while still in the egg. (This is called prenatal auditory imprinting.) Upon hatching they will creep immediately toward the source of the sound that they heard during incubation, whether it is a hen or a professor playing a saxophone. In wild nature or even in the barnyard, of course, the sound will normally be the mother's cluck. In addition to his preposterous "Cock-a-doodle-doo" (presumably a statement of territorial suzerainty or of sex status), the rooster has some useful warning sounds for the rest of the flock. His "Gogógogock" call means danger on the ground (for example, a man or a dog), while his "raaay" warns of danger from the air (most likely a hawk but conceivably a supersonic airplane). A field sparrow gives "Chip-chip-chip" to warn of a man or a crow (these animals being interestingly identified as the same kind of danger), but when it sees a hawk it gives the more desperate "Zeee" sound which causes *all* small birds, sparrows or not, to seek cover. Among many communal birds, it depends upon which particular bird gives the signal. For instance, among herring gulls, if bird A warns, they merely become attentive, evidently not trusting entirely in the sincerity or level-headedness of this particular individual, but if gull B sounds off, they all fly away in alarm. The just-hatched chicks of the prairie chicken come running to their mother if she gives her "Brirrb-brirrb" call, but they freeze on the spot when she gives her special shrill warning. In the house sparrow, there is an interesting persistence of infantile call notes throughout life. Practically the same sound pattern is used as a call to the fledgling young, as a female invitation to coitus and as a nest-relief call. (The mother, in effect, says, "It's your turn to baby-sit, daddy.") Thus, as in the Chinese language, the meaning of a given sound depends on the context.

That communication by sound is critically important in the parenthood of precocial birds is shown by the fact that deafened turkey hens peck all their children to death as soon as they hatch. The innate aggressiveness of the turkey toward anything that moves on the ground is only held in check by the cheeping of the chicks which unlocks the maternal drive.

We have noted that for efficient location of a sound source a bird likes a kind of mixed-up but repetitive series of pulses. But what if the bird, in warning its young and its companions, does not itself want to be located? This is obviously the case when the source of danger is a hawk. One can design a ventriloquist sound. It is pure tone, fading in and fading out, with no transients or discontinuities. It is pitched at an intermediate frequency between the optimum for localization by difference in place and by loudness. A number of small bird species have evolved ventriloquist sounds like this which mean "Here comes the hawk."[7] Two warning calls of birds are essentially the same throughout the world. The "Chink" call reveals the location of the caller while the "Seeet" call hides it. The high frequency of the latter prevents detection by phase difference while the slurred beginnings and endings mask the differences in time they arrive at the hawk's two ears. It is impossible even for a man to locate the position of the "Seeet" caller.

Warning or communicating in general by sound has certain obvious advantages for an active animal. While the eyes of the communicant have to be used to watch the partner during visual signaling, messages can be conveyed while doing something else, such as foraging or flocking or even copulating. We are used to being engulfed in bird songs at certain times of the year, since singing comes naturally to the passerine (perching) birds which are most likely to come to our back yard, take it over imperiously and sing their challenges to intruders of the same species. An unmated song thrush spends ten hours a day singing, nine hours roosting and five hours eating and messing around. Some species, however, have no voices at all, including storks, pelicans and some vultures. The rule that only the male sings is violated by the cardinal and the rose-breasted grosbeak and by many tropical wrens, among which the female sings nearly as well as the male when she has a mind to do it. Owls, as nocturnal lovers, have loud voices for communicating amorously in the dark. Certain hawks and crows have no courtship songs, but all crows have alarm and assembly calls. It is interesting that French crows ignore the alarm calls of American crows, but respond to the American assembly call, which is

[7] In the ventriloquist art of humans, words are formed in the usual manner, but the breath is allowed to escape slowly, the tones being muffled by the narrowing glottis, the mouth opened slightly, the tongue retracted and only its tip moved. The increased pressure on the vocal cords diffuses the sound; the greater the pressure, the greater the illusion of distance. Ventriloquism is practiced among many primitive peoples today, including the Zulus and Eskimos and for centuries was well known in Egypt, the antique Mediterranean world, in China and in Hindustan. It is probable that the Greek oracles were uttered by ventriloquism.

generally a notice that "chow's down." When birds go deaf, for over a year they may continue to sing as well as normal birds but tragedy ensues from another quarter. Since they cannot hear the hunger calls of their nestlings, the young are fed so poorly that they starve to death.

For many years there was a lively controversy as to whether singing birds learned the songs of their species by imitating their parents or were born with a gift for making the specific sounds, just as chicks are born with the simple ability to cheep and crickets to fiddle. The answer now seems to be clear that it depends on the species. The degree of instinctiveness varies from the tree pipit, in which nothing is learned (if hatched and raised separately from his family and from the sounds of all birds, he will nevertheless at the proper glandular time begin to sing like a tree pipit), through the rather susceptible chaffinch, whose general tendency is to learn only from his own species, to the skylark, who is born only with a few poorly organized clues on how to sing, finally to the linnet, in which the hormones command simply that he sings at a certain season but in which all else must be learned. In many cases, even the very young have songs, rather than mere hungry cheeps or squawks. The "subsongs" of a young male chaffinch are perfectly analogous to the sounds of a human baby before it learns to speak. A young bullfinch learns its song by imitating its father. One bullfinch that was raised by canaries learned canary song; four years later, descendants of this bird still sang canary.

One of the questions ornithologists ask themselves is: Why are there so few sham songs or mimicked sounds? If the mockingbird obtains better sovereignty by warning away all species whose songs it imitates, why do not all passerine birds sing, so to speak, multilingually? It should be noted that when birds mimic sounds, the mimicry is usually given as part of the song and conveys no more elaborate information than "Here I am" or "I own this real estate" or, in the case of amorous pairs, loss of contact. Other sounds will be made as the caller flees, attacks or attempts copulation. Perhaps we see a trend toward mimicry of dangerous enemies in the snakelike hisses made by titmice and wrynecks. That songs may change from time to time even in the same species in the same location is shown by the blackcaps of southwestern Europe. Since about 1920 a new type of song has been spreading which consists of brief notes inserted within the regular, time-honored ditty. Apparently this innovation (which, for a bird, is as serious as interpolating "Hello, Dolly" into "The Battle Hymn of the Republic") was originated by some swingers of this species in the high Alps. I have myself noted that in the course of over twenty years in Oklahoma the song of the cardinals who haunt my mimosa tree and perch on my TV antenna has changed from the previously dominant "Pretty-pretty-pretty-squee" to a commonly "squee"-less song, which constitutes an abbreviation rather than an innovation, and may signify something as simple as that they do not like my new dog or disapprove of the color of my automobile, which is cardinal red.

Since songbirds perform on an inexorable daily schedule, it is interesting to note that birds of six different species living in cities have been heard to begin their morning songs on an average of ten minutes later than the same species living on farms. This is probably not due to city smog but to the fact that the rooster on the farm is doubtless the first bird to arise and sing, thus rousing the songbirds, while city roosters are not plentiful and liable, in fact, to legal confiscation. During a complete eclipse of the sun, diurnal songbirds stopped singing entirely for about fifteen minutes during the darkest period, while nocturnal species, such as the nightingale, sang during the totality.

Even among the most advanced birds, such as jackdaws, such casual expressions as "Kia" and "Kiaw" are emotional utterances and, when unconcerned with self-assertion or warning, are communicating trivial states of their psyches, like our own yawns, brow-wrinklings and vague smiles. As Lorenz has pointed out, however, the jackdaw is perhaps the only bird that incorporates all of its call notes in its song (including "Kia" and "Kiaw,"

"Zick" and "Yipp" and even the sharp rattle used in defense of a comrade). In all other birds, sounds with "meaning" are not used in song at all. Thus the jackdaw ditty is something like the impromptu chronicle ballads of the Caribbean and even of the Deep South in which the lyrics are laced with circumstantial instances of people throwing babies off bridges or perishing in railroad catastrophes. As an exception to the rule of non-communication between the birds and humans, Lorenz genially claims that an old raven learned that "Rooh" was the call-note for Lorenz and, therefore, since Solomon's time was the only animal that has spoken a human word to a man in its right context. This achievement is perhaps equaled, however, by the crowned eagles of Africa who, according to Joel Welty, lure baby monkeys to their death with a soft whistle like the call of their mothers.

From an all-around standpoint, the greatest development of hearing, as of being heard, is found among mammals, and this is curiously true not only in the air but in the water. The development of language in man stands as the greatest biological achievement so far on the planet, while the under-water hearing, communication and sonar development of the dolphin (porpoise) represent perhaps the second most sophisticated achievement of evolution.[8] The dolphin's auditory and sound-making equipment are so specialized and subtle that we shall consider them after we have first discussed the less complex systems of the land mammals.

The middle ear of the primitive mammals contains a chain of three bones between the eardrum and the cochlea, and this curious and seemingly overfancy arrangement persists through the whole class of mammalian creatures except those that have returned to the sea. Since man is quite typical of the class, we may consider his ear as representing the ears of cats, dogs,

---

[8] When we make such statements, we are inevitably composing a manlike generalization. It is because the dolphin has so mastered arts that are, in a sense, anthropomorphic that we are dazzled and puzzled by him. In evolution's true language—that of duration of the species—*Limulus*, the horseshoe crab, is doubtless the most successful animal ever invented, although some primitive bacteria may have reason to dispute this award.

apes, rabbits and even of angels. Starting with the eardrum, we are confronted at once with an extraordinary instrument whose sensitivity men have only recently been able to duplicate in the laboratory. At some sound frequencies, vibrations of the eardrum are as small as one billionth of a centimeter—about one tenth the diameter of the hydrogen atom. Yet these vibrations are faithfully conducted by an elaborate hydraulic mechanism to a very fine membrane in the inner ear which transmits even such tenuous stimulations to the auditory nerve now at vibration levels 100 times less in amplitude. Even today we do not know precisely how these ultramicroscopic pulses stimulate the nerve endings. But let us further examine the gross hydraulic features of the ear. As we have seen, when sound waves start the eardrum vibrating, these pulsations are transmitted by a system of small bones (the ossicles) to the fluid of the inner ear. One of the ossicles, the stirrup (stapes), weighing only 1.2 milligrams, acts on the inner fluid exactly like a piston, exerting an inner rhythm. The movements of the fluid force into vibration the extremely thin and delicate basilar membrane, which transmits the stimulus to the organ of Corti, a complex structure that contains the endings of the auditory nerves.

Why do we need such a Rube Goldberg chain of gadgets to hear our wives say, "Dinner is ready"? The purpose is to conserve energy. The energy contained in sound is very pusillanimous compared to the energy in light. Even noises that are loud enough to cause us pain do not have much effect on the earless world around us. Moreover, sound is easily discouraged by barriers, and usually when it hits a solid surface, most of the energy is reflected away. In order to be effective, the ear must be a remarkably good mechanical transformer, converting the large swings of sound pressure waves in air into sharper vibrations of smaller amplitude. The mammalian ear acts like a hydraulic press, the principle of which the average person sees embodied every time his car is jacked up in a service garage for a lube job. The hydraulic press multiplies the pressure acting on the surface of a piston by concentrating the force of pressure upon a second piston of smaller area. In the same way the tiny footplate of the ear's stirrup transforms the small pressure on the surface of the eardrum into a twenty-two-fold greater pressure on the fluid of the inner ear. Still further amplification is obtained by a method so ingenious that it must have taken evolution, as a master design engineer, a long time indeed to figure it out. This final enhancement is based on the fact that a flat membrane, stretched to cover the opening of a cylinder, has a lateral tension along its surface. The more arcane fact, not realized by mankind until late in his history, was that this tension can be increased tremendously if pressure is applied to one side of the membrane. This is the job of the organ of Corti—to be the underside of a sort of fairy drum. The intricate design is such that pressure on the basilar membrane is transformed into shearing forces many times larger on the other side of the organ. The amplified shearing stress causes extremely sensitive cells that are attached to the nerve endings to be briskly rubbed. And so we hear—even a whisper which contains less energy than we receive from a distant star.

What happens to the nerve impulses? It is very important that we have two ears, for the localization process is as vital to a mammal as it is to a bird and the use of ears on different sides of the body is much more general in the animal kingdom than the implanting, in the same plane, of two eyes which can measure distance by the stereoscopic effect of image overlap. Relatively few mammals have full binocular vision, and very few have color vision, but virtually all land animals use their ears to locate the source of sound. Evolution intended the ears to be used this way after it got over confusing the ear with a gravity detector, and a wild mammal is more disadvantaged in losing the use of one ear than in having a paw chewed off. As we discussed in the case of insects and birds, each ear receives a slightly different sound pattern. In some way, which is not completely understood after 150 years of auditory research, this difference is used by the brain to fix the position of the sound source. As long ago as the days of Giovanni Venturi in the eighteenth century, it was recognized that a person with one deaf ear could localize sounds only if he turned his head while the sound continued. He simply kept turning until his one good ear was facing the source. But such a person could never localize *brief* sounds accurately. Modern civilization is perhaps cartooned most vividly by the fact that most of the information about sound localization has been developed either through the requirements of military observations or by insurance companies trying to prove malingering in the case of people claiming to be deaf or half-deaf. The Stenger test, developed in 1900 (and still in use), is used to test people who claim to have lost the hearing of one ear (presumably by factory noise or by being cuffed by a brutal foreman). Such a person, feigning deafness in the right ear, will report hearing a tone if it is presented to the left ear through an earphone. What happens if the same tone is presented to the left ear and simultaneously but more intensely to the right ear? The malingerer will give himself away by saying he doesn't hear any sound, in spite of the fact that it is just as loud as before at his admittedly good left ear. The incredible effectiveness of this naïve test makes it clear that we hear only a single localized sound and do not consciously compare separate sensations arriving at the two ears.

During World War I the location of the sound of enemy airplanes became a hectic subject of investigation on the part of both the French and the Germans. The devices that came out of these secret studies were able to locate by differences of the arrival in sound of one ten thousandth of a second at two receptors. This, however, does not equal the discrimination of the human ears, which can locate some sounds originating only five degrees to the right or left of straight ahead or straight back, where the sound reaches the right ear only four thousandths of a second before it reaches the left ear. The ear on the side more clearly opposite to a source of sound receives not only a later signal but also one of lower intensity because of the shadowing effect of the head. As happens so often and so mysteriously in the cranial nervous system, each ear is represented more strongly in the opposite hemisphere of the brain than in the same side. Wilder Penfield, in one of his typically dramatic brain surgery experiments, found that when some of the auditory areas of the brain (which are rather scattered about) are stimulated, the patients say they hear sounds, even though no sound waves have reached their ears. When the right side of the brain is thus stirred, the patient hears a ghost-sound coming from the left and vice versa. The interaction between the two ears is found to decrease steadily the lower one probes (as did Mark Rosenzweig of the University of California at Berkeley) in the depths of the old, primitive brain. Some interaction can be traced down as far as the olivary nucleus in the medulla that represents the next-to-last station before the ears. At the last station before the ears—the cochlea—there is no indication of interaction of one ear with another. In the 1930s it was reported that cats with the whole cerebral cortex removed could still localize sounds, but in those experiments the test note was sustained for several seconds and the animals were allowed to move their heads. It is now generally recognized that the higher brain centers of the cortex are required for localizing the *instantaneous* position of a sound. These cortical centers may be dispersed in the cat to as many as six different areas. But the cortex is rather impatient. If you implant electrodes in the so-called "auditory cortex" of a cat and measure the electrical impulses evoked in response to clicks (to which the cat has been conditioned, to avoid mild shocks, by tipping his cage slightly), the electric potential evoked by the clicks is at first very weak. As the cat "attends," the potential increases steadily. Then, suddenly and just as the cat has attained maximum efficiency in response, the potential drops sharply to the former level. The auditory cortex shuts down. The whole pattern of learned response to the click is apparently given over to some other subordinate brain level. Thus it seems likely that the cortex deals only with new information and delegates to lesser levels, perhaps even those of the spine, the learned techniques for dealing with situations. (In the case of men, this subordinating habit of the temperamental higher brain levels may even be involved, as we shall see later, in such colossally complicated nervous jobs as the using of a language once it is learned.)

The problem of localization by the use of two ears has become for modern man a somewhat more formidable task than simply being able to say, "The cougar that screamed must be behind that tree." It involves locating a specific voice in a background of other voices. Who said that dirty word at the cocktail party? Yet it is a curious and fortunate thing that men's ears are most delicately attuned to the frequencies of the human voice. In the low frequency range up to sixty cycles per second, the vibration of the basilar membrane produces in the auditory nerve a volley of electric spikes synchronous with the rhythm of the sound. As the sound pressure increases (or the sound becomes louder), the number of spikes packed into each period increases. Thus two variable pieces of information are conveyed to the cortex—the number of spikes and the rhythm. These convey loudness and pitch. Above sixty cycles per second a remarkable new phenomenon of hearing takes place. The basilar membrane now begins to vibrate unequally over its area. Each tone produces a maximum vibration in a different part of the membrane. At frequencies over 4,000 cycles per second the pitch is determined entirely by the location of the maximum amplitude of vibration along the basilar membrane. An inhibitory effect sets in that suppresses weaker stimuli and thus sharpens the contrast around the maximum. Thus once again we see the automatic mobilization of the working cells of a sensory organ to inhibit and thereby enhance, as the illustrious neurologist Georg von Békésy has shown to hold true also of the senses of the skin. Without the inhibition effects a tone would never sound like a *pure* tone and we would have no music. In a real sense the ear is doing, just as the retina does, some analysis and editing of its own—and this editing is further sharpened, in some manner not yet understood, by the auditory nervous system.

By means of audiograms we can now measure the threshold of a person's hearing at various frequencies. Interestingly such audiograms are usually quite similar for members of the same family, possibly due to similarity in face structure. The sensitivity of the average person's ear to a tone of 100 cycles per second is 1,000 times lower than it is to a sound of 1,000 cycles per second, and this is quite fortunate, since otherwise we would be constantly hearing the vibrations of our own bodies. If you stick your fingers in each ear, you hear a very low mutter which is produced by the contractions of the muscles of the arm and fingers. Evolution has seen to it that we are not distracted by these internal noises from our business of locating prey and mate and hearing a baby's cry. If evolution had not drawn the curtain, we would even hear the vibration of our head produced by the shock of every step we take. Nevertheless, sounds heard through our skull by bone conduction are a part of our auditory life. When we click our teeth or chew popcorn, the sounds come mainly by skull vibration. This bone-conducted noise is important to ear doctors. If a patient can hear bone-conducted sounds but is deaf to air-borne sounds, the trouble is in the middle ear, and there is some hope. If he hears no sound even by bone conduction, his auditory nerves are gone and there is no cure.[9] Using the same principle, a deaf musician can observe his rate of deterioration. If a violin player cannot hear his violin even when he touches his teeth to it, the poor fellow has had it.

The vibrations of the vocal cords go to the body as well as to the air. When you hum with closed lips, the tune you hear is mostly by bone conduction (via the jawbone). Notice that when you hum, with your ears stopped, the humming sounds much louder. During speaking and singing you hear both the bone sound and the air sound. Some low frequency waves are lost in the air. That is why you are so surprised to hear your own voice on a recording. It generally sounds much less manly (or to a woman, much more squeaky) than

[9] It has been suggested, however, that ultimately even the nerves may be susceptible to direct electronic stimulation, so that a deaf person could hear by a sort of internally established telepathic pick-up device, the carrier wave being electromagnetic rather than acoustical. Similar futuristic eyes for the blind have been proposed by the Russians.

the sound you hear as you are talking. A kind of feedback system continually adjusts and corrects one's voice. When we start to sing, the very start of our song tells us the pitch and we adjust the tension of our vocal cords to keep on key. This very swift, elaborate mechanism, which involves a billion or so neurons, is unfortunately far beyond present scientific elucidation. If we knew all about this feedback mechanism, we would be able to teach children to talk like Shakespearian actors at the age of two, whereas it now takes a child years to master this most formidable of all biological tasks, and as adults we find ourselves unable to learn to speak a foreign language without instantly being spotted as a non-native. It can be shown that if, by artificial means, the delay between speaking and hearing what we say is made long enough, it becomes impossible to speak at all. This fact is the basis of another insurance company test, this time for people who claim to be totally deaf. If the subject can continue speaking normally (that is, as normally as a deaf person usually speaks) with the delayed feedback, we can be sure he is really deaf. If he can no longer talk, however, he is given the bum's rush without the indemnity check. The feedback may be considered in sophisticated situations as comprising the whole environment—a concert hall, for example, with many human bodies in it. When a piano solo is very difficult (as are some works of Isaac Albéniz) many pianists concentrate so hard on the problem of the music that they fail to adjust to the feedback of the auditorium. The rating of pianists by this purely engineering type of discrimination corresponds closely to their reputation among musical experts or other pianists.

The sense of hearing deteriorates with age, but it is not certain how much of the damage is caused by the noise of modern living. A normal adult can perceive sounds from 66 to 20,000 cycles per second. In childhood some of us can hear well at frequencies as high as 40,000 cycles per second (which is almost high enough to hear a bat's sonar), but with age the acuteness in high-frequency reception steadily declines. In our forties over a period of five years the upper limit of perception has been found to drop by about 160 cycles per second every year. It has been assumed that this is due to loss of elasticity of the tissues in the inner ear, just as during the same period the elasticity of our skin declines. (You can readily determine about how old a face-doctored and bedizened woman is by lightly pinching the skin of her arm, if you are allowed. The rate at which the pinched fold returns to flatness is at least as good a test as looking at a horse's teeth.) However, nerve deterioration because of continual exposure to such awful noises as air-operated sidewalk breakers, jet airplane take-offs and blaring transistor radios may be more important in the long view. Dr. S. Rosen, the surgeon who developed the stapes-mobilization operation for otosclerotic deafness, reported on his visit to the Mabaans, a Stone Age people in Central Africa, who live in an environment corresponding virtually to a soundproof room. He found that even the very old people could hear as well as the young and were remarkably healthy. It has been suggested by many observers that the reason patients in first-rate European mental hospitals recover more quickly and are less disturbed during hospitalization than people in the corresponding American institutions is the absence of the typical clatter and hullabaloo of the American system. In Europe the nurses, attendants and doctors converse in subdued voices, double doors insulate each room or ward and paging is done by light signals rather than a squawk-box. (I have my doubts that any degree of training or admonition will lower the hearty decibels of the American female nurse.)

While high frequencies have been blamed for most human hearing damage, the French acoustic engineer Vladimir Gavreau of the University of Aix-Marseilles has called attention to the extraordinary and ominous effects of low-frequency sounds of high intensity. These low notes, sometimes below the level of audibility, affect organs of the body other than the ear. Gavreau first became aware of the destructive potential of such sounds when the vibrations from a defective rotating ventilator in a nearby building all but wrecked his laboratory. A sort of "sound-laser" can be easily constructed in the form of a

siren emitting an intense note of thirty-six cycles per second
(lowest E on the usual piano). This will not only cause cracks ,
in walls but can severely damage the human body by shaking
organs at their resonant frequencies. Still lower frequencies,
below audibility, produce nausea, fright, panic, chest pains,
blurred vision, dizziness and finally a profound lassitude nearly
equivalent to a coma. One of Gavreau's special whistles made
the nostrils of a colleague vibrate so suddenly that he recovered
his sense of smell that he had lost years before.

In the perception and use of *high*-frequency sounds, some
of our terrestrial mammals greatly exceed our own capabilities
and even those of the machines we have invented for making
and hearing ultrasound. The bat is, of course, the classical
example and its ability to fly in the dark, avoiding obstacles
and engulfing insects, has mystified learned men ever since
Lazzaro Spallanzani (1729-1799), who correctly deduced that
bats "saw" with their ears but presumed that they detected
the sounds of their wingbeats being reflected off nearby objects.
This hypothesis fell on its face when it was ascertained that
bats' wings don't make any sound. It was not until 1938 that
Donald Griffin, an undergraduate at Harvard, begged the loan
of some of Professor G. W. Pierce's electronic devices for
detecting ultrasound that the bat mystery was resolved. We
have seen previously, in our discussion of the eons-old war
between noctuid moths and bats, that the flying mammal uses
an ultrasonic echo-location system. That the source of the sonar
is the mouth is shown by the fact that covering the mouth ʼ
is as effective in grounding the bat as plugging the ears. Fruit-
eating tropical or "whispering" bats can generate pulses of
seven times the upper limit of frequency of human hearing. ˅
Sounds as high in frequency as 150,000 cycles per second have
been recorded, but they are so weak that even the most
sensitive microphone can barely pick them up.

Just as when a cat hears the squeak of a mouse, all his
auditory inhibition-contrast equipment is focused on this sound,
when a bat hears an interesting echo, he shoots out a rattle
of sonar beams. While on a cruising hunt he chirps at the

rate of 10 to 20 pulses per second. (This is the repetition rate, not the frequency.) When he "sees" something, however, by echo-location and proceeds to study it, the chirps go up to 250 per second. Each little cry starts at high frequency, then drops abruptly. (Presumably this helps in fixing the location of the prey by the two-ear system.) The ability to discriminate the nature of what his ultrasonic beams are reflecting from is flabbergasting to acoustic scientists. In experiments with brown bats Griffin and his colleagues found that these animals were able to distinguish between the echoes from insects and from plastic objects of the same size, even though the sensitive electronic instruments could tell no difference. When first exposed to the dummy insects, the bats would go after them but quickly learned that they were being fooled. Apparently the bat has recourse to a still more intensive inhibition-contrast mechanism that, when turned on full blast, can make incredibly sensitive discrimination in fine structure of the echo that are not within the power of an instrument.[10]

Bats in getting around can routinely fly between wires slightly thicker than a human hair and spaced just a little wider than a bat's wing span. In order to test the bat's ability to sort out his own echoes from other sounds in the same range of frequency, Griffin beamed noise from an ultrasound microphone to try to "jam" the bats. They were still able to dodge the fine wires since apparently the inaudible hiss of the microphone had some alien quality that meant simply background noise to the bat. It is apparent that we are not as good at this sort of thing as the arctiid moths. Although most attention has been devoted to the bat's hearing, we should not overlook the sleek economy of the power package that he uses for generating his sound—his "beeper." This vocal membrane weighs only a few grains, but on the basis of relative energy it

[10] The reader will note that throughout the studies of bionics experts (scientists who are trying to learn from talented animals), the emphasis has been precisely on this ability to concentrate by mutual inhibition of sensory cells. We saw this in the frog's eye and other single-minded eyes.

produces more noise than a man yelling or a woman screaming or a lion roaring.

There are other land mammals that use sounds beyond our hearing. Usually some of them are partly within the hearing range of predators. For example, an ordinary male house mouse sings, but we seldom hear it and if we do we are either very young or the mouse is a basso profundo. Cats, dogs and skunks are familiar with the mouse song. The ancient Chinese are said to have bred mouse bassos for their singing and to have kept them in cages like canaries. Actually one very small part of even the bat's echo-location sound is within the hearing of a fine young human ear under very quiet conditions. It is about as audible as a wrist watch. Assuming that the house mouse's song is similar in function to that of his relative, the golden harvest mouse, it is a song of romance. One can hear the harvest mice bugle during the mating season. The wild rodents are far from bashful in making noise, since they are the natural prey of so many beasts. All three members of the woodchuck tribe whistle but the hoary marmot is the champion. If a golden eagle appears overhead, this western woodchuck lets loose a shrill blast which is not made by his lips but formed in the throat. He may also bark, yip and yell. He also grinds his teeth when angry.

Members of the cat family are, as we know too well, very noisy about their amours. The female cougar screams at mating time, while the male answers with a surprising little whistle, like that of a bluejay. When mating during the winter, lynxes carry on in screaming fits that have to be heard to be believed. French-Canadians, who call the lynx "loup-cervier," have a folklore about this caterwauling that reminds one of the stories of Irish banshees. Hunting cries, like the brain-paralyzing roar of the male lion, have a more practical purpose, to terrify the prey and thus immobilize it and to let the silent lioness know where he is, since she is almost invariably expected to do the dirty work of the kill.[11] Aside from mating calls, in

[11] It is interesting that in the reserve animal parks of Africa, the automobile of a tourist or an official has now served as a sort of substitute

fact, most mammalian noises in the wild are those of the threatened or the despairing. When alarmed the wood rat thumps with his hind feet and, when seized by the enemy, will give a heart-breaking shriek of terror. The beaver is an exceptionally versatile sound maker. When angry he hisses. When frightened or hurt, he cries like a child. By slapping his tail on the water he expresses warning, anger, disgust and probably exuberance. One of the most peculiar and somehow lovable sounds is made by the porcupine at night who seems to be saying "Dear, dear, dear." Nobody has figured out exactly what this means; and it may be the equivalent of an unafraid man talking to himself.

As might be expected, the primates have a broader repertoire of sound than most land mammals. The vervet monkeys have at least six sounds for predators, each call identifying not only a different enemy (snake, eagle, leopard, etc.) but often the posture of the enemy. For example, there are separate signals indicating a flying eagle and a perched eagle. The "snake chutter" from one vervet monkey demands that all monkeys in the vicinity approach and examine the snake from a prudent distance. When the "Chirp" sound for a leopard is uttered, all the monkeys run to trees and climb to the top. Upon hearing the "Rraup" call for a hovering eagle, the monkeys scramble out of the open into thickets and descend from the tree tops. (One can readily see from this that, if leopards and eagles were smart enough to co-operate in their hunting, they would really raise hell with the population of vervet monkeys.) The howler monkey communicates his individual reactions with nine distinctive cries, each with meaning to his society, some of them specific enemy-naming sounds, like those of the vervet monkey, but some of them simply phatic communications that spread information about an individual's state of mind or a generalized emotional tone throughout the monkey band so that

---

for the male lion. The lioness uses the car as a visual and odor screen between her and the prey that the sound of the motor has baffled, thus waiting for the most opportune moment to make her run and spring.

all its members have the same attitude toward a situation. Some of this "talk" is on the level of our automatic clichés about the weather. As we shall make plain later, such monkey talk is not to be compared, however, with any human language. It is perhaps not coincidental that the gibbon and the siamang of the Far East also have a nine-sound repertoire, although the sounds are not the same. The call for help among primates seems to be necessary and specific. In a chimpanzee group studied by Wolfgang Köhler, mutual assistance came only if the threatened chimpanzee gave a definite, characteristic cry. The same behavior has been noted in baboons who are notably loyal gangsters. The band would rush to the rescue, but only after a special cry.

In approaching the unparalleled hearing and communication talents of the dolphin, we had perhaps best sneak up on this overheated subject by way of the seals. The earless, or "true," seals have no external ears, but they can nevertheless hear very well. Tiny channels to the inner ears open when they are out of the water and close tight when they dive in. This is an automatic valve system. Thomas Poulter in 1963 found that California sea lions send out beams of sonar-like properties for echo-location, as do dolphins and (in the air) bats. Underwater recording of captive sea lions swimming in a concrete pool at night showed that when pieces of fish were thrown in, the signals the sea lions gave met the criteria of a pulse-modulated sonar system of considerable sophistication. It was later shown that stellar sea lions, sea elephants, harbor seals and fur seals also make use of pulse-type sonar signals. Further studies of the remarkably vociferous California sea lion showed that, in spite of a much smaller brain, its power of modifying its vocalizations may be comparable to that of the much more publicized bottlenose dolphin, although the dolphin buffs would hardly ever be expected to admit this. In an oceanarium in California a sea lion was recently put in the embarrassing position of competing vocally with the pulsing squeak of a water pump. After a few wary attempts to broadcast over and through this noise, the sea lion suddenly figured out the answer and sent out a brilliant sequence of echo-location clicks *between* each stroke of the pump. This is the kind of ingenuity expected of a native Californian and the question is whether the dolphin can do any better.

Let us then finally consider the dolphin, more popularly known as the porpoise. About twenty-five years ago two eminent Canadian psychologists, Edward McBride and Donald Hebb, pointed out that the brain of *Tursiops truncatus* (the bottle-nose dolphin) is similar to that of man in both size and development, and thus this species, and other cetaceans, probably possess a high degree of intelligence. Some years later the echo-location abilities as well as the lower frequency communication sounds of dolphins with one another were discovered. A great many scientists as well as entertainment entrepreneurs entered the arena of delphinology, with the result that we wound up with permanent dolphin circuses in California and Florida (*Flipper* on national TV) and a public relations problem. Although it was now realized that if the Japanese continued to catch and eat dolphins, this would be regarded as equivalent to Hitler's crimes of genocide, the truth was that the public was satiated to the point of total boredom with dolphin or porpoise news and free-lance writers were being advised by their literary agents to find something else to write about. The American public is well known for its great swings in taste in the entertainment field but, as Dr. John Lilly, the most active of all delphinologists has pointed out, it is something akin to racial discrimination to regard the dolphin as an entertainer in an aqueous minstrel show. Lilly does not even dare to call them "animals," in the usual dichotomy of man versus the animals. So for the next few pages let us discuss dolphins as soberly and realistically as possible, while the reader who simply cannot stand any more dolphin lore is advised to skip ahead to the discussion of the language of the human animal.

The dolphin belongs to that group of aquatic mammals known

as the toothed whales. These vary in size from the "true" porpoise (*Phocaena phocaena*), whose brain is about the size of a human child's, through the different species of *Tursiops*, about adult human size in body and brain, to the killer whale (*Orcinus orca*), seventeen feet long and with a brain three times human size, and finally to the sperm whale (*Physeter catadon*) whose brain of 9,200 grams is the largest on the planet. Most of the scientific work has been done with either the Altantic bottlenose dolphin (*Tursiops truncatus*) or the Pacific bottlenose dolphin (*Tursiops gilli*). Most of the careful studies have been done either by Lilly and his assistants at the Communications Research Institute in the Virgin Islands, by Kenneth S. Norris of UCLA at Oahu, Hawaii, by U. S. Navy investigators at Point Mugu, California, or by various government contractors such as the Lockheed California Company. One might say that the purely bionic interest of the Navy in the dolphin as a sonar-equipped animal developed naturally from naval experience during World War II in mistaking whales and other cetaceans for enemy submarines, from which it quite understandably concluded that if the toothed whales had better sonars than we did, we'd better see how their sonars work. On a brilliant and somewhat erratic tangent from such pragmatic considerations, Dr. Lilly had burning in his mind the notion that the toothed whales, with their somewhat larger brains, were at least our equals in intelligence and that if only we could learn to communicate with them, we would find a new window to the universe. Since our own abilities to hear and be heard under water are less than the abilities of the dolphins to hear and be heard in the air, although it is foreign to them, the approach was by air-borne communication. Lilly's experiments so far have culminated in having a young woman spend virtually every hour of the day and night for six months in a pool with an adolescent male dolphin. It cannot be said that the lady was able to teach this dolphin (Peter) how to converse in English, nor was he able to instruct her in delphinese, but it soon became evident that, like all like-sized mammals, they got to understand the common language of sex. If one is to take Peter's message to the world, it would seem to be "Love conquers all" in the most Polynesian sense of the word "love."[12]

Although we shall return to Lilly's dream of establishing a common language with which men and dolphins can exchange thoughts, we should first see how they apparently communicate with each other and how they locate fish and other prey by sonar. Before systematic hydrophone recordings were made, people described the underwater sounds of dolphins that were perceptible to the human ear as "rasping," "grating," "filing," "woodpecker sound," "clacking," "knocks," "snarls," "sputtering," "whines," "a rusty hinge," a "creaking door." It was first believed that the dolphin made such sounds by expelling air and making air-borne signals. In his head the dolphin has a complex system of valves and air sacs connected with the air passage leading from the blowhole to the lungs. The clicking occurs when the valves are closed and they may vibrate like human lips. However, no air leaves the system under water; after being used to cause a whistle or click, the air is re-circulated to be used again. It is extremely complicated sound-making equipment. The clicks "shock-excite" resonant frequencies and harmonics of the air-containing cavities, such as the variable sacs, the fixed sinuses and the fixed nasal passages. One or more of the sacs can produce whistles, and others can simultaneously click-resonate during or between whistling periods. Changes in frequency and resonance correspond to change in size and shape of the sacs. Besides these sound producers which may roughly be classed as "nose emitters," the dolphin produces ultrasonic pulses for echo-location with his larynx up to 150,000 cycles per second. All head sounds, both for communication and for sonar, are emitted from the forehead through an amplifying membrane called a "melon." Sounds are picked up apparently by the lower jaw and transmitted to the inner ear. (The dolphin has no outer ear, or pinna.) However, low-frequency sounds, at least, may also be

[12] In view of the normal, sexually aggressive nature of the male, it might have been preferable to choose a female dolphin for this live-in, but apparently Lilly was also obsessed by some Freudian coyness.

received, as some sharks receive them, in the "lateral-line" organs of the skin. This is important in locating sources of low-frequency sound, since there is a peculiar difficulty (as previously noted) in the localization of sound under water because of its high speed. The two internal ears of the dolphin are about twelve inches apart, but the dolphin under water does not have the inherent advantage of the habit of air-borne sounds of going *around* the head rather than *through* the head. Since the head conducts at about the speed of water, the difference between arrival time at one ear and the other is very small. Difference in phase at the two ears can only be perceived if the waves are very short or if the dolphin uses the length of his body (skin receptors) rather than the distance between the ears for sound-fixing. In echo-location he has no trouble, since he is measuring the difference between the arrival of very rapid, patterned pulses. Seville Chapman of Cornell has estimated by the use of acoustical mathematics that with a reasonable signal-to-noise ratio (and biological systems are always able to get better ratios than artificial machines by reason of the inhibition-contrast effect), the dolphin at pulses of 150,000 cycles per second should be able to obtain a three-dimensional image of an object under water at least as clearly as we can *see* an object on land. The world of the dolphin is thus a remarkably sophisticated auditory world, embracing the sound range from about 500 to 250,000 cycles per second.

While our optimum range for communication by language is about 1,000 cycles per second, the dolphin's best communicating whistles and clicks (but not his echo-location pulses) range from 2,000 to 80,000 cycles per second. Through his eyes the central nervous system of the dolphin receives only about 10 million "bits" of information[13] per second while we receive ten times as much. However, when it comes to sound information, the situation is reversed. The dolphin receives at higher

[13] In the theory of communication, a "bit" is a unit of information equivalent to the result of a choice between two equally probable alternatives. Thus a nerve fiber conveys a bit when in effect it can ask the brain to decide what to do next. Since the answer may be to "shut up," this can be the beginning of central inhibition and attention.

frequency about 40 million bits in one second while our ears get only about 2 million bits. The dolphin's brain structure reflects this disparity. His acoustic cortex, the central hearing center, is much larger than is man's. Although the dolphin has no sense of smell, his skin is much richer than ours in pressure, touch, temperature and pain nerve endings and his tongue is specialized to pick up the ocean's tastes and carry them to deeply buried sensory organs which are quite different from our tastes, being of course totally unrelated to odor.

The versatility of the dolphin's marine sound-making apparatus can be only dimly appreciated and it is quite evident that attempts to make him oracular in the air are like trying to make W. H. Auden recite his poetry while bobbing for apples in a tub. Consider, for example, that the right and left phonation apparatus in the nasal passages are *capable of independently operating*. Thus a dolphin can carry on a whistle conversation with the right side and a clicking conversation with the left side, simultaneously and independently, using the two hemispheres of the brain. In this context the dolphin is "liberated," as we can see the promise of liberation of two human brain hemispheres occupying the same skull. The dolphin can control the two airflows separately and the two membrane vibrations separately. If two dolphins are in different tanks but connected with a hydrotelephone (so that they can hear but cannot touch or see each other), the conversation is very polite. When one is talking, the other keeps quiet. They can talk with whistles and trains of clicks at the same time. Thus one pair of dolphins can sound like two pairs of dolphins, one pair exchanging clicks, the other pair whistles. This is as if we were able to talk perfect English and Chinese simultaneously. No wonder we feel astounded, like Dr. Lilly, and wonder what in the world they are talking about. That it is a true conversation seems proved by the fact that if the telephone is disconnected the couple either stops talking or one or the other gives a personal "signature whistle" which is characteristic of a solitary dolphin. Because of Lilly's unabashed enjoyment of the constant and hearty sexuality of dolphins, he usually has a boy and girl dolphin on the telephone line, so one might guess that the conversation is not unlike that to which any parent of teen-agers has been exposed—a kind of extension of dating or date-making. When Lilly separately recorded the female part of the conversation and later played it back to the male, Peter (or whoever he was) listened briefly, then, so to speak, hung up the phone and swam away. He had heard her say all that before.

Yet the dolphin's phonation capability is, uncannily, still more complicated, since it can not only speak two languages simultaneously, but can also modulate between the two in a process, apparently unique in the animal world, which has been called "stereophonation." The source of the voice can be moved from one side to the other and very rapidly varied to and fro so that a Doppler effect[14] is added to the speech. Thus complexity is piled upon complexity. And still we have no idea why such an extraordinarily elaborate vocal apparatus, backed up by such a ponderous nerve-pack of a brain, was put on this planet. Norris' studies of the Pacific bottlenose dolphin shows a gay but rather hysterical animal, almost piteously subservient to man. Once he had been trained in captivity to eat tiny killifish, he would eat nothing else, even if live, plump halibut were put in the pool. In preparation for a test in the open sea, in which he would be taught to return to an artificial sonic signal, he was obviously afraid to leave the lagoon. His jaws chattered, his tail slapped and he showed the whites of his eyes, like a whipped dog. In all of the dolphins Norris studied, there was a marked disinclination to sever social ties with other captive dolphins or even with humans and there was a fear of facing unknown waters alone.[15]

[14] The Doppler effect is the apparent change in frequency of a sound as the source moves away from the hearer. Thus when a train whistles as it goes away, the whistle seems to the observer left behind to grow lower in tone.

[15] This behavior is in line with the pedamorphic nature of young dolphins, who are like human children in remaining associated with their mothers or "aunties" (any adult female and not necessarily the mother's sister) for an unusually long time. The toothed whales, although

The Lockheed California Company studied the behavior of a school of the same species when it was confronted with a ship-to-shore fence of aluminum poles. One scout left the group, detected and thoroughly analyzed the fence by sonar from a distance of 500 yards and returned to inform the others. Hydrophone recordings showed sixty-six separate whistles, sixteen different patterns including eight identical to those emitted by the Atlantic bottlenose dolphin. (Thus the generic relationship is shown in "language.")

It is probably unfair to draw conclusions on the basis of attempts to make the dolphin talk to us in the alien air in humanoid syllables, as Dr. Lilly attempted in his experiment with Miss Margaret Howe and Peter. Within the strangulating limitations of trying to talk at frequencies much below his wont, he did at least repeat the *number* of sounds made by his teacher, often accurately making more sounds than she realized she had made. A Southern girl (like Miss Howe) in saying "it" makes two syllables out of it—"iy-(pause) it"— and Peter responded with two syllables. Moreover the dolphin can understand when you are telling him to listen ("meta language") and will obediently attend. When you say "One, two, three, four, five" the intonation of "five" is different. The dolphin detects this and knows that you have finished a sentence.

Critics of Lilly's mystique have pointed out that all the dolphin has done so far is well within the capacity of an animal somewhere between a smart dog and a dumb chimpanzee. The elephant has a much larger brain than ours; yet, in spite of Romain Gary, a long acquaintance with this noble animal has not convinced mankind of the elephant's intellectual superiority. But Lilly sticks to his guns. The whales and their relatives, with their large and convoluted brains, have not conquered the world, because this is not within their ethic. Lilly would like to talk to a sperm whale before they are all

---

large enough to defeat most sharks (and certainly, as the killer whale, ferocious enough to burst up through thick ice and seize an Eskimo's dog), are mama's boys.

exterminated, because he believes the whale, no species or genus of which, unprovoked, has ever attacked a man, possesses an ethic that may include the Golden Rule only as a corollary to a vast and brilliant morality. He supposes that the best way to communicate with the giant central nervous system of a sperm whale would be to play for him one of Beethoven's symphonies. Then he would savor each of its notes and harmonies and perhaps in his silent plunges would even meditate upon the masterpiece, and within his great brain would even improve upon it for his own pure amusement and edification. Unhappily there is no sign that the cetaceans that we know best, such as the dolphin, appreciate music more than the dog who either regards it as irrelevant noise or howls at it.[16]

So far Lilly's doctrines have attracted only people who (like myself) *wish* that they were true. In the meantime at Point Mugu, Tuffy, an eager young bottlenose dolphin, serves as bodyguard for swimming sailors and as a delivery boy, and those performing at Miami shout in ducklike accents something reasonably close to "All right, let's go" as they dutifully dive through hoops. I think the truth of the matter is that the dolphin can technically never teach us anything except sonar and how to swim, because evolution, which cheated the octopus out of a higher status by allowing him no hearing, cheated the toothed whales by allowing them no hands or tentacles. A dolphin with the eyesight and suction arms of an octopus would be something else. The nexus of things that we vaguely call "Western thought" or "technology" might then have started 100 million years ago in the sea. It is always tempting to look at vague alternatives, as Lilly does, and point out, as did John von Neumann, that such things as arithmetic are accidents of evolution, and perhaps unfortunate accidents. If we had developed a sort of biological calculus that allows no process of enumeration or classification, perhaps we would understand better both the dolphin, ourselves

[16] Curiously enough, the only mammal who seems to be susceptible to music and is soothed by it is the rhinoceros, whom everybody regards as a singularly stupid and even mentally retarded animal.

and even the primeval protoplasm. But that is not the way we evolved. To maintain, as does Lilly, that because of a large brain and a goblin's deftness with the ways of sound, the dolphin must have a message of portentous significance for us, is equivalent to joining the parade to the Gurus—to pretend, for example, that all of Western thought must submit itself humbly to the fake "Wisdom of the East."

Lilly just may be right in one sense. He points out that the dolphins first came to man about the time of Aristotle and enchanted the superb cultures of the Mediterranean with their debonair friendship. Plutarch best expressed the dolphin's attitude at this time: "To the porpoise alone, beyond all others, nature has granted what best philosophers seek: *friendship for no advantage*. Though it has no need at all of any man, yet it is a genial friend to all, and has helped many." The dolphins left man about A.D. 52, according to Lilly, and only in the twentieth century have returned once more. Perhaps it is no great and subtle missionaryship, as the great physicist-turned-biologist Leo Szilard painted in his satirical fantasy *The Voice of the Dolphin*, but maybe they turn to us in the same spirit with which another of our mammal friends wags his tail and bestows his simple gift of love. It does not seem to me that we can have too many friends like that.

Although Plutarch did not mean his words in this sense, appropriately the dolphin's most pragmatic skills for application to the human scene have been in helping the hopelessly blind. Winthrop Kellogg has shown that blind people can develop an hitherto unsuspected talent for echo-location and that this can be encouraged to remarkably fine discrimination by using dolphinlike techniques. By making clicking sounds, a blind boy can avoid obstacles when riding a bicycle, and indeed most of the blind now can be taught to get around quite comfortably by tongue-clicking, although some blind prefer to snap their fingers, hiss or whistle. Some use a singsong voice in the diatonic scale. Some speak explorative sentences such as "Now, now, now, this is the . . . this is the . . . uh . . . let me see now, this, I think. . . . uh. . . . is . . . er . . . a smaller dish."

One blind youth, who was studying Russian, repeated the word "*gdya*" (where). Each of the successful blind moves his head from side to side while uttering his echo location sounds, precisely as the dolphin does in turbid waters. The distance or depth perception of a typically sonar-trained blind individual is capable of noting the four-inch movement of a one-foot dish placed two feet in front of his head. Actually this compares favorably with one-eyed visual depth perception. Blind subjects could also distinguish between targets of the same size made of metal, wood, denim and velvet: "They sounded different." In comparison, the judgments of normal people with their eyes closed were never above the level of pure chance.

Lockheed scientists have been able to increase the blind person's ability to echo-locate by substituting sounds imitating the bat and dolphin cries (but at a lower frequency). So far the blind have not taken willingly to these rather complex gadgets, but the British engineering professor Leslie Kay has a new model that may be more acceptable. It is a small transmitter carried in the hand and aimed like a flashlight. It is effective up to thirty feet and can readily detect poles, steps, curbs, and manholes and the difference between a gravel walk and a grass lawn.

When we come to study the origin and nature of human language we are up against a stifling wall of conjecture and prejudice. The question of the nature of language has, in fact, engendered a new philosophy (Wittgensteinism), and from the works of the mathematical logicians, such as Kurt Gödel and Alfred Tarski and others, it would seem possible that language can never be explained from within its own bounds, just as Gödel proved that the axioms of logical arithmetic can never be established within the system of the arithmetic itself. A mess of more or less classical theories have been presented over the years and given nicknames, but these are hardly so much theories as they are points of view or suggestions. For example, the "bowwow" theory emphasizes that primitive man might have imitated the noises of an animal to warn his companions of the approach of that animal. This may have taught him that his gift of imitation could be extended to all things that

make a noise and his use of onomatopoeia could include the
rain, the wind and the sea. (It is convincing that perhaps
one of the oldest words we know of is the ancient and vivid
Sanskrit expression for an arrow whizzing through the air and
striking its target: *chish-chá*.) Still, although our language and
others are stocked with animal imitations, these do not persist
in the naming of the animal in a classification. When we speak
to a child about the "bowwow," the child is temporarily impressed but soon learns that this is not what dogs are called,
but what dogs say. And the imitations of animals sounds, as
Mario Pei has emphasized with graphic instances, vary wildly
from one tongue to another. (An English pig says "Oink," for
example, while a French pig says "*Oui-oui*.") An Eskimo accurately imitates a whale's sound but would not dream of calling
the whale by that sound. Then there is the "pooh-pooh"
approach, suggesting that language originated from interjections
or grunts of emotional significance; the "ta-ta" theory, calling
attention to the probable accompaniment of patterned gestures
by patterned sounds (raising the hand, for example, along
with some primitive vocal equivalent of "Be seeing you"); the
"singsong" theory, pointing to the possible priority of the chant,
especially in courtship; and the "goo-goo" theory that has elements of all the others.

We do not know how we imitate sounds, and in fact decade
after decade of intensive studies of imitative birds, such as
those of the parrot family, have not taught us even how or
why these animals imitate human words, which certainly they
have not the slightest intention of using symbolically as we
do. Eric Lenneberg in his *Biological Foundations of Language*
concludes that the human gift for language cannot be explained
by the anatomy or the physiology of the vocal apparatus or
even by the size of the brain. There are no specialized speech
organs and the gift of speech is one ability that is not inherited. The muscles and membranes that are used to talk or
to sing with are the same used in respiration, swallowing or
grimacing. But timing is crucial and no matter how many
sneezes one sneezed or how like a sneeze some languages are,

we would never converse by sneezing or by coughing at random or by yelling in pain. One anatomical advantage *Homo sapiens* has over other hominoid animals is the relative smallness of his mouth. A container with a small mouth, like a wine bottle, resonates better than a jelly glass. We arrived at small-mouthness in our slow switch to the upright posture (where our muzzle became divorced from the things of the ground), the transfer of grasping and manipulation from mouth to hands, the enlargement of the skull, the advancement of the forehead, the recession of the jaw and the reduction in size of the teeth, perhaps partly as a result of the invention of cooking. Often anthropologists have made guesses about the possession of speech on the basis of sociological deduction. Thus *Sinanthropus* (or the Peking-type of ancient man) is assumed to have had language because so many skeletons of old people are found. In primitive societies old people are assumed to be tolerated only if they can talk. The use of tools may be much older, according to Lenneberg, than language. Tool-making and tool-manipulating tend to give an asymmetry to the two sides of the body and in developing right- or left-handedness, for some reason, the brain is conditioned also toward speech. The left temporal lobe seems to be the center of speech comprehension and this makes direct connections with the right ear. If you present the word "cat" by microphone to the right ear and simultaneously present the word "bat" to the left ear, all normal people will perceive only the word "cat." During the years of childhood, when language habits are being established, this language dominance of the team of the left brain and right ear is not a dictatorship. Before puberty the child is sufficiently flexible so that if the left temporal lobe (the speech center) is damaged, the right lobe can still take over. It has recently been ascertained that in the case of music, radar signals and the like, it is the right brain and the left ear that are dominant.

A baby first cries, then coos, then learns how to babble. This is a true language because the phoneme units can be distinguished, although it is not a symbolic language, because the baby does not know anything to symbolize. True, single words are spoken between twelve and eighteen months, followed by two-word combinations, not random, but in a primitive subject-predicate grammar. If the brain is injured or the baby is deaf, the rate of language learning is slowed down but he goes through the same *order* of learning. Thus development of language is proceeding rapidly at two years and in fact is irreversible. It is next to impossible to stop a normal infant from learning to talk after the two-word phase. If, however, under some unusual conditions (such as being brought up by apes, like Tarzan) a child is restrained from learning to talk until early puberty, it is then too late. The inexorable stations have been established. He will never learn to talk.

The actual sound of speech in any language has the wildest range of variations, but the objective—the target of what is being said—remains discrete and finite. There is no such thing in any language as an indefinitely small difference of sound. The perceptions of sound differences of course vary. In the Athabaskan system of Indian languages there is no distinction made between the sound of "b" and the sound of "p."

It often seems to those of us who live commonplace lives that we are always saying the same thing. To some extent, this is true. The clichés of everyday talk about the weather, the things we say to dogs, the things lovers say to each other, advertising, political arguments, theology and even the common man's philosophy—all are cheerful repetitions. But it is unrealistic to imagine that our everyday language consists in only such parrotings of ourselves. By calculation and by actual recording it can easily be shown on the contrary that the overwhelming majority of sentences that are understood and produced have never been heard or uttered before. To explain all our speech by conditioned reflex is to hide from the problem; there are not enough reflexes to go around. The crucial question is how we generalize.

The very understanding of language introduces a mystery of perception. Take the vowel sound of "o." It is made differently (as can readily be shown in audiograms) by a man, a woman and a child. Moreover, by the same person it may be kicked around into various forms and clang-tints, depending on context and emphasis. Yet through all these ranges and changes, the essential o-ness is perceived. What mechanism in the brain can be assigned this brilliant yet automatic detective job? At Georgia Tech it was found that a tiny switch of vowel sound can often obliterate a consonant from a test syllable or to cause it to sound like a different element of speech entirely. If a person's cortex did not respond to one or several of these infinitesimal clues in consonants, he would be virtually speechless. In most languages 80 per cent of the knowledge is carried by consonants. In the Semitic languages with "trilateral roots" the vowel is shaded in rather sneakily between forbidding consonants, thus flicking the root back and forth between noun, verb, adjective, etc. It is impossible in such a language, as Claude Lévi-Strauss has shown, to express so essentially an Indo-European concept as Platonism. In Arabic, even at the time of Arabian efflorescence, when the center of the world civilization could be accurately located in Baghdad, Platonic metaphysics translated only as bad grammar. This would be true of the Eskimo language and of most of the enormously complex polysynthetic languages of the American Indians. Yet oddly enough the Eskimo grammar (in which the protean root word is exploded brilliantly by qualifying affixes into whole sentences) is peculiarly fitted for dealing with the world of atomic physics. The Eskimo language has no word for "snow" per se. But this is paralleled by the fact that the Basque language has no word for "tree." Both are richly supplied with names for different kinds of snow and different kinds of trees. There are Eskimo words for wind-driven snow, snow on the ground, snow packed like ice and a dozen other snows that are important to a man of the Arctic, but no word for snow as a Platonic idea.[17]

[17] According to H. L. Mencken's *The American Language*, a somewhat similar situation exists in the professional jargon of experienced prostitutes. The ancient key word, going back to the most primitive of Aryan roots, is seldom used, not because of fastidiousness, but because the variants (like the different kinds of Eskimo snows) are more meaningful than the basic idea.

Early in the comparative study of languages, it was realized that, in spite of the fallacious notions of sixteenth-century European savants who imagined that "savages" spoke in grunts and snorts, even the forlorn and diminished little tribes of California were likely to be in possession of speech so complicated and so subtle that it was almost impossible to parse them and adequately to translate them. Perhaps the most complex of all well-known American Indian languages is Comanche, in which some letters are whispered and some are sounded with the larynx. In World War I this was used with confidence in tank warfare by the Americans, since it was known that no enemy linguists had been able to master it. Navajo was sometimes similarly used in World War II, but with less assurance. Of all Indian languages, the most suited to metaphysical thought is probably Hopi, in which an affix to any word can mean that whatever is being described is *characteristic*. This power is not possessed by any Aryan tongue. We cannot, except in special context, express, for example, the idea of "running" as an abstract idea. If you say, "Now I am going to talk about running," your audience will think "Running for what? Mayor, councilman?" or "Do you mean jogging every morning?" or "You mean horses?" But the Hopi word "*warikugwe*" means "running, characteristically" by virtue of the affix "-*gwe*."

As the precise obverse of such languages, the Chinese dialects are almost completely simplified down into separate words with a variety of intonations. Thus "*ma*" in the Mandarin dialect may mean "mother" (rather surprisingly), "hemp," "horse," or "scold," depending on whether it is spoken with a high-rising, low-rising or low-falling pitch or intonation. In Burma a famous sentence is made up entirely with "*ma*" to mean "Get the horse, a mad dog is coming." The curious analytic property of Chinese shows up in pidgin English. For example, the word "b'long" is not really a word at all. It is what linguists call an "empty word." It is possessivizing in grammar, which means "the word that follows is the possessor of the word that precedes." Thus "b'long" is really the grammatical equivalent of the English apostrophe. Classifiers are the catalysts of the Chinese tongue. They are necessary to cause full words to combine meaningfully into a sentence and are usually translated in pidgin into "one piecie." The innate requirement for such words is shown in the original Chinese where you cannot say "*i jeu*" to mean "a man" but must say "*i go jeu*," or in pidgin "one piecie man." Yet Chinese is a tremendously comforting language and the Chinese have always been sound-minded. The classical Chinese thought that the inner secret of reality was the *huang chung*, the note sounded in the mysterious "Yellow Bell," which classical Chinese sought as the medieval West sought the Holy Grail. Because of the great significance of intonation to the Chinese, even those who are academically well versed in English are shocked when they hear the typical emphasis of native English or American speech. For example, the sentence, "She's the *sweet*est girl" means to the Chinese listener that the speaker is passionately angry.

One should emphasize that English has an enormous ability to form sublanguages, not necessarily as exotic as pidgin, but using grammatical changes that are in themselves truly formalized. "Black English" within the American cities is such a sublanguage in the sense that it is not only thoroughly understood nationwide (mainly by the efforts of such geniuses of language as Bill Cosby of television, whose personal powers of innovation and evocation may fairly be compared with those of Mark Twain), but has even been considered as approved language in schools. For example, an acceptable black version of the beginning of *The Night Before Christmas* is:

> *It's the night before Christmas and here in*
> *our house*
> *It ain't nothing moving, not even a mouse.*
> *There go we-all stockings, hanging high off the*
> *floor*
> *So Santa Claus can full them up, if he walk in*
> *through our door.*

In one sense English has the disadvantage of languages, such as Chinese, which rely on a limited number of sounds and, unlike the "synthesizing" languages, such as Eskimo, cannot automatically clarify the difference between what are known as "homophones" (e.g., *pair, pear* and *pare*). One of the peculiar small pleasures of such languages, including all those deriving from Aryan roots, is however the *pun*. It would be impossible to imagine a pun in Alaskan or in any of the highly synthesizing languages of native North America. (I may be wrong on this, but I have been told by an anthropologist that even natives of a synthesizing language cannot understand the humor of a pun, even in an adopted Aryan language.)

In simple non-synthesizing, non-Aryan languages, such as the Polynesian, the pun is not as common as might be expected because of the use of the "glottal stop." The seemingly fluid flow of vowels is not as fluid as you might expect from merely having been to a *luau* and quaffed a good deal of Navy grog.

Another curious property of English, which perhaps derives from the fact that England in the sixteenth and seventeenth centuries had either a population explosion of poets or a peasantry of unexampled word-inventiveness, is the richness of collective names for animals. Although I am reasonably familiar with Russian, German, French, Italian and Spanish, I know of no equivalent words in these languages as:

An *exaltation* of larks
A *murmuration* of starlings
A *leap* of leopards (obviously not concocted by an English peasant)
A *skulk* of foxes
A *banquet* of pheasants
A *richness* of minks
A *cowardice* of cur dogs
A *clowder* of cats
A *kindle* of kittens
A *pride* of lions (also not of peasant origin)
A *convocation* of eagles
A *sloth* of bears

A *shrewdness* of apes (also not of peasant origin)
A *labor* of moles
A *barren* of mules
A *murder* of crows
A *charm* of goldfinches, et cetera

In spite of the delicious research on this subject by James
Lipton, I suspect a good proportion of these words were invented by some sly men like Oliver Goldsmith or even Lewis
Carroll. It is notable that few of these appear in Dr. Johnson's
dictionary, but the question is not closed by this fact, since Dr.
Johnson did not approve of such language. (There are a good
many expressions used by Eudora Welty's Mississippians which
smack of Elizabethan English, yet Dr. Johnson did not see fit
to place them into his lexicon.)

To show how much essential trouble we are in about the basis
and structure of language, the average professional linguist, if
asked to define a "word" in a given language, would never dream
of trying to do so without first thoroughly mastering the
grammar of that language. Yet, as John Pierce, the well-known
communications theorist of Bell Telephone Laboratories, has so
cogently pointed out, we do not really know even the grammar
of English. This dismaying fact came out recently when the
machine-translation of English into Russian was attempted. It
immediately became apparent that to do this an accurate grammar would be necessary by means of which a computer could
phrase a sentence with no ambiguity. It became distressingly
clear that linguists could not supply even a reasonably satisfactory grammar for *any* language—at least a grammar that a computer could use. As Pierce points out, the grammars we have
are like tips for playing good golf. With the aid of their tips
and with the use of our mystifying, hidden and unformulatable
skills of speech, we can construct grammatical and meaningful
sentences and the teachers can interpret and parse such sentences. But because we don't consciously understand how we do
this, we cannot tell a computer how to do it. This is a hell of
a mess and has greatly strengthened the case for the Wittgenstein
philosophy.

As time passes, we find language problems accumulating at a terrifying rate. The problem is not to cope with a foreign language but to handle English, which has a habit of proliferating like a virus across the world but, in the process, forming a host of impenetrable sublanguages. Thus the jargon of scientific disciplines explodes into subjargons and no scientifically minded person can ever hope to understand them all. There is an exasperating pride-of-jargon involved, which used to be only the pride of medicine, with its preposterously latinized and grecianized words that made even the description of a boil on the big toe safely beyond the comprehension of a layman. But such hollow vanity now infects all areas of intellection. Bertrand Russell in his autobiography tells how he was invited to hold a seminar at the University of Chicago and proposed the subject "Words and Facts." However, he was told that Americans would not respect lectures titled in monosyllables, so he regretfully changed the title to "Correlation Between Oral and Somatic Motor Habits." This is a vicious and overwhelmingly paralyzing trend. In order to make Ludwig Wittgenstein acceptable for a grant at Cambridge, Russell had to translate one of his own typically fluent and thoroughly vivid thumbnail letters into gobbledlygook. It is ironic that most British philosophers now speak to each other in the cryptic language of Wittgensteinese. The danger of this kind of thing is not that the truck driver or the congressman cannot understand scientific jargon, but that a scientist in one field cannot understand a scientist in another, even closely related field. Harold Orlans has warned justifiably that if this trend continues, the intellectual society of the world will come to resemble the uncommunicating tribes of the New Guinea highlands.

CHAPTER 3

Signaling with Molecules

THE CHEMICAL SENSES, which in mammals are referred to as "smell" and "taste," are much older in the planet's animal history than vision and hearing. They may be older even than the sense of touch. This is because a very small animal is on "speaking" terms with large molecules separately, and when something brushes against him, his tiny cell membranes tell him whether it is something he can eat, something that will poison him or something with an indifferent grandeur outside his consciousness, like a transatlantic cable. Even protozoans choose their prey with regard to digestibility or flavor, and if we plunge down still further in the ladder of life, we can only suppose that bacteria and even viruses must be guided to their target hosts by a chemical instinct. Indeed, even the plant kingdom is based to a large extent on chemical signals. The lowly slime molds, studied by John Tyler Brown of Princeton, form societies that are held together by an odorous gas which attracts the faithful and repels the foreigners. The weird arum family of tropical plants, which includes the calla lily and the philodendron, also contains the voodoo lily and the lords-and-ladies, which lure flies and scavenger beetles (to accomplish pollination) by a most perverse trick. These plants heat up their floral parts to as high as 27° Fahrenheit above the temperature of the air by a mystifying acceleration of metabolism which makes them smell like the inside of an old sewer. Compounds known as "amines" are evaporated from the hot, passionate surfaces and these bring such of the insects who like carrion or fecal odors from miles around.

In the animals of the sea it is difficult to distinguish smell from taste until we get as far upward in evolution as the fishes. We speak for the most part of "chemical receptors." In the jellyfish and other coelenterates there is an undoubted reaction to small concentrations of chemicals from a prey, especially one that has been snagged by the dart from the nematocyst. Is this taste or odor? Because we, as land animals, cannot taste from a distance, we are prejudiced in favor of calling chemical senses that result in orientation for the pursuit of prey or the avoidance of predators "organs of smell." However, a current in the water is analogous to the wind on dry land, and just as many land animals are skillful at detecting extremely small molecular clusters coming downwind from an interesting source, so aquatic creatures can sense the taste of food or danger borne to them on an oceanic current or the stream of a river. The tiny lobes on the heads of some flatworms are true organs of chemical sense. As it travels along, a planarian worm delicately waves the projecting flaps of these lobes, tasting the water as it goes. The tentacles of the garden snail have competent olfactory organs. If you wish to recapture a snail that is running wild and free some place in your house, the best thing to do is to put a dish on the floor with a piece of boiled potato on it. He can smell this at a distance of at least seventy-five feet and will come running. He will also be greatly attracted by a piece of suet. In most marine gastropods, however, the organ of smell is associated with the breathing apparatus.

Currents in the water made by threshing tiny cilia in the case of flatworms and other marine animals of modest stature may be important in telling the worm where the food is. In general, neurologists cannot tell whether a small primitive animal who lives in the water is using taste or smell. In a general way, smell is supposed to be useful at longer distances, for seeking and detecting and especially for pushing the panic button. Taste is regarded as primarily a contact sense, for testing and controlling eating movements. In the crayfish, single chemical-receptor units can be isolated from tufts on the chela (jaws) and walking legs, which are sensitive *only* to amino acids. Since these comprise an extremely crucial primary food, such little organs are obviously useful but the remarkable selectivity is not understood. All scavenging marine animals, such as most crustaceans, are also very sensitive to a particular chemical given off by decaying fish muscle—trimethylene oxide.

In the fishes, olfaction is quite well developed and is remarkable in some kinds, such as the Pacific salmon, who return if possible to the ancestral stream where they were spawned, in turn to spawn and die. Arthur Hasler of the University of Wisconsin has made a good case for this uncanny homing instinct's being seated in the sense of smell. When salmon have their noses plugged they show no such nostalgia. A sort of olfactory imprinting process occurs just after the fishes are hatched. Each part of a stream has a unique symphony of odors because of the particular kinds and relative number of plants that grow by that stream, the essential oils from the shrubbery identifying this place of water as indelibly "home." If the little salmon as fingerlings are caught and transplanted to another stream, the smell will be different and they will grow up regarding that stream as home. This childhood memory of the salmon persists through his adventurous life in the salty ocean, and when it is time to spawn he is led by his nose (although first guided roughly by some rather obscure compass navigation sense) to the right river, the right tributary and ultimately to the spot whose odor memories have haunted him all his life. It is not a matter of feeding, since during the spawning migration the future parents do not eat. It is purely an instinctual drive based on evolution's teaching that the only place to spawn is where one was brought up.

Fishes become conditioned to many scents other than place-of-origin odor and food smell. Notably they react to odors of alarm, to recognition of sex and to the body odor of their

schoolmates (in the schooling species of fish). Fishes that have
elaborate barbels, such as catfish and bullheads, generally also
have a sharp sense of taste. These barbels are used primarily
for touch, and in combination with taste, fishes that feed in
the dark can thus find food. The barbels are waved about, not
only to seek out tangible objects, as a cat's whiskers do, but
to get a fix by taste nerves located at different places on the
fish. Usually the fishes with luxuriant barbels have puny eyes.
The bullheads (genus *Ectalurus*) have taste cells scattered on
the head, flank, on the fins and barbels themselves and even on
the tail, all sending branches of fibers to the cranial nerves.
The brown and yellow bullheads have thousands of external
taste buds on the body with especially dense concentrations
on the barbels. The experiments of J. E. Bardock and his associates at the University of Michigan have shown that these taste
buds act as unerringly to locate food as the sense of smell
does in most animals. The fish needs no current in this job.
He operates on what is called a "true gradient" principle; that
is, he continues swimming ahead as the taste grows stronger
or turns, as the fast taste senses on one side send more powerful
messages to the brain. In contrast to the classic lopsided search
of a shark when one nostril is plugged, the one-sided elimination of smell in the bullhead does not in the least weaken his
single-minded seeking of the chemically desired prize. But when
all the barbels and also the flank taste buds are paralyzed by a
drug on one side only, the fish tend to circle toward the intact
side. (This is precisely analogous to a one-eared man turning
until his good ear faces the sound.) It is thus evident that
in such extremely well-endowed gustatory animals, taste can
be used not only for detection but also for orientation. It is not
known what the bullhead uses his nose for, but probably it is
for the detection of members of the opposite sex or of predators.
Actually it is not experimentally possible to eliminate the taste
sense of bullheads in order to study the sense of smell alone,
since the taste nerve fibers are distributed in the widely branched
seventh, ninth and tenth cranial nerves and extend to taste
buds in the mouth, pharynx, gill cavity and all over the head

and body. It is, in fact, not certain that this fish *has* a sense of smell. In the red mullet the barbels can be drawn back into a groove under the throat, just like the retractable undercarriage of an airplane, when the fish is not searching for food. When he stops to feed, out come the barbels again, and he can use them not only to taste with but also to dig with.

We noted that the dolphin has no sense of smell, although he can taste. The octopus and squid have extremely well-developed chemical receptors and in their isolated arms (malacologists use this term rather than "tentacles") they still respond, so that the surface of even the amputated arm of such an animal reacts to the smell (or taste) of food and can do everything but eat it. Most mammals, such as the dolphin and seal, who have returned to the water for a livelihood, lose their sense of smell. The ferocious water shrew, for example, depends almost entirely on its whiskers for contacting prey. In hunting, the water shrew is guided only by the sense of touch in the snout whiskers. Certain free-swimming species of catfish find their prey by the same method. When these fishes swim fast and straight, the long feelers on the snout just drag along, but, like the shrew's whiskers, are stiffly spread out when the fish senses nearness to his dinner. Like the shrew, the fish begins to gyrate blindly in order to establish contact. Perhaps at close range, water vibration means something. All such action is too quick for the human eye.

In another evolutionary switch, the birds, although descended from reptiles who had good noses, did not require or could not, as a general rule, use the sense of smell. Lizards and snakes use the so-called "Jacobson's organ." A turtle's sense of smell is very good at close range. The humble little newt (an amphibian, belonging to the salamander family) is able to use its nose to find its way home from distances as great as eight miles. This feat—a very respectable one in view of the newt's pitiful size and its ancient primitive place in the vertebrate phylum—is apparently accomplished by much the same technique used by the salmon, although it is air-borne rather than water-borne odors that it detects. The odd complex from trees, small plants and decaying plant material, maintaining a collective identity for a large time in a newt's life, leads him, after a period of scouting with his nose, to his homesite, usually a special place by a special creek. If you paralyze his nasal membranes with formaldehyde he nearly always fails to make it, but the fact that sometimes he still does indicates that, similar to the salmon, there is some other internal compass at work. We shall postpone for a while a discussion of such unknown senses that many animals possess and which we have all but lost.

We should mention some more about the peculiar connection between the snake's tongue and its Jacobson's organ. Most snakes, with the possible exception of the pit viper, whose organs of radiant heat perception will be among the *outré* subjects to be discussed later, find their prey by flicking their tongue. The tongue is really homologous to a trunk in an elephant. It flicks out along the trail and molecules picked up are carried to the Jacobson's organ of smell, located in a cavity far forward in the roof of the mouth. The tongue itself has no taste buds but is a kind of vacuum accumulator for the Jacobson's organ. This is why it flickers constantly, taking its direction from the motor centers of the brain working with Jacobson's organ.

Most characteristic animal odors are caused by rather large molecules that do not get very high up in the air. Nevertheless some birds can smell. It is noteworthy that these (ducks, kiwis and snipes) make their nests on the ground. In the nocturnal kiwis, who actually find their food by scent, the nostrils are located at the very tip of the beaks. Vultures, being high-flying, are insensitive to odors—the black vulture is one of the few animals that will attack, kill and eat a skunk.

All land mammals, including man, have some sense of smell, and to what extent we shall discuss later. But it is to the colonial land insects, who have developed chemical signaling as a means of communication and even of government, that we look for the most sophisticated organ of both smell and taste. It was for this fantastic ability in throwing chemicals around and detecting them that in 1959 the word "pheromone" was coined to indicate a chemical signal used in communication among members of the same species. It is quite evident that none of the advanced social insects, such as ants, bees and termites, would have been able to form their complex and rigorous societies without the use of pheromones.

Although we have noted in the preceding chapter that insects are often responsive to sound, the colonial insects might, if misfortune deprived them of hearing vibrations in the ground, get along very well. This is probably true even of the honeybee, where the much disputed ballads during the wagging dance might easily be dispensed with and the hive could revert to the primeval chemical medium, representing perhaps no more a shattering blow to the civilization of bees than would be to us a sudden failure of all the television sets in the world. We have mentioned the tooting of queen bees and the quacking of their rivals, but it is possible that these too are luxurious redundancies, since it is now known that a queen honeybee carries a minimum of thirty-two separate chemicals in her head which can be released to convey certain messages and accomplish decisive effects. We don't even know what some of these substances do, since our own chemical consciousness is so degenerate that we have only lately been able to appreciate the enormous voice with which the odors rule a society.

This society is based, of course, upon the queen mother concept, although among most termites (an order far older and immensely removed in phylogeny from bees and ants) the queen is allowed a permanent consort, much as Victoria was allowed her beloved Albert. In primitively socialized insects which, in their evolution, are really tens of millions of years away from the sophisticated welfare state of honeybees, ants and hornets, control by the queen has an air of precarious adventure. In some *Polistes* wasps and some bumblebees, the queen differs only slightly in appearance from other adult females. She dominates by bluster and by the fact that her more intense femaleness is distinguished by sharper body odor. In the just barely socialized *Lasioglossum zephyrtum*, there is an unstable situation which certainly cannot last for more than a million years more without the society exploding into solitary families or, alternatively, voting the straight Socialist ticket. In this case, there is a sort of uncontrolled caste or gang of several queens who do not have the grace even to fight each other to the death, but go around removing each other's eggs from brood cells and substituting their own. The evolution from this sort of aristocratic sexual anarchy (which would appear inconceivably shocking to the advanced *Hymenoptera*) to the rigorous patterns of behavior in which the workers of the hive unite in regulating the reproductive habits of the queen is arrived at by inventing chemicals by which the queen not only controls the workers but also dictates that they control the queenhood. This is indeed a constitutional monarchy but there is only one party. If the chemicals fail to be secreted, the hive is just a box of insane, starving insects.

Some students of the social insects have detected nine different categories of chemical communication (pheromones). They may be oral (taste) or olfactory, according to what part of the body receives them. There are pheromones of alarm, recruitment, grooming (including assistance at moulting time), exchange of oral and anal liquids, exchange of solid food particles, facilitation (teamwork or help in carrying food, common among ants), recognition (of nest mates and castes) and, most important of all, caste determination by inhibition or stimulation. A worker honeybee is restrained in her serfdom and maidenhood by means of at least two chemicals released from the queen, which are powerful enough to paralyze the worker's sex endocrine gland system. One of them (the relatively simple compound *trans*-9-keto-2-decanoic acid) is produced in the queen's jaw glands and released as she opens her mouth. This chemical alone is enough to inhibit to some extent any queenly behavior and ovary development in the worker. It works in conjunction with a second inhibitory scent produced in some other part of the queen's body to keep the worker on the job as a toiling virgin. Several other scents, which merely command attention or special treatment, are also released by Her Majesty. When the mother queen of the honeybee colony is removed or dies, the workers within half an hour change from their usual superorganized activity to a mood of profound restlessness. In a few more hours the workers set about to alter one or more worker brood cells into emergency queen cells. Within a few days some of the workers (but, for some poorly understood reason, not all of them) begin to show increased femininity—their shrunken ovaries start to bloom. It has been found that coincident with this change, the corpus allatum (the essential gland), which had been suppressed by the regal odors when the queen ruled, starts to grow and to send out a "gonadotropic" hormone into the blood. The hive thus prepares for another tournament of fighting queens and for a new autocratic and reproductive regime.

In some incomparably more complex termite societies, the construction and control of several castes are under chemical control. Starting with the more primitive termite organizations, the key caste is the "pseudergate," a large nymphlike stage that performs the tasks of the workers in other insect communities. It is a sort of all-purpose living robot that can be transferred, through chemical command by royalty, into a soldier or into one of two reproductive castes. Here again the pheromones act by influencing the endocrine glands. Soldiers can be produced from or changed into reproductives. In the higher termites, reproductives, however, can be derived only from nymphs. A true worker class exists that lacks the potential for caste alteration, but that a caste system within a caste may exist is shown by the incredible specialization of jobs in certain Mediterranean species. There may be as many as fifty-six different types of trades—harvest workers, water-bearers, fungus gardeners, alarm-sounders, nurses for the young, builders, soldiers, police, preparers of the queen's food, chamberlains and valets for the king, etc. All of these are controlled in their situations in this steely all-class society by chemicals—presumably—that are absorbed to affect the gland system (if we regard the central nervous system in this case as a sort of gland) or by the kind of food they are compelled to eat. But who does the compelling? Who balances the society into its over half-a-hundred trade unions and keeps them balanced? The mind becomes dizzy at the intricate computerlike parceling out of body- and soul-molding substances that assures not only the continuity of the reproductive monarchy, but also the availability of all the specialists at just the right time and the right number. No wonder that Eugene Marais conceived of the "spirit of the colony"—a sort of infallible *E pluribus unum*, but we must invoke for such biological chemical magic the same principle that we have found (in other books) necessary to summon for the general processes of tissue differentiation and for cell operation—the law of transcendental memory. The termite establishment acts in this infallible way because for hundreds of millions of years and a billion or so generations it *has* acted in this way. Social and molecular memory persist by the same rules and with the same inevitability.[1]

In somewhat simple termite kingdoms, such as that of *Kalotermes flavicollis*, the king and queen produce substances (pheromones 1 and 2) which inhibit the development of pseudergates into the royal caste. It is known experimentally that these inhibitory pheromones are passed directly (through the air or by contact) and *also* indirectly through the digestive tracts of the pseudergates. Another kingly substance (pheromone 3) stimulates the female pseudergates to transform into the reproductive caste, but the queen does not have this prerogative. When there is an excess of males present in the colony, they reorganize each other through pheromone 4 and promptly fight to the death. The same is true with supernumerary royal females, in which pheromone 5 is the agent. Finally, by some unknown chemical signal, the royal males stimulate the production of pheromone 2 in the royal females, while the queens stimulate the production of pheromone 1 in the kings. In spite of this reciprocal chemical equivalence, one must not imagine the king and queen as sitting side by side on tiny thrones. The queen swells into a huge, balloonlike paunch about four inches

[1] It is now suspected that termite castes owe their continuity chiefly to the food their members eat. The role of the recently discovered vitamin T is thought to be crucial in determining whether a termite becomes a soldier or, say, a mason. This substance is contained notably in the fungi which were cultivated in undergardens by gardener termites. But the question remains as to who decides which young termite shall eat what.

long (roughly ten thousand times the size of an ordinary termite). She is an absolutely immobile reproduction machine, laying an egg every two seconds. The king can hardly be discovered as he crawls microscopically around, pausing in his agitated revery occasionally to fertilize her. In some termite colonies of a million or so individuals, which are distinguished by modern architectural novelties such as automatic air-conditioning and which consist of innumerable labyrinthine passages and suites, the queen, in the inmost chamber like a pharaoh in a pyramid, is fed by a ceaseless parade of workers who stuff predigested food in her mouth and carry away the freshly laid eggs to the nursery. (The food that termites eat consists of wood pulp brought in by the harvest hands and passes through some ten stomachs and several guts before all the nutrition has been wrung from it.)

If the queen dies (and in her dropsical gigantism, it is a wonder that she lives at all) the other million or so members of that colony do not perish mystically at the same time, as the science fiction of Maurice Maeterlinck would have us believe. Some of the brood spectrum of sexless workers (and how they are selected is as obscure as the similar choice that has to be made in a queenless bee hive) are fed, probably with vitamin T-enriched rations. Their sex hormones are revitalized by this diet, transforming them into supple young queens, ready for the inevitable elimination tournament.

We have been discussing up to now only those pheromones that act on the inner glandular structures of the insect and that might be regarded as government edicts. In every society as intimately bound together as that of the colonial animals, there must of course be signals for communal effort, for alarms and excursions. The infamous fire ants leave an odor trail to a food source. When a scout finds a likely new nutritional object, such as a dead beetle, or a better nest site, it runs homeward, laying a trail of minute secretions from its Dufour's gland located on the belly, which scrapes the ground. As this chemical tracer diffuses, it forms a tunnel of active space, the maximum radius of which is approximately one centimeter. During the lifetime of the odorous tunnel—about 100 seconds—recruited workers dash away from the nests following the tunnel of scent to the food source. The amount of information provided is certainly comparable to that of the honeybee's waggle dance and does not have so many entomologists arguing about it.

Chemicals used as recruitment calls are often used also for alarm signals, possibly varied in chemical compositions by amounts too small for us to detect. The reaction to alarm smells may be cautious in some species, but in others the soldiers and even the workers may recklessly sacrifice their lives in defense of the realm or at least of the queen. In some kinds of ants the alarm secretions act as attractants at low concentrations.[2] In the fire ant an unidentified chemical from the glands of the head causes frantic alarm whatever the concentration. The number of alarm chemicals identified so far among social insects far exceeds all other kinds of pheromones. There is a simple reason for this. The alarm substances must be quite volatile, conspicuous and stored in readily accessible glandular reservoirs. From the standpoint of chemical analysis, it is usually small in size and uncomplicated in structure. Typical alarm signals are given chiefly by those compounds known as "aldehydes" and "ketones." Of significance also to a chemist is that the insects' chemical receptors are so constructed that in the course of evolution they tend to respond more efficiently to molecules of increasing size in a homologous series of compounds, such as ketones, esters or aldehydes. Thus an alarm chemical should be large enough to be specifically recognizable yet not so heavy as to fail to diffuse rapidly. For obvious tactical reasons, it is best to have a chemical that gives a short, sharp signal and then vanishes. The insect colony then is able to localize the alarm communication in time and space. If it were not so, some spot near the nest would continue to be cursed with the sour odor of fear and would cause indefinite uneasiness among the apart-

[2] This double meaning of a chemical, according to concentration, is quite familiar to us. Few people could tolerate the odor of straight, undiluted musk, although it is a reinforcing ingredient of most perfumes. Only people of great fortitude would chew on garlic, yet as a trace flavor it is delicious to most of us.

ment house dwellers. It is true that three kinds of alarm substances (citral, 2-heptanone and methylheptanone) are found in more than one species of ant, but this has proved to be a nuisance rather than a help, and the colonies of these species avoid each other as much as possible and even move their nests to get away from one another.

Medleys of chemical odors may have more than one meaning, according to the composition or to the context of the emission. The worker control chemical of the queen bee (*trans*-9-keto-2-decanoic acid) is used as a sex attractant for the drones when the queen makes her nuptial flight. (As we shall see later, there is a wonderful distinction, even in human beings, between the male and female susceptibility to certain odors.) The same chemical from Dufour's gland in the fire ant, used routinely as a trail blazer to food sources, is used under different situations as a sort of assembly call in preparation for a mass emigration and, when mixed with an odorous secretion from the head, is a red alert to imminent danger. The workers of the ant *Pogonomyrmex badius* react to low concentrations of a certain chemical from a gland in the jaw by approaching each other and waving their antennal noses interrogatively. At high concentrations they become extremely agitated and run around in circles, smelling for danger, and if a high concentration is maintained for over a minute, many of them stop wringing their hands and start digging furiously. This behavior is aimed at getting at the source of the odor and perhaps rescuing a comrade who has been injured or trapped. The "wring-the-hands" behavior which I have mentioned is identified by ethologists more drily as "unoriented alarm," but some secretions from an excited worker evoke "oriented alarm" such as ganging up around the alarmist, then taking off in one direction in a soldierly manner, presumably to meet the enemy. Honeybee workers who have been confined closely with the queen for hours, feeding or grooming her, acquire temporary queenly scent which, in combination with their own workers' recognition smell, cause them to be attacked by their nest mates. This unfriendly attitude could be regarded in the same light as that presented by the servants of a great house to a personal maid who emerges from her mistress's dressing chamber smelling of Chanel Number 5. The worker is literally "putting on airs." The males of the ant *Lasius neoniger* discharge most of the jaw-gland contents during the nuptial flight as weapons of aerial courtship. There is, however, a chemical problem of greater genetic significance involved here. Two species of *Lasius* and one species of the related genus *Acanthomyops* are found to have many courtship chemicals in common. Yet it is forbidden to breed outside the species. The problem is solved by mixing the ingredients in quite different ratios so that the appropriate queen is charmed only by the perfume of a male of her own species.

In the colonial insects, we have only investigated, so to speak, the outer layer of odors. The "surface pheromones" that are emitted and perceived only in close bodily contact are so complicated and so much higher in molecular weight that their nature has eluded us so far. These include colony odors. An ant community has its own smell which is perceived when one individual gets within antennae distance of another. If the odor is the right one, the mutual response is "Pass and go with God." If the odor is the wrong one, it is "Cry 'havoc' and let slip the dogs of war!" and the ensuing mass battle may be indescribably ferocious. Thus nations of ants of the same species (notably the harvester ants) may fight each other close to mutual extermination. They may have their Thirty Years' Wars. Even Thoreau referred to historic battles of ants and concluded mournfully that this was not what the Scriptures had in mind in recommending that we imitate their behavior. In one of his early science-fiction stories H. G. Wells conceived of an ant state that had invented subtle weapons, including tiny artillery and death-rays, and was prepared to challenge man for the suzerainty of the planet. Quite evidently, if we extrapolate the fierce xenophobia of the ant to man size, we get what we have got—modern man—an animal specifically organized for mass murder by governments.

It is not only the advanced colonial insects that are gifted in emitting and detecting odors. Moths are notoriously keen smellers, especially in detecting sex odors, and there is a significant reason for this. In many moths, including that of the silkworm genera, the adult flying stage is simply a brief foodless honeymoon. The adults, after having emerged from the pupae with a store of food in their blood, do not seek food or ever eat again. Their only mission in their brief days of wine and roses is to find a mate before they die. Since this can be a hard thing to do in a non-colonial insect, they are provided by evolution with extraordinary techniques. The female silkworm moth informs males at distances of a mile or more that she is ready for mating by exuding a definite perfume from her abdominal glands. To determine the distance from which this sex lure can get results, scientists have released specially tagged silkworm males from a train at regular intervals. Some at least found their way back to the caged female from seven miles away. Yet the female has stored up only one millionth of a gram of this perfume and exudes it only in small installments during her short life. Thus the concentration that the male can perceive and follow to its source may amount to only one molecule in a cubic foot. (But without the stimulation by this one sexy molecule, the male remains as unresponsive as a stone. He can be surrounded by females beseeching his attention, but if their odor glands have been removed he regards them as mere dummies of delusion.) This is enormously greater sensitivity than any analytical instrument designed by man. For this the moth has some 200,000 sensory cells of twelve different kinds located in his frondlike antennae, but the nature of these remarkable cells—the details of construction that make possible this unbelievably delicate feat of olfaction—have not told us yet how to do likewise. It is an important ability for bionic reasons, since we would like to be able, for instance, to sniff out the hidden enemy. We would like to be able to detect a few molecules of gunpowder from a gun hidden in an air traveler's briefcase or the trace of nitroglycerin or TNT from a bomb in his luggage. We should also like to lure the male of many moth pests to his death. For this assignment, the scent glands of literally millions of female moths have been ground up and extracted to yield a few drops of essence; this material has been identified chemically and, in many cases, synthesized artificially. If the synthesis of the original perfume is cheap enough, or if effective substitutes that still do the job can be made economically, this offers a better way to get rid of such pests than with some harsh, all-purpose club like DDT, which not only poisons our friends and enemies alike, but to which insects also rapidly develop immunity. The silkworm moth is not a pest, but there are the gypsy moths, the vine moths, the fruit moths, the nun moth and others, whose caterpillars cause grave agricultural damage. If the females are left without males, they lay only infertile eggs from which no voracious caterpillars can emerge.

Martin Jacobson, the foremost American expert on insect sex lures, points out that, aside from the urgent dilemma of the moth who is living on borrowed time, specific sex attractants are almost a necessity because of the extremely crowded nature of the insect class. Hundreds of thousands of species are found living together at single localities. In the swarming mass of predators, parasites, competitors for the same food, mimics, commensals, symphiles and sibling clusters, privacy is unknown, unless you have some freak habit such as boring into hardwood like a deathwatch beetle or inhabiting the lips of a liverwort that eats all other insects except you. Although it was not until 1960 that the first female attractant, a complex alcohol produced by the gypsy moth, was identified and duplicated by Jacobson and his associates, sex attractants have now been found in virtually all insects where they have been sought, including the housefly and at least one species of mosquito. *Male* sex pheromones are also shown to be commonplace. Some are aphrodisiac in action and are taken, as some human females smoke marijuana, to make the sexual experience more intense (or rather, from the insect point of view, more productive). But some perfumes emitted by the male are panted after at great distances by the female, who arrives at the male's room just as he has finished applying his irresistible shaving lotion. Although, as mentioned, the colonial insects are careful to brew their scents to avoid a mix-up in species, other insects, untrained by the rigors of the socialist state, are not so careful. Many female substances are so powerful that they can attract males of another related species who will attempt to get fresh, although in 999 cases out of 1,000, such attempts at interspecific rape are foiled by engineering incompatibility of the sex organs or by the realization on the part of the female that she is in the clutches of a horrid alien and she will *not* relax and enjoy it.

In some cases a delicate co-operation with a plant is necessary to achieve an olfactory honeymoon. Lynn Riddiford and Carroll Williams of Harvard noted that the males and females of the polyphemus moth would fail to mate in a laboratory cage, even though the temperature, the time of year and the soft music were all correct, and learned observers were at hand to cheer them on. Miss Riddiford finally got the bright idea of putting some oak leaves in the cage. The moths immediately proceeded to engage in the acts of love. It seems that some unidentified emanation from the oak leaves is necessary to trigger the female's exudation of sex lure. Alcohol or water extracts of oak leaves will do the same thing, but no other plant has this aphrodisiac property. If all the oak trees were killed off by a blight, there would be no more polyphemus moths. This is a strange and fatalistic connection, since, although oak leaves are a favorite food of this moth's caterpillar, other common foods such as the foliage of maple, birch, chestnut, horse chestnut, elm, hickory and beech have no sexual effects.

The chemical relations of insects with plants are often very complex. Although the flowering plants usually need insects to assure pollination, they do not need *all* insects, and some of the larval feeding forms are a plant's worst enemies. A plant would prefer that pollinating insects be reliable and well-behaved, like bees, and that the pollinator's voracious children be kept out of the act. For the good offices of such insects and for their orderly behavior, the plant is willing to produce nectar for them and to greet them with fragrant smells and a pretty face. To protect themselves against the destructive and hooligan element in insects, plants have evolved special repellent odors. The odor which we know as catnip, a strong-scented extract of a special mint plant, is one such insect repellent. The main ingredient is a terpene nepetalactone, and if you let fall a drop of this on the carcass of a curculionid beetle being carried away by an ant (an animal for which most plants have little affection), the ant will promptly drop his enormous load and proceed furiously to wash himself while all ants that touch the soiled ant with their antennae will also go into furors of washing. There does not seem to be any good reason why the mint plant would want to make a cat rapturously playful, but it is now believed possible that something like catnip may be present in the pheromones of cats themselves. The terpenes are very widely distributed in the animal kingdom, and indeed even some insects use them as defensive odors, imitating the strategems of the plants. If the cat uses them during urination, for example, the meaning of the pheromone is obviously quite different, communicating sexual allure or perhaps simply the pleasure of being a cat. Obviously the meaning of a smell is in the mind of the smeller and across the phylogenetic gulfs the same molecules may speak quite different languages.

One of the most serious of all forest pests is the bark beetle which gives off a witch's brew of scents, mainly to lure other bark beetles to new feeding and breeding grounds. Since bark beetles cause more damage to timber forests than fire (over $100 million a year), the U. S. Forest Service has been encouraging chemists from the University of California and Stanford to identify these pheromones so that the beetles can be led astray. The beetles usually attack after a fire, when the trees are weakened through lack of sap. It is a much tougher job to develop a specific lure, because it is not simply a matter of sex pheromones but of generalized tribal olfactory yells, such as "Burn, baby, burn" or "Come onna my house."

One question that has puzzled entomologists is why mosquitoes alight on stagnant water to lay their eggs. It has now been demonstrated that mosquitoes choose their brooding-ponds by odor. It is the sweet smell of bacteria and of bacterial products that attracts them to a given piece of water. The killing of mosquitoes thus essentially involves the sterilization of standing waters.

Since the intensity of the search for pheromones was stepped up in the 1960s, certain odd-ball applications of the sex-lure principle have been suggested and tried. The attractant idea has certain weaknesses. What would you do, if you attract all the male moths of a given species to a false rendezvous? You still have to kill them or outwait them until they die of starvation or of a broken heart. This is a messy and vague business. One possibility is to confuse them to death. If the breeding environment can be so saturated with the female attractant that the small additional amount from a real female is imperceptible, the male has the equivalent of a nervous breakdown. Surrounded on all sides by seductive smells, he knows not where to turn. The insect mind (held together by a slender thread of behavior patterns) breaks down and thus the insects do what virtually all animals except man do in the face of an insane predicament—they die.

We have mentioned the powerful taste sense of certain fishes and should also point out that many insects have delicate tongues, although they are located on their feet. By means of these feet organs, the housefly strangely rates various sugars in the same order of sweetness as the human tongue. (This is determined by testing the most dilute water solution of the sugar in which the fly will dip his proboscis.) The red admiral butterfly can distinguish sugar in solutions two hundred times more dilute than are detectable to man. The spider has chemical sense organs in its feet, which may be for smell or taste, but chiefly for the latter. The male spider becomes aware of the female through the touch of her thread, the trail she leaves or the odor of her body, but seldom if ever is he able to see her or hear her.

The chemical gifts of insects have been taken quite seriously by research organizations that are looking, not so much for ways of foiling or destroying insects as for learning from them. The Aeroneutronic Division of Ford Motor Company, for example, set up an ambitious project to study odor reception in the green-bottle fly, which is capable of discriminating a large number of chemicals which are imperceptible to human beings. The olfactory organ and the antennal nerve attached to it are removed and set up in moist chambers with odorous substances. Microscopic probes are attached to the nerves through electrometers and an amplifier with an oscilloscope measure the nerve's electrical response to whatever makes an impression on the sensory organ. These electrical engineers believe that such tests may open up a new oscillogram or perhaps even a sound pattern will be able to perceive what their noses cannot tell them.

As mammals, we ourselves doubtless started out with the ability to perceive a chemical universe that has been mostly lost to us when as primates we took to the trees to get away from the rodents. Now we use rodents to study, among other things, their chemical senses. Rats ordinarily use their senses of touch and smell to solve a problem and do not bother to use their eyes unless absolutely necessary. Note how completely reversed this is to our attitude. A man sees a wild rose and may approach it to smell it. A rat can smell the same fragrance, but to him it is a completely meaningless and neutral odor as it is to a dog or a cat. They say, "To hell with it," while the man may take it to his wife or even write a poem about it. Rodents in general have powerful but rather strange taste as well as smell senses and there is a sex difference in their response to sweetened water. Although females don't drink any more water than males, they will consume greater amounts of water sweetened with glucose and water sweetened with a non-caloric material such as saccharin. After several days males will switch from saccharin to sugar, while the females not only continue to prefer the saccharin, but will take it in much higher concentrations of absolutely sickening sweetness which the males refuse to touch. (This seems to be true of humans to some generalized extent, since men prefer peanuts to the chocolate-covered sugar that some women devour by the ton. On the other hand, one cannot overlook the cream pies that have ruined the average American man's figure and probably shortened his life by more years than the cigarettes he smokes.) Actually rats are not so attracted to sweet tastes as their relatives the hamsters and guinea pigs. Cats are not attracted at all to sweet food. All rodents are much more sensitive to potassium chloride than to sodium chloride. Carl Pfaffmann of Rockefeller University, in studying the taste senses of rats and hamsters, made some rather fundamental neurological discoveries. He found that a single nerve fiber could respond to more than one kind of basic taste stimulation. Some single fibers are sensitive to such widely diverse tastes as those of sugar, salt and quinine. A small number of fibers, on the other hand, respond only to one kind of taste quality, such as salt. Pfaffmann was unable to conclude that the actual taste receptors (carried in the taste buds) varied in any important way from one chemical to another. Since, however, one nerve fiber innervates several taste cells in a taste bud, it is still possible that the receptors may differ in their individual response to chemicals and that the final sensation in the rodent's brain is the result of a sort of majority poll. When the rat perceives that something tastes sweet, this is by no means a simple and categorical feeling. The nerve fibers intercommunicate through fine branches near their roots and there is evidence that a preliminary processing takes place at this nerve level. The taste nerves ask each other, "Is this salty or what?" and then send on to the central nervous system a kind of coded message, a compromise between the opinions of a good many receptors and fibers. Recent analyses of the rat's taste nerves come up with the conclusion that the responsiveness of the taste receptors to different chemicals is determined by the inherent properties of the tissue from which the receptor cells are formed rather than by the taste fibers that innervate them. All the nerve fibers of the chemical senses in mammals are so extremely fine in size that they have been hard to examine and, moreover, because of small diameter, they conduct very slowly. The acuity with which a mammal detects a chemical seems thus to depend on how well he has been able to solve a difficult problem in nervous communication. Often the chemical sense organs are in the position of a political convention with only one telephone line to the outside and that one usually full of static. However, when the nomination is made, the rat does very well. Certainly he can tell the difference between a female in heat and a female who is not, and if you remove the olfactory bulbs in his brain, he will be unable to mate.

Like the dog, the wolf marks his property with a squirt of urine, the fragrance of which is reinforced by the output of a special scent gland. When we see a dog conferring deliberately around a prominent pissoir-post or fire hydrant, he is trying to find out who claims to own it and later he may be able to make an intimate inspection by his nose of the producer of the original odor—the claimant. This is important social business for a dog, since he no longer commonly runs in packs, as his ancestral wolves did, and the matter of territorial claims via the lifted-leg route has become a complicated problem to him. Your dog knows he owns your back yard, and if other dogs approach this territory he will noisily warn them off. But beyond that, the question of territorial rights is so ambiguous that a good many claims must be made and disputed. Luckily for the underdog in a fight, the top dog, having won his victory, feels an irresistible urge to leave a sign on the battlefield that this is his property, which he does by lifting his leg against the nearest complete object, which may be as modest a thing as a pile of horse turds. Wolves recognize each other by the scent of urine marks, and it would at once be clear to the members of a pack if a non-member—a foreigner—presumed to lift his leg in their hunting grounds. When strychnine is used in the cruel and absurd wolf-control projects, the adults that survive learn to shun the bait. They recognize that the sweetish smell around a carcass means death. (Domestic cats living free in open country can share the same hunting ground by arriving at a mutually satisfactory timetable. One cat hunts when he knows the other one is asleep. A cat finding another cat's signal on the hunting path can assess the other cat's age and, of course, its sex and can then decide whether to continue on the same route or to choose another.) Practically all breeds of dogs, except the age-old, peculiar saluki, have magnificent senses of smell and, aside from helping a man to hunt, many uses have been made of their sensitive noses. By experiment it has been amply proved that a dog can readily identify any piece of clothing as belonging to a particular person. There is an exception to this rule, and it tells something about the nature of the human body odor. A dog cannot distinguish between the clothes belonging to one or the other of identical twins. That this is not due to environment or diet was shown in a given case when the twins were both married adults living apart. Thus human odor patterns must depend on genetic factors. You smell like your older brother but not so much like him that the dog cannot determine the difference between two dirty socks within the family. But if it is your twin brother, you were both born to smell alike and even the dog is baffled. This individuality of human odors has been used in chemical setups, where a gas "chromatogram" of odors from the body is recorded, something on the order of a chemical fingerprint.

One exceptional use of the dog's nose has been made in the Russian metal prospecting industry. Dogs are trained to sniff out ore deposits containing iron sulfides. In Siberia one dog discovered a sulfide ore deposit of from ten to twelve feet thick that was buried beneath seven feet of clay-type earth. The technique appears to have been invented actually in Finland in 1962. A Finnish dog was reported to have found 1,330 ore-containing rocks in a three-kilometer area, while a trained prospector was able to locate only 230 pay rocks in the same patch. Although a dog can quickly detect the scent of a rabbit, it is probable that the rabbit can even more quickly detect the dog's odor. An ordinary cottontail has over 200 million odor-receptor neurons in its nose. The rabbit's relative the arctic hare has an even denser and more sensitive apparatus. He can readily detect food buried two feet deep in the snow. Not only this but the rate of reaction is marvelously instantaneous. Sometimes a hare, running at full speed, will jerk to a stop as though pulled by an underground magnet. Burrowing frantically, he will come up with a succulent willow twig (a hare's basic diet).

There are some colonial mammals who, although not quite so dependent upon chemical signals for regulating their lives as are ants, bees and termites, nevertheless establish certain rules of social conduct by means of odor. This is true of prairie dogs, the unhappily disappearing rodent species whom the ethologists

John A. King and his wife studied for three years in the Black Hills country of South Dakota. Like a human community, the prairie dog town is divided into districts of which there are about thirty, each inhabited by a clan of around forty members. These districts are separated from each other by invisible walls of scent trails marking the boundaries. Although, unlike most of our towns and cities, there is no ranking of districts into ghettos and white middle-class suburbs, nevertheless it is forbidden to cross the boundaries, which are fiercely patrolled by the leading male or alderman. One goes across only by a regrettable mistake or with deliberate warlike intent—when, for example, one of the younger males, feeling his new manhood, has decided to try to take over. Females are also expected not only to respect the scent boundary but also to drive other wandering females away. John King describes one typical encounter in which a female feeding on grass was apparently not certain about the exact course of the boundary which she overstepped by a foot or so. A female from the district thus unlawfully trespassed upon approached cautiously, showing her teeth and, in effect, said "Whatcha doing here?" The stranger, still confident that she was within her rights, turned around and raised her tail, exposing her behind with the anal glands, and allowed the other female to sniff. This is a common way for a prairie dog to say approximately "Go ahead and have a smell and you'll see I belong here." The other female then showed *her* buttocks. This display was repeated by each female several times, until one of them lost patience and suddenly bit the other in the behind. The bitten one started to run away but anger conquered fear and she returned to the dispute. The two kept running backwards and forwards, biting each other mildly and displaying their scent marks every now and then. Finally both of them picked up the scent of the boundary line, which had obviously weathered and grown faint, and went their separate ways, paying no further attention to each other.

In animals with a highly developed sense of smell, both the olfactory mucous membrane and the entrance to the olfactory organ are normally deeply pigmented. In the genetic accident or breeding practice that produces an albino, the total lack of pigment in these areas prevents the animal from smelling at all. White hogs in Virginia commonly die because they cannot discern through smell the difference between the poisonous *Lachnanthes* root and other roots they feed on, though pigs ordinarily have such a good sense of smell that in France they are used instead of dogs to sniff out underground truffles.

Although man is not as clever at smells as a dog or a pig, he is by no means an olfactory cripple, as witness the fact that in 1966 man's grooming aids alone represented a $500 million business. A very great amount of money has been spent on investigations of the human sense of smell, not only for purposes of perfumery development but because odor is such an important part of the combination sense of flavor, which determines whether people will take to a new food product or not. Odors perceptible to man (or at least European man) were classified pretty well as long ago as 1895 by the Dutch physiologist H. Zwaardemaker, and very few changes have been suggested since then. The classification includes nine categories as follows: *ethereal* (fruits, raisins, ether), *aromatic* (camphor, clover, lemon, bitter almonds), *balsamic* (flowers, vanilla), *ambrosial* (amber, musk), *alliaceous* (hydrogen sulfide, arsine, chlorine), *empyrematic* (roasted coffee, benzene), *caprylic* (cheese, rancid fat), *repulsive* (deadly nightshade, bedbugs) and *nauseating* (carrion, feces).

Since it has been recognized that some of the components of odor, although present chemically in very small amounts, may be significant for the total effect, great efforts have been made to develop microanalytic chemistry, and new techniques have been applied to the problem, such as mass spectrometry, infrared and ultraviolet spectroscopes, nuclear magnetic resonance and gas-liquid chromatography. Under the best conditions, the mass spectroscope can detect close to quantities of one picogram, which is one trillionth of a gram. But this really isn't good enough. The average human nose can detect skatol (3-methylindole), the offensive chemical from excrement, at concentrations of 3×10^{-11} per cent by weight in air, but unfortunately this was recently found not to be the offensive odor. Skatol, when completely purified, is odorless. Hence what we smell in an old outhouse is not skatol but some unknown chemical that goes along with it in analytically indeterminable traces. If 99.999 per cent humulene (wood odor) is mixed with 0.0001 per cent of ionone (violets), the mixture will smell only of violets when diluted with air. This is because the olfactory threshold (or amount just necessary to cause a reaction) is only 10^{-14} grams for ionone, while it is 10^{-7} grams for humulene.

"People-sniffers" consist of analytical instruments that are sensitive to very small amounts of ammonia arising from the decomposition of sweat. Honeywell Company's "electronic bloodhound" uses the principle of preferential ultraviolet radiation. But even oil companies will trust only the human nose in regard to customer reaction to a new product. (I can recall when one oil company for which I worked brought out a new polyethylene plastic and employed whole panels of human noses to detect whether a given batch of product possessed a stubborn fecal odor or not.)

The olfactory membrane is always covered by a thin layer of fluid. Chemicals that expect to be smelled must dissolve almost instantaneously in the tissues of this nasal mucous membrane. That this is not a sufficient condition for being smellable, however, is shown by the fact that carbon dioxide, which is both volatile and soluble, has no odor. (It is probable that the common compounds with which life has been surrounded ever since its inception, such as carbon dioxide and water, are not smelled because evolution decided that this would be too confusing. It is better that they provide an odorless *background*.) Practically all the pure elements, except chlorine, bromine and iodine, are odorless. Compounds with a molecular weight of over 300 are generally imperceptible by odor.

For a long time the most plausible theory of smell was one that goes back to Lucretius (50 B.C.)—the idea that odors are like keys that fit certain locks. The odor-receptor cells are regarded as fashioned to receive and to be set off only by molecules of a certain size and shape. A refinement on this theory, which suggests how the setting-off is done, has been proposed by John T. Davies, a British chemical engineer. According to this idea, the odorous molecule is adsorbed on the olfactory nerve ending, which it then penetrates, forming a small hole. An instantaneous exchange of sodium and potassium ions takes place through this momentary window, which would cause the discharge of a nerve impulse. For a strong odorant, such as ionone, the act of adsorption of just one molecule on a receptor site would be enough to cause membrane puncture. It appears from the work of Piet Stuiver, a Dutch physiologist, that the threshold of one human olfactory cell for causing an odor sensation is at the most about eight molecules. If only one molecule in a thousand that enter the nose excites a receptor, the amount of material needed to produce a response is 50,000 times less than can be detected by such sophisticated physical techniques as gas chromatography.

Although it has been very difficult to count the number of olfactory nerve fibers, because of their small size, they seem to be capable of conducting to the brain about 10 million bits of information per second. However, some people have better noses than others. Professional odor technicians in the perfume trade can distinguish 19,000 different odors at twenty levels of intensity each. According to one of Freud's theories, man's sense of smell became repressed along with his sexuality as civilization advanced. Children do not distinguish between agreeable and disagreeable smells until they are about five years old. Recent studies have shown, for example, that three- to four-year-old children actually find the odors of sweat and feces to be pleasant, but at five, under parental instruction, they learn that these odors are supposed to be disagreeable.

Musk is one of the oldest perfume constituents that we know of. The best natural musk is extracted from certain glands of a tiny male musk deer native to the high Himalayas. It has always been associated by the Chinese with sexual attraction and was regarded as an aphrodisiac. Now there are many different kinds, classified as macrocyclic, steroid, nitro, indane, naphthalene and benzene musks. The fact that the odor of musk is somehow of sexual significance to humans, and probably always has been, is shown by the remarkable sex differentiation in ability to smell musklike chemicals such as pentadecanolide. Over 50 per cent of men cannot smell this substance at all and the rest cannot smell it in dilutions of more than one part per million of air. Yet all normal women are sensitive to it in dilution of one part per billion. During the course of the menstrual cycle the women's sensitivity increases so that during ovulation some women can detect one part per *quadrillion,* an almost unbelievably small concentration, comparable to the dilution at which the male gypsy moth is able to smell his lady's lure. Although the reason for this unique female ability to perceive musk is not clear, it is obviously related to hormones. Women whose ovaries have been removed are about 1,000 times less sensitive, but when given estrogen treatments they regain their normal sensitivity. It is possible that if we were not drowned in an olfactory flood-wave of artificial smells, such as those of air pollution, cosmetics and cigarette smoke, the sexual facets of natural musklike odors might be of clearer importance to us. Several years ago, in a marketing study, a large number of women shoppers were offered a display of stockings of the same make, half of which, unknown to them, had been faintly perfumed. The overwhelming majority of them bought the perfumed hosiery, although when questioned, they mentioned quality, texture and appearance, but never odor. Probably this is a subliminal effect. That Neanderthal man 60,000 years ago was attracted by flowers, probably both because of their pleasant smell and their pretty color, is shown by a recent discovery by Arlette Leroi-Gourhan in Iraq. A funeral bier was excavated which was found to be covered with pine boughs and by the relatives of the present grape hyacinth, the bachelor's button, the hollyhock and the yellow-flowering groundsel. It is even deduced that this heavy-faced ancient man occasionally went around with flowers in his hair.

Our scientific study of the chemical senses is handicapped by the fact that, unlike sound and light, odor or taste intensity cannot be amplified, since no wave motions are involved in the message. However, it is regarded as possible that the *consciousness* of chemical messages can be increased (an internal amplification) by the use of drugs such as LSD. It might thus be possible to reinforce the effect of those odors that result in definite nerve impulses but in no impingement on cortical awareness (subliminal perceptions) so that they come in clear and strong. Everyone could then be a true wine connoisseur instead of merely pretending that he makes the delicate distinctions of the professional wine-taster between "full-bodied," "velvety," "virginal," etc. That we are mainly dependent upon odor rather than taste in distinguishing between the flavor of various foods is shown by the fact that a man without a sense of smell cannot tell whether he is eating an apple or an onion. The aroma of coffee was once attributed to 30 chemical compounds, but the list of probable ingredients has now gone as high as 150. The flavor is still elusive. The fact of the matter is that the sense of smell, although very primitive, is simply not understood.

The olfactory cells are primary neurons. The nose epithelium is separated from the brain by only a thin plate of bone. The epithelium, as well as the entire nasal cavity, contains bare nerve fibers from the trigeminal cranial nerve, not all of them giving odor messages. It was once assumed that such companion cells participated in odor detection solely by evoking a *pain* response (in other words, the central nervous system was supposed to say, "Ouch! That smells dangerous!") but according to modern evidence these non-olfactory receptors may simply participate in mechanical sense impressions, such as detecting the presence of inert dust. The sensory endings of all the true olfactory cells have tiny cilia that wave in the breeze of the nose. There are half a dozen cilia per cell in man, compared with up to fourteen in the rabbit. These are kept moist with mucus from adjacent cells. The total surface of these microscopic hairs is enormous. Many of the extremely fine axons from the receptor cell bodies group together in bundles and pass through the cribriform plate separating the nasal chamber from the brain cavity and enter the olfactory bulb. Within this bulb the axons terminate in many small bodies called "glomeruli." Thus each smell nerve fixer leads directly from the point of stimulation to the bulb and only one nerve junction in the glomeruli separates the receptor from the olfactory *lobe* of the brain. This is the most direct path from the outside universe to the brain of any of the senses and emphasizes the importance that evolution at one time attached to chemical signaling.

That the olfactory bulb with its glomeruli must be an autonomous and frantically busy sorting-center is shown by the fact that, although about 20,000 incoming axons enter each glomerulus (in the rabbit), only twenty-four mitral (or secondary olfactory) neurons lead out to the brain. The messages coming in thus undergo a brutal censorship and classification. It is as if the messages of every Mrs. Smith calling into a telephone exchange were lumped together and the resulting chatter channeled simultaneously into the home of one Mrs. Jones. Actually the situation is less confusing, since it is the nature of Mrs. Smith's message and not the marital accident of her name that is sorted. The signals from *one type* of sensor are fed into the mitral funnel. Retaining the telephone exchange simile, it is as if an alert phone operator of the old-fashioned type listened to Mrs. Smith's whole message, which included a list of her ailments, gossip about Mrs. Brown, miscellaneous talk about her own children, et cetera, et cetera, and an invitation to dinner, and transmitted to Mrs. Jones only the invitation to dinner. The residual message is subliminal and presumably what we would pick up in the form of nose chatter if we lifted the bulb's censorship by some such expedient as a special drug. This can be afforded only by animals like man that can afford the luxury of experimentation. In a wild animal who needs his nose to earn a living, it might be catastrophic if his olfactory bulb suddenly became non-discriminatory and passed on the messages of flowers, of insecticides, of gasoline fumes and of other purely esthetic background odors when he is interested only in tracking down a ground squirrel.

We can readily see from neurological studies on animals that the olfactory bulb does not and should not reproduce faithfully all the processes at the olfactory epithelium. Different classes of receptor sites may be distributed in different ratios over each primary olfactory neuron, thus providing some specificity. It has been found that in the olfactory bulb of frogs over one half of the olfactory neurons responded to a given chemical but only two responded in the same way. There seems to be some indication of spatial localization in the bulb. In cats, for instance, the back region of the bulb is particularly sensitive to the smell of decayed meat or fish—an important smell for a cat. In other animals, water-soluble compounds at low concentrations stimulate the *front* of the bulb, while water-insoluble hydrocarbons excite the *back*.

On the whole it now seems doubtful that highly specific receptors for particular chemical compounds exist or indeed that chemical specificity alone can be the basis of odor discrimination. A biologically important smell is more likely to be a complex pattern of chemicals and it is the pattern to which both the bulb and the brain respond.

We know much more about the chemical sense of taste than about odor. In particular we know more about the taste behavior of the blowfly than of any other organism, including man, because it depends upon such delightfully accessible organs of taste reception, which consist of hairs. Through the work of V. G. Dethier (then at Johns Hopkins) and of Edward S. Hodgson of Columbia University and of others, it was found that hairs on the proboscis of flies are housings for living taste-receptor cells. Thus, the fly can taste with the hairs of his little elephantlike trunk before he goes all out and decides to slurp up what he tastes through the trunk. (This gives him an advantage over us, since it is inconvenient or at least boorish for us to stick our tongues way out and lick everything before we put it in our mouth and, besides, even a dirty tongue has to return ultimately to the mouth.) Each sensory hair on the blowfly's proboscis has three receptor cells at its base. Two of the cells send thin filaments through the hollow shaft of hair to its tip. These are the taste receptors. The third cell is a touch receptor, sensitive to the bending of the hair.

The first question to be answered by the investigators was: Are both the taste receptors sensitive to the same kind of chemical? The answer is "No." Salts, acids, most alcohols and other compounds *except* sugars cause an electrical impulse with a constant amplitude of about 300 microvolts. Solutions of sugars and other things that the blowflies like to eat gave an amplitude of 200 microvolts. One sensory call responds to the sugars, etc. (the signal means "Good stuff"); the other cell responds to the other things (the signal is "Ech!—Bad stuff"). In a natural environment when the chemicals available, either for eating or for rejecting, are mixed, the feeding behavior of the fly depends on the proportions of "good stuff" and "echs" in impulses reaching the brain. Mixtures seldom evoke impulses that are simple sums of the two opposed reactions. For instance, the addition of table sugar to a salt solution not only activates the sugar-sensing receptor, but also lowers the frequency of the salt-sensing receptor. This tends to increase the discrepancy between the frequencies of the two messages. Since it is good for a fly to eat sugar plus a little salt, the message says "Very good stuff." If, however, quinine is added to the salt solution, the discrepancy is in the direction of "*Very* bad stuff." (Here again we see the ever-present tendency of sense receptors to build up a contrast that is useful to the behavior of the organism. The fly has to have some very positive report, for after all he is either going to dip his proboscis in to slurp or he is not. He needs very positive encouragement or very positive inhibition.) However, time must be allowed for a proper decision. Receptors in some hairs of the fly are slow in responding to stimuli and are relatively inexcitable, while those in other hairs always fire rapidly. Thus strong stimulation that would quickly inactivate the sensitive receptors because of fatigue would still be affecting the more sluggish receptors. There is reason to believe also that the fly, in contact with a heated syrup, can receive from a single hair the message that the prospective food is not only strong and very acceptable but that it is warm and sticky.

For every million smell receptors in man, there are only

about a thousand taste cells, and it has been agreed for a long time that there are in man only four basic tastes: sweet, salty, bitter and sour. All the other distinctions are distinctions of *flavor* which includes odor, roughness or smoothness, hotness or coldness and pungency or blandness.

All mineral acids have a sour taste, which is really the taste of the hydrogen ion. Organic acids, however, may have additional tastes. Acetic acid (vinegar) actually tastes more sour than it should given the concentration of hydrogen ions. But in more complicated organic acids, the hydrocarbon part of the molecule gets into the act. Citric acid tastes both sweet and sour, while citraconic acid tastes both sour and bitter.

Most all the single mineral salts, such as sodium chloride, sodium sulfate, potassium nitrate, etc. taste simply salty, but potassium and ammonium bromide taste both salty and bitter. Curiously enough, the salts of beryllium and some salts of lead taste sweet, a bad thing for the safety of children since they are poisonous. Low molecular weight salts are usually salty, but with increasing molecular weights the trend is toward bitterness.

There is no chemical guidance as to what ought to taste bitter or sweet. Thus both saccharin and cyclamate, once the most widely used synthetic sweeteners, were purely accidental discoveries. Differences in chemical structure, which are hard for even a chemist to determine, make all the difference in the world to the taste buds. Thus D-glucose (a sugar in which the molecules are the same in number and size of atoms as in L-glucose, but in which a slight difference of geometry causes an optical difference in the way the beams of polarized light are rotated) is sweet, while L-glucose is slightly salty. The anomers (or *almost* identical siblings) of D-mannose have different tastes. The compound 2-amino-4-nitropropoxybenzene is 4,000 times as sweet as table sugar while the very similar 4-amino-2-nitropropoxybenzene is tasteless.

The taste receptors are believed to respond in much the same fashion as odor receptors. The first step is for a compound to be adsorbed on the surface of the receptor, then to puncture the membrane. Sodium ions move in, potassium ions move out, the resting potential of the nerve fiber drops and the wave of electrical impulses passes along to signify to the brain that something has been tasted. The impulses last only a few milliseconds at a maximum frequency of from 100 to 200 per second. Frequency signals the intensity of the taste.

The taste receptors in all mammals, including man, are located on the tongue and soft palate. The papillae (which are little fingers that make the tongue feel rough) at the back are each surrounded by a trench into which a watery fluid is secreted by nearby glands. Along the walls of the trench we find the taste buds, and within each bud ten to fifteen taste cells are arranged like the segments of an orange. The taste receptors are like little walls with microvilli (or tiny fingers). The number of taste buds decreases with advancing age, which is one of the reasons why parents and grandparents cannot understand some of the finicky food objections of children. Adults have about 900 buds, chiefly on the upper part of the tongue. There are few in the center of the tongue. The sensation of sweetness is signaled mostly by buds at the tip of the tongue, sourness at the edge, saltiness along the edge and tip, bitterness at the back. Thus if solutions containing both chemicals that are bitter and chemicals that are sweet are placed in the mouth, we taste the sweet before the bitter and the bitter lingers after the sweet has disappeared. However, we should avoid false simplification, even in this relatively simple domain of the senses. It has been found that taste buds by themselves do not really show specific responses. However, one nerve fiber innervates several taste cells within a bud and possibly single taste cells may respond to only one chemical stimulus. There is also evidence that a single taste cell may respond to more than one of the categories of taste that we have set up. As we have mentioned already in the case of the taste of rodents, there is much preliminary classification at the papillae level involving consultation between different nerve fibers. Since there is no reason to suspect that humans have a more refined sense of taste than rats, our taste sensations probably also involve such peripheral conferences in which the decision is made as to what encoded message to send to the brain.

Although taste is simpler than smell, there are more nerve trunks associated with taste. Three of the cranial nerves contain taste components. One of these, the chorda tympani, can be studied by electrophysiological methods. It is found that the integrated response in this nerve sums up what is being tasted in the front two thirds of the tongue. The glossopharyngeal and the pharyngeal nerves innervate the rest of the tongue and the soft palate. By a cryptic freak of evolution the fibers of the chorda tympani leave the main nerve stem and pass through their own bone canal into the middle ear, then join the facial nerves to the brain. The chorda tympani is thus near the surface and it has been easy to tap it. The result is that most of what we know about taste is from the messages that go through the chorda tympani nerve. Even in man the nerve can be reached in the middle ear after the eardrum has been removed, as in ear operations for otosclerosis.

Some chemicals have paralyzing effects on the sense of taste without affecting smell, the paralysis affecting only certain sensations. Thus gymnemic acid, which is contained in the leaves of the asclepiad (a member of the milkweed family) completely abolishes the sweet taste. If one chews these leaves, sugar tastes only gritty—like fine sand. Bitter sensations are also repressed but salty and sour tastes remain untouched. The natives of Nigeria chew the "miraculous fruit," a wild berry that abolishes the response to sour tastes. After eating this berry, a lemon tastes like a sweet orange, but more importantly to the Nigerians, their humble acidulated cornbread and their sour wine taste lovely. Western civilization has played around for many years with flavor enhancers. Monosodium-L-glutamate has been common since 1909 and more recently disodium-5'-inosinate and others have been used in the attempts to make cheap meat cuts taste like filet mignon. It has been found that single nerve fibers of the chorda tympani respond to the presence of these chemicals, indicating that they are actually tasted, rather than that they modify the chemistry of the food to which they are added. They may also have a secondary effect of reacting with metal ions to make additional receptor sites available to normal taste stimulation.[3]

The subject of the flavor of foods has not only received enormous research expenditure on the part of the intensely competitive packaged-food industry, but more recently has become something of a planetary problem. Flavor, being cultural, depends on geography. Whereas in the early history of the exploration of the planet, a big drive was on to reach the spices of the East so that the foods of the West might be made to taste better, we now struggle with the flavor prejudices of the Easterners to prevent them from starving. It is no use to ship them wheat if they will eat nothing but rice. The rice-eating Bengali proved in 1944 that they would rather starve than use wheat flour. Riots broke out in Kerala, India, in 1966 when people felt that the government was forcing them to eat wheat. In a world where two thirds of the population may be facing famine before the end of the century, it is probable that, to survive, they may have to stomach not only wheat but fish flour and perhaps flour from cultivated algae and proteins from petroleum. If one could make all this "taste" like rice, presumably the problem would be solved. Large chemical and food organizations, such as Monsanto Chemical and General Mills, have concentrated their best flavor chemists on such problems.

An example of a reverse problem that was solved by flavor chemists is the favorite Hong Kong soft drink based on soybeans. Monsanto a few years ago joined forces with the Oriental firm of K. S. Lo, who invented the drink. The problem was that, while this concoction was popular in the Orient, just

[3] Such flavor enforcers, when used in excessive amounts, have recently been found to cause a mysterious sequence of allergic symptoms known in popular medical language as the "Chinese restaurant syndrome." It turns out that thousands of Americans have suffered this agony in silent fortitude, believing that they were shamefully unique in responding with dizziness, burning sensations in the neck and headache to bird's-nest soup and other delicacies containing as much as two spoonfuls of monosodium glutamate. The glutamate additive is also under the gun because it is found to tend toward infant deformity in the brains of rodents.

because it tastes strongly of soybeans, nobody outside the Orient seems to like the taste of soybeans. The Monsanto chemists succeeded in developing a new beverage with the same base which now, however, tastes somewhere between "nutty" and "custardy." The consistency, the color, the odor and the "mouth feel" all had to be adjusted too, so that the Westerner thought he was drinking something on the order of malted milk.[4]

Even in South America it has been very hard to get poor people to pay for wholesome high-protein foods imported from the well-fed nations. They will not even pay the nominal price that would partly cover the transportation costs. If the food is free, they will eat it, but with lack of enthusiasm. If it costs anything, they will buy coffee instead, because, they say, the "children like coffee." The truth of the matter is a bitter axiom known to food exporters and to people in the Peace Corps: "If the mother doesn't like it, she will not pay for it or feed it to the children."

We see in all these cases of food prejudices among people who cannot afford prejudices, an insane result of what is known as "cultural evolution." Just as certain arctic foxes will die rather than eat anything except lemmings, most of the Eastern people will die rather than eat anything except rice. Just as man evolved from a vegetarian primate into a powerful omnivore, mainly because he learned to eat so variously, so in the East and to some extent in Africa and South America, he has passed through a process of devolution in which only certain species of grains will satisfy his remarkably fastidious nose and tongue. Although an emergency solution may lie in chemically doctoring up other available foods so that the flavor is acceptable, the long-term remedy is obviously to change the culture. The Western mother teaches her child that sweat and excrement are bad things to smell and that spinach is good to eat. The Eastern mother must teach her child that wheat, for example, is good to eat. And there are many more Eastern mothers than Western mothers.

---

[4] Malted milk is not acceptable in the Orient, since it has been discovered recently that practically no adult Oriental is able to digest milk. After weaning, his intestinal tract can no longer handle lactose, or milk sugar.

CHAPTER 4

Touch, Temperature and the Mystery of Pain

ALL one-celled animals may be regarded as having a sense of touch, even though a conservative biologist may deny that this is actually a sense, since he does not admit that they can have a nervous system. This is a wrongheaded point of view, since such animals not only behave as nervous creatures but anatomically they can be seen to have miniature connective threads within this single cell, and they have the chemicals associated with nerve activation and conduction. However, we are here at the brink of a profound distinction that applies not only to the sense of touching but to any sensation. As we shall soon emphasize with respect to the skin organs, the functioning of all the senses of a metazoan, such as an insect or a man, are like the process of producing a first-class movie. The producer and director preside at the taking of thousands and thousands of feet of film but show to the audience in the end only a selected fraction of this footage. Similarly, although the sense receptors are always grinding away, only a few of these grindings are intense enough to cause nerve fibers to spike a coded message inward, and because of the hierarchical and mutually inhibiting character of the nerve fibers, the representation of the external world is not what the world is like but a cartoon of the world simplified and exaggerated so that the owner of the senses can best arrive at a life-preserving or life-enhancing strategem.

In a one-celled animal, the sensations (perhaps only of chemicals, of water pressure and of contact with meaningful objects) obviously are not subject to the multitiered editing and threshold restrictions of multicelled animals. Every foot of film is printed and exhibited. This is philosophically interesting in a rather mournful way, since it means that only the simplest animals perceive the universe as it is. All the rest of us are bound by the well-meant but sometimes (as in man) anachronistic internuncial editors, translators and censors.

Perhaps simply because it is so primitive, the sense of touch or pressure is in all higher animals including man very poorly understood, but it is notably subservient to the sense of vision and mixed up in a most vexatious and subtle way with the sensation we call "pain," which is perhaps not a sensation at all; it is a concerted *act* of nervous emergency.

Even in a protozoan, which is so poor in equipment that it does not have cilia or hairs, touch may involve bruising or pricking the external membrane of the cell. This causes an electrical potential charge, since there is at least an infinitesimal leaking in or out of ions. The amoeba perceives it has touched something because its skin has been penetrated enough to cause the movement of water-soluble ions. An enormous refinement and perhaps the greatest early invention of evolution —and one that has not perished even in man—was the construction of cilia or hairs to mediate this membrane reaction. The cilia could feel something coming before it hit the precious membrane with a thud. Now when evolution arrived at animals in which certain cells were specialized for receiving touch signals on the skin, it had also been decided to give most of such animals muscles and organs. Thus *internal* touch senses (proprioceptors) had to be provided to tell an animal whether it was defecating, whether its stomach was moving and in what position the joints of its legs were disposed from one moment to another. These touch (pressure or tension) receptors, whether on the skin or attached to voluntary or involuntary muscles, can be regarded as "transducers," just as can all sensory receptors. They convert one form of energy into another, in this case mechanical into electrical energy. The transducer effect in mechanoreceptors was first shown by Bernhard Katz of University College, London, who discovered in 1950 that the stretching of a muscle spindle (the mechanoreceptor built into skeletal muscle) generates a local electric current in what is called the "Pacinian corpuscle." When the current reaches a certain intensity, it triggers the firing of an impulse in a nerve fiber leading from the muscle spindle to the higher nerve centers. In a man this message may say, "Left arm is drawing back preparing to give opponent the old one-two punch." Similar Pacinian corpuscles are found in the skin. As a sense organ it is impressive and a delight to work with because it is so large that it can be seen with the naked eye, but, like some of those Chinese box-within-a-box puzzles, it is deceptive. Most of its substance seems to be padding. It is constructed along the lines of a little onion from which one layer of skin after the other can be peeled away. Werner R. Loewenstein of Columbia University found that 99.9 per cent of the onion could be removed without impairing the transducer function of responding electrically to touch. Apparently all these layers are cushions to prevent the nerve ending itself from being weakened by sudden impact or riotous vibrations. The membrane of the nerve ending, constituting the working core of the Pacinian corpuscle, is the seat of the generator potential that may or may not trigger a nerve impulse. Under resting conditions (and it is hard to imagine true resting conditions for a skin organ unless the body is suspended naked without tension in still air) the membrane resistance is so high that no appreciable net ion current leaks through it. Distortion, as by contact with something or someone, produces a decrease in resistance which allows ions to move across the membrane, causing the resting potential to drop—along with the local flow of current. This is the *generator* current and, although it is probably sensed in protozoans, it is not necessarily felt in animals with multiple cells. In order to make an impression on such animals, the generator current must be large enough to excite in turn the action current in the nerve fiber connected with the Pacinian corpuscle.

Loewenstein's precise experiments proved that excitation in the receptor membrane is confined to the mechanically distorted region. The summation of two or more currents each generated at a separate active site on the membrane may explain why the intensity of the generator is proportional to the strength of the stimulus. Neurologists now believe that one can picture the touch receptor as a membrane in which there are a number of tiny holes, or at least potential holes, like a piece of Swiss cheese covered with cellophane. In the resting state the holes are too small or the cellophane too thick for certain ions to pass through. Mechanical deformation opens up these holes. When the generator currents are being formed here and there over the membrane by a strong pressure such as a pinprick, the currents are strong enough to trigger nerve impulses and the intensity of the prick is signaled by the frequency of the impulses, since this is the only way nerve fibers can code intensity. (Along with this may go the pain sensation, but that is a more complicated and mystical story.) The touch receptor itself may wind up in a refractory state. This means that it reduces its responsiveness or "adapts" to a given touch pressure after a time. A stimulus that produces a generator current of 100 units in a fully rested receptor yields a current of barely 10 units after the application of 5,000 stimuli (at the rate of 500 per second) and none after 7,000 stimuli. Something, we are not sure what, has been depleted and has to be restored. This development of refractoriness is also shown by other touch organs such as the hair follicles, Merkel's disks and Meissner's corpuscles. This adaptation to a sequence of small stimuli is a good thing for humans because otherwise we would be driven wild by the breeze and the water and would find clothing intolerable. No such fatigue or refractoriness is shown by the internal Pacinian corpuscles and Ruffini's organs which send information about closure of the joints or by the Golgi's organs which respond to tension in the tendons. This, too, is lucky, for if these receptors started to take coffee breaks, we would never be able to drive a car to work or play a round of golf or swim across a lake.

As mentioned, hairs as touch organs are used by predatory single-celled animals and are especially sensitive to prey. The cilia respond differently to noxious stimuli, although it is doubtful that a ciliate feels the sensation of pain, which seems to be reserved by evolution for more complex animals. In general, in the evolution of the sense modalities the trend has been from few to many, from the general to the subdivided and from the mixed to the pure. Thus the sense of touch in some lower animals may be confused with the sense of cold and carried by the same fibers. When we get to the highly sensual insect class, we find over a hundred times as many input nerve fibers entering the central nervous system as output fibers for action. The factor is only five in man, indicating not so much a degradation in sensory yield as an enrichment in efferent nerves which respond by commanding some act of behavior. It is much easier for evolution to pile up sensory devices than it is to find something to do with the signals. Perhaps this is one of the reasons why some web spiders build a new web every night. They have nothing else to do.

Even sponges have a sense of touch. In the colonial hydroids, touch is about as sensitive as it is in some insectivorous plants. Small disturbances of the water are felt. If a copepod is brought near the polyp (one colony) of a hydroid, it causes no response until it moves. Then the polyp bends down like a graceful flower and devours the small animal. Flatworms have touch receptors and also specialized ones called "rheoceptors" to detect currents in the water. Tapeworms are believed to have *only* a sense of touch, although somewhere in their complicated life cycles chemical receptors must also be involved. The nematodes are peculiar. There is a remarkable fusion of nerve fibers, so that a nematode senses something that may be indistinguishable as a separate modality (touch, smell, temperature) but adds up to a pattern that in his exceedingly well-nerved body is sufficient to result in appropriate behavior. His specialized nerve endings and sense organs (sensory bristles, papillae, amphids, plastids, etc.) give an integrated message, the like of which we cannot imagine, because our perceptions are *sequential*. We see in the distance a four-legged animal. As he gets closer we hear a "Baa"; closer still, we smell a goat. But, supposing there were goats in a nematode's world, several senses would instantaneously combine, not to give a visual, chemical or tactile image but simply the one message "goat." Another possibility should not be overlooked. The nematode may be one of the only multiple-celled creatures in which *graded* responses, rather than the familiar all-or-none nerve messages, are the rule. The nematode thus may have a more complete picture of his little universe and may operate on sensory cues that are too small for a more conventional animal, such as an insect or a crab, to bother with. Perhaps this is the secret of the nematode's success. Figuratively he sees all, knows all. He finds margins of profit by which to make a living that the more coarsely quantumized senses of other animals in the same ecological niche have overlooked. Like a good businessman he is quicker to act—to close a deal—because he perceives more fully and more clearly.

Cuticular hairs are the commonest touch receptors in the arthropods, especially the crustaceans. The localized control is outstanding. If you touch the protective hairs of an arthropod's spiracle, just the spiracle that is touched will immediately close. Myriopods on the other hand rely on more central control. They will close *all* of the spiracles. Among insects the cockroach is a common laboratory animal for demonstration of the sense of touch (by the startle response) just as the fly is a model for chemical receptors. Among pelecypod mollusks, such as clams, touch receptors are sufficiently sophisticated for the sorting of particles of food. The gastropod (snail) has a tremendously dense enervation in his foot, which is supposed to be associated with a versatile tactile sense, although careful observation has uncovered no remarkable powers or activities. It is conceivable that this fantastic nervous richness of the foot may be connected with a sense other than touch but, as in so many cases of animals that are utterly alien to our ways, we have not discovered the modality. We can only admit with a respectful sigh that it is a mighty peculiar foot for all those nerves and let the problem slide to other generations of malacologists with more sympathetic interphylum insights.

The reptiles have a rather luxurious sense of touch. It is seldom realized that the shell of a turtle is tactually very sensitive. Large sea turtles like to have their shells scratched lightly. They can feel the tip of a straw dragged across. Birds inherit the reptile's tactility and often in unexpected parts of the anatomy. There are pressure-sensitive corpuscles situated on a duck's back and the cere (the forehead adjoining the beak) is also well supplied with corpuscles of touch.

All nocturnal and digging mammals are especially equipped for touching. In mice and cats the vibrissae, or nose hairs, are used to feel out objects in the dark. Rats like constantly to touch each other. (Thigmotropism, the tendency to touch things, is greatly developed in all mammals.) Within a pack of normal rats there are touch games, sometimes quite violent, but no more deadly than touch football as played outside a college dormitory. There is boxing with the forepaws, kicking with the hindpaws, but never any intrapack biting. The fighting of strange mice can be prevented by handling them just before they are put together. Not only are the gopher's whiskers responsive, but his hairless tail also has sensitive tactile nerve endings to help him when he wants to back up into his hole.

From the sensory point of view the evolution of primates depended upon hitherto unexploited techniques of teamwork between touch and eyesight. Touch in the hands (or in the tail) became so important that it began to occupy a very considerable part of the brain. If the digits' surfaces are roughened by fingerprints and by lack of glands that exude oil or sweat, then one's grasp is firm and one's tactile discrimination is improved. Furthermore, one no longer needs claws but can get by merely with flattened nails.[1] Some primates, however, have residual claws on one or more digits and nails on the rest. Neither the lemurs nor the order of *Lorisiformes* have separate control over

[1] Except for the human female, no primate would seriously consider using its digital nails for harming or defending itself against another animal.

individual digits. Their grasping ability is superb, but they have little ability to manipulate. The spider monkeys of South America have no thumbs but the tail is grasping. These and a few other primates have hairless areas on the tails with dermoglyphics such as our fingers. An individual of such a species could thus be readily identified by a "tailprint." On the hairless parts of the human body, such as the lips, palms and soles, the density of Meissner's corpuscles and Merkel's disks of touch are very thick. A surprisingly large part of the brain in man represents touch sensations from the lips. It is perhaps for that reason that we find kissing such a natural and satisfying activity and why oral eroticism is so popular.

The longest kiss in history is probably represented by a picture of a stringy-haired, mustachioed violinist grasping his piano-playing accompanist in a passionate embrace while lifting her off the piano stool. The origin of this obviously Victorian depiction of "masculine passion," which no doubt would even have titillated such sexual skeptics as Jane Austen, is something of a mystery. About thirty years ago a perfume company began featuring this as an advertisement, and it has since been published over 10,000 times in print reaching at least half a billion people. The framed reproduction is called *Kreutzer Sonata*. Somewhat tentatively the original is attributed to an obscure French artist, René Princete, but it was unknown and unsalable until the perfume company picked it up, and none of the officials of this concern know the whereabouts of the original and don't even know whether it exists. It is rumored that the original resides in some English bank's vaults along with other "art treasures" of unknown but probably substantial value (including the obscene master sketches by Turner and others, when they made artistic visits to whorehouses).

Georg von Békésy has recently shown that the tactile sense, like sight and hearing, is also subject to intricate processes of mutual inhibition and enhancement. In the "Mach bands" of visual sensation a softly graded distribution of light is transformed by such processes into a much sharper (and actually falsely representative) distribution of internal sensation; and Von

Békésy has established the existence of analogous Mach bands perceived by the organs of the skin for both direct pressure and vibration. The simultaneous action of inhibitions and summation funnels spreading stimulations into a localized nervous pathway. The filtering and amplifying and shuffling that go on increase the signal-to-noise ratio, so that, although we do not perceive the world around us as faithfully as an amoeba or a nematode, we do feel what evolution has considered it most important that we feel. Von Békésy has especially studied the sensory impressions we get from two points of stimulation on the skin as the points are removed from each other. Adjacent stimuli are summed or reinforced, while more distant ones are inhibited in such a way that one can definitely conclude that every point stimulus on the skin produces an area of sensation surrounded by an area of inhibition. If tactile Mach bands are to occur, the inhibitory area has to be larger than the sensory area and moreover this discrepancy must increase with the intensity of the stimulation. When you poke me with your finger, I feel the poke more sharply and resent it more fiercely when more of my sensory nerve endings are telling my thalamus that they have nothing to report. This makes the message from their neighbors ("Strong poke here") all the more serious. It is relayed to the cortex, which concludes that a serious incident has occurred, calling either for reprisal or withdrawal. I decide to poke you back.

The localization of vibrations on the body may be shifted by introducing delays in two vibrators. This acts in somewhat the same way as localizing a sound by two ears, although the skin receptors, unlike the sound receptors, have "local signs" that indicate position in space. Even when two vibrators are placed in the vertical position on the same side of the body, it is possible at least to feel the sensation as coming from the place on the body that was vibrated first. There localization is not tied to interaction between the hemispheres of the brain, as it is in hearing. It is significant that both sound and touch localization are best when the onset of the stimulus is abrupt. Von Békésy has found it possible to establish some rather surprising and new numbers in rate of nerve conduction. Since we don't perceive a large area over which the traveling waves move when the body is stimulated by vibration, the funneling process in localization must be in the range of thousandths of a second. The change in localization as the result of delay in vibratory stimulation provides a means of measuring the true speed of nerve conduction. In his classical nineteenth-century experiments Hermann von Helmholtz used reaction time to estimate the speed of tactile nerves, finding it to be from 50 to 60 meters per second. Reaction time, however, involves a whole complex of messing around in various circuits. When localization is used, as by Von Békésy, the speed of transmission for vibrations on the skin is estimated as high as 208 meters per second.

It is evident that there are two speeds of nervous conduction: a fast process for the inhibiting interactions that produce localization and a slower process for the growth of a sensation, this sensation ("My belly is being vibrated right near the navel") coming only after the local processes of inhibition and enhancement had a chance to agree upon a coded telegram to the brain. Whereas localization is determined within 2 or 3 milliseconds (thousandths of a second) after onset of the stimulus, the time necessary for the growth of a sensation may take from 20 milliseconds in hearing to over 1,000 milliseconds in taste, smell and vibrational touch. Furthermore, the speed of the transmission of sensation is greatly disturbed by unusual temperatures or by pain. If an electric shock is given to an experimental animal 10 seconds before measurements of nervous speed, this speed will be reduced. Lower speeds of nervous transmission reported from animal studies, according to Von Békésy, may often be due to the effect of anesthesia, unusual temperature and pain, all of which disturb the nervous system. One rather odd effect is observed where you study the sensation of vibration in the human knees. When there is a time interval in stimulating the two knees with vibrators, the sensation jumps from one knee to the other depending on the time interval. When the knees are vibrated simultaneously, however, the vibrations seem to be located in free space between the knees.

Asenath Petrie has built up a curious relationship between certain tactile discriminations and other psychological and even psychiatric aspects of human personality by a simple test. She asks the subject to rub his fingers along the edges of a 2½-inch-wide block for 60 seconds and then to judge, by touch alone, the width of a 1½-inch block. Some subjects will guess that the latter block is wider than they would have judged, without the preliminary rubbing, and some will guess that it is narrower. The wide-guessers she calls "augmenters" and the narrow-guessers "reducers." She finds that augmenters have a lower tolerance for pain than reducers. They also have high scores for hypochondria on the scale of the Minnesota Multiphasic Personality Inventory—an indication that they are highly aware of their bodies. Reducers, on the other hand, often have painless peptic ulcers. Reducers also tolerate sensory isolation much more poorly and seem to prefer pain to being left alone. If Miss Petrie's tests prove repeatable, it appears that even the workings of as elemental a sensory modality as touch are co-ordinated with that ghostly concatenation of all the nerves that we call "character" or "individuality."

A rather antic group "happening" during the years 1967 and 1968 was established by various "free universities," essentially a group of students, occasionally joined by the younger, more kittenish professors, on or near existing campuses. The "feelies" was one of the courses preferred at the free schools and was designed to exorcize the hang-ups of the young. The teacher or leader orders blindfolds put on a dozen students. They lie on their backs. "Now feel your head," they are ordered. "Your neck. Your left leg. What does it feel like? Now touch the person on your left. Is it a boy or a girl?" At this point, or shortly thereafter, the hang-ups are supposed to disappear.

The body's sensations for hot and for cold depend on two quite distinct receptors, Krause's end-bulbs for cold and Ruffini's corpuscles for heat. It is a scientific scandal that so little is known about the way in which these organs work. One of the most curious situations is that receptors for touch, heat, cold and possibly pain (although we shall consider that undecided for the moment) seem to be quite uniformly distributed over the surface of the skin, but particular spots nevertheless seem highly sensitive to one sensation and much less to others. When such spots are microscopically examined, there appears no difference in kind or density of sensory endings.

Each kind of skin sensation is handled by a separate set of nerve fibers, both myelinated and unmyelinated. The channels for temperature are not very clearly worked out, but it is believed that a drop in temperature is recorded by large myelinated fibers while a rise in temperature is reported by small unmyelinated axons.

Until recently it was assumed by many that the sensation of pain depends, like all the other modalities, on the existence of specific nerve endings (which, however, did not elaborate into distinct organs, such as those of touch and temperature). These branched endings cried "Ouch!" and the message, given priority over all other incoming communications, went straight to a "pain center" in the brain, which demanded an instant meeting of all cortical areas to decide what to do about the emergency. It was even assumed that the very small unmyelinated fibers that are found in all regions of the body are the ones assigned to pick up the dolorous message. Pain results from extreme stimulation of any kind, such as high temperature or high pressure. Many years ago Sir Charles Sherrington first pointed out that pain only results when there is danger of damage. At a steady temperature of 94° Fahrenheit, damage to the skin will start, but it is not until about 113° that a surface actually becomes painful to the touch. Some biologists have suggested that all painful stimuli cause a chemical to be released from damaged cells, but no evidence to support this oversimplified solution to the problem has ever been obtained. According to modern exponents of what is now known as the "pattern theory," the sensation of pain is by no means a specific sense modality, like sight, hearing, touch and temperature, but is a sort of concerted nervous reaction. The sensation of pain is the act of reacting to dangerous stimulations. In this sense, pain is something that happens interiorly as the organism responds as a whole. It depends no more on specific pain fibers than does the pleasure of sexual gratification depend on "pleasure" fibers in the sex organs. Recent research by investigators such as Ronald Melzack of McGill University, Patrick Wall of MIT and W. K. Livingston of the University of Oregon Medical School have focused a bright new light on the whole rather terrifying problem of pain.

That pain is a valuable event if an animal wants to survive is shown by what happens to people who are occasionally born without the ability to feel pain. If they survive their childhood at all, it is with a mosaic of burns and bruises and often they bite so deeply into their tongues while chewing food that they are unable to learn to talk. But even when an animal is able physically to detect pain, it appears that he has to learn what it means. Avoidance of pain has to involve a nerve-education process. Melzack and William R. Thompson raised Scottish terriers in complete individual isolation, from infant pups to mature dogs, so that they had none of the usual body buffets and scrapes and falling-over-each-other play of normal puppies. When they had grown up, they failed to back away from a flaming match. They poked their noses repeatedly into the flame. They would barely respond to pricking with a pin. In contrast their littermates, who had been reared normally, showed commendable alacrity in jumping back from a flame at the first sight of fire and one could not approach them pin in hand more than once. The senseless behavior of the artificially retarded dogs was not because of a general failure of the sensory nerves and their messages of pain. An intense electric shock caused violent excitement in them as in any animal. Moreover, their reflex movements in contact with the flame or the pin showed that they felt something. But somehow this "something" had not been connected emotionally within the nervous system as a whole. They were like small towns equipped with adequate sirens to warn of the approach of a tornado, but in which nobody in town has been informed what the sound of the sirens means. It is evident that in the higher species of animals, pain is thus *not* (as Sherrington believed) simply an automatic sensory response to bodily damage. The amount and the quality of the pain are determined either by previous experience or an emotional teaching which involves the higher centers of the brain.

In Western culture childbirth is widely regarded as painful and at one time was fraught with all manner of ominous forebodings. An expectant mother was supposed to go down "through the valley of the shadow of death" every time she had a baby. There are other cultures in which women during parturition show no distress at all. The woman may have the baby in the midst of tending a crop of yams. Often in the same tribe the husband stays in bed to recover from the terrible ordeal *he* has just gone through, while the new mother returns to harvest the yams.[2] Since there appears to be no essential difference between the relative size or innervation of the reproductive organs of civilized and primitive females, the difference in pain may in this case be simply a matter of emotional education.

The extraordinary degree to which the general nervous *attitude* of people can influence pain was perhaps most graphically shown by the observations of Henry K. Beecher of the Harvard Medical School during the Anzio beachhead landing of World War II. Only one out of three severely wounded soldiers complained of enough pain to require morphine. That they were not in a state of shock was shown by the fact that they would still gripe snappishly at a clumsy hypodermic puncture of a vein. In the case of civilians with surgical incisions similar in depth and nerve involvement to the soldiers' wounds, four out of five claimed to be in terrible pain and pleaded for morphine. What was the difference? Every man who has stood in battle could tell you. The wounded man's overwhelming response was *relief*. He was still alive and on his way out of the war. He had it made. The euphoria took the play away from the pain apparatus. There

---

[2] This custom, called the "couvade," is seen variously in primitive peoples throughout the world. There is some dispute among anthropologists as to just what the man thinks he's doing. Lévi-Strauss contends that the husband is not trying to imitate his wife (or rather an imaginary action of his wife) but is trying to imitate *the baby*.

are numerous other examples. Men in furious preoccupation with an enemy or even an opponent in sports action commonly feel little or no pain. It is common experience that prize fighters and football players can sustain severe injuries without being aware that they've been hurt.

As shown by certain of Pavlov's experiments, pain can even be turned into a conditioning event. Dogs normally feel highly insulted and grieved when given a strong electric shock in the paw. However, Pavlov found, if he always presented food to a dog after each shock, the dog developed a new response. After a shock the dog would salivate, wag his tail and turn eagerly toward the food dish. This conditioned behavior persisted when Pavlov increased the intensity of the shocks and even when he supplemented them by actually burning and wounding the dog's skin. Using the same incentive of food, Jules H. Masserman of Northwestern University trained cats to administer shock to themselves by walking up to the switch and closing it with their paws.

It is apparent that the psychic factor in pain is quite complex and elaborate. It is perhaps not unrelated to the still mysterious and completely unexplained phenomenon of hypnotism. If hypnotism had to be explained in a few words, the hypnotic state could be defined as a trance in which the subject's attention is focused rigidly on the hypnotist while paying little or no attention to other stimulations. But what is a trance? Nobody can say. However, it is significant that a certain percentage of people can be hypnotized deeply enough to undergo surgery without anesthesia. The religious fanatics of India who walk with bare feet on hot coals are obviously in a state of self-hypnosis, although it is hard for us to say just what this means and how it is achieved. The skin of their feet smokes and one can smell flesh cooking (there is no interference with the ability of fire to burn), but the nerve apparatus of pain has been paralyzed by a self-inflicted trance.[3]

[3] With some fakirs, advantage is taken of a peculiar nerve geography in the human body. The skin just below the shoulder blades, back of the arm over the triceps muscle, over the forearm in general and at the side of the

Anticipation of pain often determines its intensity. Investigators in England found that the simple appearance of the word "pain" in a set of instructions made anxious subjects report as painful a degree of electric shock which they did not regard as painful otherwise. There is a peculiar psychic problem in connection with morphine. It now appears that one of the chief benefits obtained by morphine injections is merely the quieting of anxiety. (This may be the reason for its addictive properties.) Morphine diminishes pain if the anxiety level of a patient is high but has no effect if anxiety has already been dispelled by some other means. Of course, anxiety as a basic skeleton for the whole complex of pain has for years been recognized by physicians and that was why the placebo was invented. About 35 per cent of patients in severe pain show marked relief when administered placebos (which may be milk sugar or some other artless material). Since morphine, even in large doses, will relieve pain in only about 75 per cent of patients, it can be seen by simple arithmetic that nearly half of this drug's effectiveness is of a placebo or anxiety-dispelling nature.

Since it has become obvious that brain functions are able to modify the patterns of nerve impulses produced by an injury, it is natural for neurologists or psychologists to look for some tangible communication system by which this modification is brought about. Research studies in a number of countries during the past decade have shown the presence of hitherto overlooked networks of fibers that run from the higher brain centers downward to make connection with the familiar message-carrying nerve trunks in the spinal cord. These down-going systems are not the usual efferent axons carrying muscle commands. They might be regarded as special emissaries sent out for purpose of mediation. If electrical activity is induced in the higher brain areas, the emissary group of nerves may suppress or modify the incoming message. It may never get beyond

---

chest at the level of the lowest rib, is singularly insensitive. It is also loose enough to be pinched up roughly without causing pain. Here insertions of needles and all the other armament of the fakir can be made without noteworthy distress.

the lower levels of the central nervous system or it may be changed into an entirely different message as it reaches the sultans of the brain. The emissaries reflect the mood of the sultans. The sultans may be with their harems and cannot be disturbed. They may decide that this message is not one of body damage but one promising food. It is true that the precise origins and terminations of these emissary fibers have not been established. Yet, if we are to preserve the notion of physical strands of communication rather than resort to some sort of mystical extrasensory perception in the body itself, we must assume a physiological model that accords with the unquestioned fact that psychological events play an essential role in fixing the quality and intensity of pain and of other perceptual experience.

Let us follow what happens when we burn a finger. Heat energy is converted into a code of electrical nerve impulses in the skin receptors (although it was formerly popular to identify one of the unspecialized nerve endings as specific pain receptors, it is now thought that the receptor mechanisms for pain are more complicated). It is generally conceded that receptors that respond to "damage" or "noxious stimulation" are widely branching, bushy networks of fibers that penetrate the layers of skin in such a way that their receptive fields widely overlap with one another. Thus damage at any point on the skin will trigger at least two or more of these networks and start the transmission of nerve impulses along bundles of sensory nerve fibers that run from the finger to the spinal cord. Before the impulse pattern can begin its climb to the brain, part of it at least must check in with crowded offices and assembly yards of short, densely packed nerve fibers that are all interconnected in one way or another. To the impulse pattern this may be like getting through a Russian customs nexus. Auxiliary fibers of these nexuses are found throughout the length of the spinal cord and are called "internuncial neurons." Here is where the pattern may find itself modified or its passport taken away. Patrick Wall found that in humans normally painful electric shocks and pinpricks are not perceived as painful when the surrounding skin is stimulated with a rapidly vibrating device. Athough it has classically been assumed that pain impulses have absolute priority, here is a case where they get lost in the shuffling of nervous red tape.

With W. K. Livingston, Melzack found that electrical impulses that do get through the minor bureaucracy to the spinal cord are transmitted through the lower parts of the brain along at least five different and mostly alternative routes. Three of them (the spinothalamic tract, the central tegmental and the central gray pathway) are obviously major conduction systems for sensory pain patterns, since their electrical activity is completely wiped out by analgesic agents such as nitrous oxide, which are able to erase the awareness of pain without affecting such senses as vision and hearing. Analgesics are also able to calm greatly the electrical furor in the fourth route—the central core of the reticular formation, which has the role of arousing the whole upper brain. The fifth pathway—the lemniscal tract—plays an ambiguous but viable role in the total process of pain and is notable for the fact that it cannot be blocked out by the usual anesthetic or analgesic drugs. A good deal of work has been done with cats, who are at least as complicated as monkeys or men with respect to pain. Cats with lesions that make the spinothalamic or the central gray pathways inoperative fail to react to normal pain stimulation. On the other hand, cats with the lemniscal tract inactive still respond immediately. Lesions of the central tegmental tract had the unexpected effect of making cats oversensitive to some kinds of painful stimulus. In fact, many of these cats showed "spontaneous pain" in the absence of any external stimulation at all.

The awful pains of certain kinds of terminal cancers have, of course, continuously been under study, since quite frequently they are not relieved even by the most powerful drugs. Frank Ervin and Vernon Marl of the Massachusetts General Hospital found that patients with unbearable cancer pain can get relief by means of a small surgical lesion in that part of the thalamus that receives fibers from the spinothalamic tract as well as from pathways that start elaborating in the reticular formation. If the lesion by mistake is made just a few millimeters in front of this area, destroying the thalamic fibers of the lemniscal pathway, the pain remains unabated.

Much clarification as well as some additional mystification has come out of studies of that weird and terrible thing known as "phantom-limb" pain—pain from a leg or arm that is no longer there. About 30 per cent of amputees develop pain in phantom limbs and in about 5 per cent the pain is excruciating. The agonizing sensations seem to come from particular places in the part that has been cut off. One young woman described her phantom hand as being clenched, the fingers bent over the thumb and digging fiercely into the palm of her hand. She moaned that all she wanted was to be able to unclench her imaginary fist. When, as the result of specialized drug treatment of the stump, she was convinced that she could do this, the pain disappeared.

Symptoms such as these are not explained by any of the classical theories of pain, especially since the realization of the presence of the haunting leg, arm or hand and its hurtfulness may be brought about suddenly by emotional aspects, such as seeing a television show or a movie in which there are violence and sharp or brutal conflict. The usual emergency procedures, such as severing the spinothalamic tract, fail to bring relief. Since quite obviously the central nervous system is involved in these seizures, one would think that hypnosis might be effective, but it is seldom realized that only a very small percentage of people in the world are susceptible to hypnosis. Livingston suggests that during the amputation and the trauma associated with it, the usual patterns of the internuncial offices and assembling junctions in the spinal cord have been thrown into unnatural reverberation. Thenceforth impulse patterns that would normally be interpreted merely as touch may now trigger these neuron collections into greater activity, causing them to shoot volleys of abnormal patterns to the upper nervous system and bringing about a sense of pain.

The presence of the two dimensions of pain, the purely sensory and the emotional, is shown by the results of prefrontal lobotomy, in which all connection between the prefrontal lobes of the cortex and the rest of the brain are severed. The typical patient, after this operation, will cheerfully report that he still has pain but it doesn't bother him. Yet, like the wounded soldiers at Anzio, these people are still quick to complain about a clumsy hypodermic jab, a pinprick or a mild burn. It is simply that the larger anxieties, including the fear of death, have left them and whatever painful disease they have they accept with pride of ownership rather than with morbid pre-occupation.

Thus pain more than ever now appears to be a complex nervous act or performance of the whole organism and can no longer be regarded as simply a specific sensory impulse to which an animal appropriately reacts. It is the reaction or the behavior of the nerves, rather than the stimulus, that we feel as pain. Although normally the reaction (and thus the pain) will increase in proportion to damage to the body, this does not have to be the case, as we have seen above. From consideration of pain in this light, we should not conclude that pain is not an essential evil—perhaps the primary evil in the world. Its complexity does not mitigate the suffering, and perhaps in many cases makes it more hopeless. In her essay "On Being Ill," Virginia Woolf said, "English, which can express the thoughts of Hamlet and the tragedy of Lear, has no words for the shiver and the headache . . . The merest schoolgirl, when she falls in love, has Shakespeare and Keats to speak for her but let a sufferer try to describe a pain in his head to a doctor and language at once runs dry."

At the same time I believe we should not assume because pain is a complex nervous phenomenon that it is the privilege only of highly developed animals such as man or other mammals. The neurologists who specialize in the study of the invertebrates are very cautious about this matter. Since a lobster or an octopus cannot tell you when you are hurting him and cannot scream in agony like a human being burning at the stake for some idiotic religious reason, most people therefore blandly assume that a lobster or an octopus suffers from neither religion or physical pain. The invertebrate neurologists infer that something equivalent to pain is present if an animal shows "behavioral reactions resembling those of a man under pain." What does a live crab or lobster do when he is being scalded to death? He goes through hideous convulsions of movements exactly like a man being scalded. He doesn't scream because he doesn't have screaming equipment. Yet people who ought to have more sense and sensibility, such as the unflappable Julia Child, maintain that a large crustacean is put to a painless death by scalding. Heaven knows what excruciating torments of how many lobsters and crabs she now has on her conscience! This sin of torture is all the more inexcusable, since it can be avoided by another means of killing the crustacean that gives no visible sign of causing any pain at all. Nearly all marine animals are living in water in the summertime which is very close in temperature to their lethal upper limit. Just as certain antarctic fishes cannot even survive in what we would regard as cool water, the crabs and lobsters that we eat cannot survive water at 96° Fahrenheit. Thus if you put the crustacean in the pot with a low burner under it and heat slowly, the animal will die a painless death (rather similar, apparently, to death by freezing in warm-blooded animals) before the water has scarcely become more than lukewarm. The dead crabs and lobsters are perfectly limp, because death from the heat has occurred before coagulation of the proteins that takes place at a much higher temperature. The contention that crabs are not good unless they have been scalded to death is ignorant superstition and, in fact, the situation may be the precise opposite. Agony in any creature with nerves and glands may suffuse the flesh with the poisons that the extreme emergency of dying a horrible death calls forth. It would be deserved retribution for the lobster or crab, having been mercilessly tortured to death, if he could give you at least indigestion in return for your senseless cruelty.

CHAPTER 5

How to Get Around

Traveling Light

BECAUSE modern man is a sensory creature, he is prejudiced in favor of the primacy of seeing, hearing, smelling, tasting and feeling the world, rather than in simply moving around in it. Yet, as an exercise in practical epistemology, the question is still open as to whether these explicit channels to the outside universe are more than conveniences or luxuries, telling us no further truths about existence than does the squirming of a senseless creature who knows the world only as a place to crawl in and who translates his squirmings as information by reason of the proprioceptive nerves that tell him not only how far he has gone and in what direction, but also if he has come up against the barrier of a rock or a phagocyte in a man's blood. It was presumptuous of John Locke to assume that consciousness is simply a memory of past, explicit, sensory experiences, since the proprioceptive world may in the end turn out to be not only the most basic but the most subtle world. Certainly it is a phase of being that has been least exploited scientifically and in consequence offers the most cheerful solutions of problems that beset us the more pressingly because we are not even aware of them.

If this sounds like obscurantism, let me specify by a single example. Certain ants can be taught to follow an invariable and odorless path away from home and back to home, because they have an unerring capacity to store up in neuromuscular memory the various zigs, zags and serpentine routes on which their legs have carried them. This we accept as an antlike talent, somewhat akin to the dead reckoning of a mariner or to the inertial guidance systems of missiles. But go one step further. Suppose in this ant path there is a large rock that the ant walks around, much as we would walk around a mountain rather than ascending and descending it. Now remove the rock. Is the ant now confused or does he continue in his stubbornness to make the circuit to avoid a mountain that is no longer there? The ant patters unhesitatingly across the site of the rock, making a perfect geometrical short cut to intersect the familiar path beyond, saving a few seconds thereby in his total journey. Although one might say, "The ant saw that the rock was gone and simply did what comes naturally," all the evidence points to the fact that the ant did *not* see the rock or notice its absence visually, since ants do not operate in such a clumsy fashion. The decision to cut right across the site of a former barrier to save time was a proprioceptive decision of a most mystifying subtlety. As a topographer the ant is a master, because *getting around* from here to there on the complicated surface world has been his problem—his "thing"—for millions of years. It may be that in our own expanded universe there are many rocks and mountains that actually are only imaginary barriers and which we could cut elegantly across if we had the proprioceptive insights of the ant. One of them may be our supposed limitation to a universe of three dimensions. If we are going to get out of this present artificial box, perhaps what we need is not so much a more elaborate topology (the mathematics of geometrical transformations) as a more canny exploitation of our own proprioceptions. Let us, in the meantime, review not only proprioception but also locomotion throughout a representative cross section of the animal world.

The embarrassing truth of the matter is that when we observe simple one-celled animals getting around in their world, we are helpless in trying to explain clearly how they do it. The simplest of ambulating creatures is one that is not even provided with oars or whips, but moves by the method known as "amoeboid." At one time it was thought that an amoeba moves in a manner that can be simulated by a drop of oil or of mercury. It is possible to make an oil or mercury droplet move in a singularly animalistic fashion by touching with a slender probe one spot on the surface, which lowers the surface tension so that this inorganic blob of matter extends a tiny finger, much as the amoeba projects its "pseudopod." It was quickly realized, however, that a profound and practical difference exists between the two locomotive phenomena—between the dead and the living. With drops of oil or mercury, a particle of dirt that happened to be stuck to the drop's surface would be pulled away by the contraction from the advancing edge of the artificial pseudopod. But this is not true of the living animal, who likes the dirt. Either the dirt moves with him or, if some other surface has more dirt appeal, the amoeba loses a brief tug of war. Under the microscope the difference in behavior is unmistakable.

One classical theory is now based on the intrinsic contractility of protoplasm and is not so much a theory as an educated observation. It states simply that an amoeba is like a piece of muscle, but what is a piece of muscle? When the animalcule *Arcella*, which lives in a little shell, moves, its rodlike pseudopod contracts and pulls the body of the amoeba and its shell toward the point of attachment. There are heliozoans and foraminiferans which send out many thin threads of cytoplasm like the rays of a little symbolic sun. If the long end of an amoeba's pseudopod is cut off, the cut surface will heal together by means of a microscopic glass thread, leaving the severed end as a miniature amoeba composed of merely the cytoplasmic membrane. It includes no nucleus, no granules. Yet this orphaned fragment will itself crawl around by amoeboid movement for many hours. Contractile proteins like those found in the muscle of larger, multicellular animals have been extracted from some of the giant amoeboid organisms known as *Mycetozoa*, which have thousands of nuclei and spread themselves out over rotten wood as a thin plasmodium sometimes the size of a half dollar.

More explicit is the reversible "sol-gel" theory which views amoeboid motion as the result of alterations between the condition of being a jelly (gel) and being a soup (sol). If the advancing pseudopod of an amoeba like *Amoeba proteus* is watched under high magnification, one sees in the center of the pseudopod a stream of flowing, granular protoplasm. Tiny crystals, mitochondria, food vacuoles and nucleus are carried forward in this stream like junk in a sewer conduit. Around the edges of this flow and completely enveloping it as a tube or sleeve is a continuous layer of protoplasm in gel form, in which the granules remain stationary. At the advancing edge of the pseudopod, the central core of flowing protoplasm spreads out sideways and solidifies, thus elongating the sleeve of gel. German biologists have likened this process to a magic fountain in which the water freezes as it falls and so instead of splashing builds up a collar of ice. At the hind end of the amoeba the inner surface of the gel can be seen becoming fluid and adding itself to the liquid stream, thus making the process of locomotion a continuous alternation of sol and gel states. But what starts the flow? What stops it in an instant of meaningful coagulation? What co-ordinates the process so that the organism is rhythmically liquefying and solidifying? Here we stare at a miracle of life, as strange and mechanically inexplicable in its tiny way as the building of a spider web or the birth of an idea. One can only say that this supple cycling of colloids, in which the net result is progression of the amoeba from one place to another, is an act of fundamental behavior—recalled in transcendental memory—and that the communication system that binds the acts together is proprioception at its most basic level. Of course we can further theorize about the mechanism. The contraction of plasma membranes obviously plays the part of muscular contraction in higher animals. The pseudopod may adhere to some object, say, a leaf or a glass slide. A wave of

constriction (obviously a proprioceptive act) then passes backward, squeezing the cell's contents forward. Possibly in an
intact amoeba the gel contracts as well as the membrane. We
know that calcium is essential to the process—a fact easily
shown in marine amoebas by placing them in sea water from
which calcium has been removed, whereby they are rendered
immobile; it is noteworthy that calcium is also essential for
muscular contractions in multicellular animals. (One notes also
the loose similarity of the whole process to the gelation of
adductor muscle tissues in bivalves, which makes their closure
so fierce and final, when attacked.) When the contraction wave
ends at the "tail" of the amoeba, it often leaves a little irregular
mass of cytoplasm called a "uroid." It is important to animals
that have white blood cells or leucocytes, as does man, that
these constituents of the blood are little individual animals
and move on their duties as a wild amoeba moves, and they
also form uroids. From time to time the uroid is completely
pinched off (possibly as an act of excretion) and a new one
begins to form.

When we step slightly upward in evolutionary sophistication,
we arrive at protozoans, such as the flagellates who have little
whips to lash themselves around their universe. There is fundamentally no good distinction between a flagellum and a cilium,
except that the former is usually scarcer and longer. Most
flagellates have two whips, one that extends forward as the
animal moves ahead and one that trails, beating, behind, although
some species have only one flagellum and others a great number.
These things seem to grow out from a basal granule in the
cytoplasm, indicating again that single-celled creatures are far
from being simple blobs. In structure the whips are microscopically complicated. Under the tremendous magnifications of the
electron microscope, all flagella appear virtually identical and
the distinction between flagellum and cilium has vanished. There
is a central core of two strands surrounded by a tube sheath.
Outside this there is a circle of nine strands in turn enclosed
in another sheath. Somewhere, probably in the sheath, an intrinsically spiral structure persists, like a Pythagorean ghost.

The action of the flagella is complicated and hard to follow. In *Puranema* the simple flagellum is poked forward as a stiff rod, but the tip dances like a snake's tongue as the animal makes its way. In *Euglena* the whip is extended backward at an angle of 45 degrees to the long axis of the body. The threshing of the flagellum pushes *Euglena* forward and sideways and causes it to rotate on the long axis. The result is that the animal gyrates forward as though following the path of a corkscrew.

In still more sophisticated protozoa, such as the ciliates, the animal is propelled by the beating of thousands of little oars (cilia), but the beat is far from random, being as orderly as the military leg drills of a centipede. Successive "metachronal" waves of action sweep smoothly along each row of cilia. The co-ordination is assured by a fibrillar system called the "neuromotor apparatus." The central structure from which the fibrillar strands radiate is the "motorium." Thus an animal consisting technically of only one cell may nevertheless be literally as nervous as a witch. The fibers may be too small to be called neurons by the neurological Puritans, but they result in nervous activity and are co-ordinated by what in multicelled animals would be called a "ganglion," or nerve center. (However, pieces of an advanced ciliate, such as *Paramecium*, without nucleus or endoplasm, will still show metachronal, or rhythmic, waves of beating.) Such animals, with the controlled timing of their thousands of little oars, have quite a repertoire of motion. In creeping they can go straight ahead, can suddenly back away and can turn to the right (but not to the left). In swimming they can advance slowly, go forward in fast spiral revolutions, make either a sharp turn to the right, make a circus turn to the left (but not a sharp one) and withdraw rapidly backward.[1]

---

[1] The lack of parity between left and right is curious, but should not be compared with dexterity in man. It is true, however, that many higher insects (such as ants) and crustaceans (such as sow bugs) have preferences as to which way to turn, probably induced by the position of the sun or the rotation of the earth. As far as I know, nobody has investigated the influence of latitude on such preferences.

As the Worm Turns

ONE WOULD think that worms would move like snakes, but of course they do not possess serpentine subtlety. Flatworms and most earthworms move mainly by a kind of peristaltic action, much like a little piece of intestine. The back part is squeezed together while the front is poked out, sometimes lifted, in blind groping for a new purchase. When the purchase is decided upon, the rest of the body is hauled up an inch or so. If we analyze this peristaltic contortion a little more closely we observe that from a resting condition (when the worm is digesting or thinking about his problems) the peristalsis always begins as a wave of thinning (circular muscle contraction) at the front end and proceeds to the tail, the worm's progress going in the opposite direction to that of the peristaltic wave. Polychaetes, or bristle worms, who can boast of several points of social and structural superiority to their relatives the earthworms, have learned two kinds of locomotion: creeping on a solid surface, using the parapodia (or "side arms") alone, and more rapid ambulation grading into swimming, with the lengthwise muscles acting in co-ordination with the parapodia. Unlike the earthworms, the polychaetes' alternating muscles are left and right and the wave moves forward in the same direction as the locomotion. (If one ignores the wavelike motion, this means of getting around is not unlike a man whose hands and feet are bound hitching himself along the ground by alternate movements of the right and left sides of his body.) From a motionless state, movement begins with contraction of the forward segments (parapodia alone or with lengthwise muscles, the two sides of a segment always in opposite phase). Then occurs a very rapid spread toward the tail, activating every fourth to eighth segment, establishing the number of waves—typically many instead of one as in earthworms. Finally begins the slow, effective wave, successively activating more forward segments one by one. There is greater reliance upon central nerve centers and independence of re-flexes than in earthworms. If you cut the nerve cord, you destroy all co-ordination between regions of the worm, but even short pieces can show all the phases of normal locomotion and loss of several adjacent parapodia does not interfere with pro-gression of the wave.

In the well-studied bristle worm *Nereis* swimming is similar to the rapid, undulatory creeping described above but highly speeded up. Actual propulsion through the water is due to the parapodium acting as a paddle. If *Nereis* had no parapodia, it would swim actually in the other direction, that is, opposite to the direction of the waves over the body. This is an em-barrassing thing to a worm and it illustrates the difference between making one's way around in a liquid and on a solid surface surrounded by a compressible fluid like air. The leech *Hirudo* swims in a different manner. The lengthwise muscles contract symmetrically, but alternately on the belly and back sides, so that a wave passes backward, opposite to the direction of locomotion. Pieces of the leech's body can also swim. After cutting the nerve coil, one half of the leech may swim while the other half walks, or both halves may swim independently, making over-all very little useful progress. The leech responds proprioceptively, since it knows when it is swimming in viscous mud rather than in clear water.

In all crawling worms, removal of the brain brings about one peculiar deficiency. With a brain, a worm, sensing no surface blow on its front segments, stops crawling immediately and wonders what topographic catastrophe has occurred. Without a brain, the worm continues crawling and falls off the table. One can say in this case that the brain's chief function is to inhibit against rash adventures.

In conformance with their insistently busybody, ubiquitous and pushy mode of life, the nematodes as free-living species have many tricks of getting around. Since they are not seg-mented but are rich in lengthwise muscles and nerves, some can swim like a snake, by undulation. Some glide with the aid of purchase of a surface, like an ice skater. Some crawl by alternate lengthening and shortening, with sinuous curving during the abbreviation cycle. Some crawl with the body straight, gripping the surface seemingly by sheer force of will power. Some walk on stiff bristles like caterpillars, with peristaltic waves progressing forward. Some loop like a leech or an inchworm, using adhesive bristles. Some very small species simply advance by a fierce sort of end-to-end thrashing. All of this gigantic phylum of fearsome little creatures seem to arrive where they want to go.

Tiptoeing Through the Waters

THERE are many beautiful show-piece animals that evolution has kept in a room for the retarded, who practice the same way of life that they did in pre-Cambrian times and, if they are promised no glory in the future, they have on the other hand an almost limitless and languid past to swim around in. The ctenophores (pronounced with a silent "c") are such a phylum. Their lovely, lazy method of propulsion is to wave their combs through the water, a kind of extrapolation of the metachronal waves of the ciliated protozoa, and in fact as a locomotive animal in many respects they resemble a ciliate blown up in size by a very large factor. The sea cucumber, almost as ancient an animal, moves by extending little tube feet, attaching the terminal suckers and dragging itself along. It can climb up the glass side of an aquarium. The crinoids, or sea lilies, which look like the small animated trees that Walt Disney used to draw, are in actuality quite complicated animals, when it comes to locomotion. When swimming they alternate their ten leaflike arms, so that five are beating downward while the other five are floating up. An isolated ray of two arms behaves as a functional swimming unit, the stimulation of one arm evoking a contrary movement in the functional twin. When not swimming, they go forward typically in two ways. In one pattern a single arm leads, another trails, and the others act as oars. In a daintier pattern, which might be called "running," the central disk or head is held high between two flexed arms and the crinoid moves on tiptoe on the other arms in ballerina fashion. In starfish, as in the sea cucumber (also an echinoderm), tube feet extend by hydraulic pressure, attach themselves by suckers and then move forward by muscle contraction. Hundreds of these organs have to be co-ordinated— a tough job—and occasionally a tube foot will cling too long and be left behind. The starfish can travel in any direction and no arm or ray assumes the leadership more often than the others. Necessarily there is co-ordination and at one time or another one arm may happen to be the one to move first, triggering a concerted action of the rest. Changes in direction of pointing or stepping tend to occur spontaneously either in a clockwise or counterclockwise direction. Light falling on one arm may induce it to lead, while too strong a mechanical stimulation, such as in electric shock, will throw this arm into a trailing position. When the direction of pointing is being changed from one arm to another, all stepping ceases. When the new direction is "agreed upon," stepping resumes at a brisk pace, slowing down for the next change in direction. It appears that each foot of a starfish is nervously equipped for independent action. Neurologists have been unable to figure out, however, how this capacity for independent assertion is keyed into the organism as a whole. This mystery of co-ordination extends to the action of righting or getting oneself right side up. It is a true locomotive piece of behavior, since one arm (perhaps the first to think of it?) starts the turning maneuver. But to achieve righting, the other, temporarily subordinate, arms must detach their feet from the surface and must stay inert until the active arm has pushed hard enough. If all arms independently pushed and wriggled, there would be no resultant torque and the starfish would remain helpless on its back. How this co-ordination is achieved is neurologically also a mystery.

Although we seldom think of mollusks as a notably locomotive phylum, the fact is that within this vast animal grouping are some of the masters of underwater propulsion. The scaphopods (which include bivalves) have only one foot, but it is a powerful one (scaphopod means "boat-footed"). The broad sole of the foot in abalones, limpets and chitons enables them to secure a firm hold on a surface and to move about by alternate suction and contraction. The motion that most scaphopods are chiefly interested in, however, is burrowing. As Professor E. R. Trueman of the University of Hull, England, has shown, a burrowing clam is a rather ingenious hydraulic machine. It had long been known that the water contained in the bivalve's mantle cavity is used as the fluid in a hydraulic system that enables contractions of the shell-moving muscles to extend the siphon or to retract the siphon and to open the valves. Burrowing movements of the foot represent the action of the foot muscles together with a sudden inflow of blood. When the valves (shell parts) are closed, high pressure occurs in both the blood and the mantle cavity and this is the hydraulic pressure used in burrowing. By using electronic recording, Trueman showed that all bivalves that live in sand or mud go through the same sequence of digging movements. The foot is extended, the siphon is closed, the valves are closed, the foot swells and its muscles contract, causing the shell to move into the sand, and a period of relaxation takes place with the valves open, as the animal prepares for another digging cycle. The foot may probe on its own, without hydraulic control, in an effort to find out if the hole is a good one. When the shell closes the hydrostatic pressure is increased not only in the foot but also through the whole body enclosed within the shell. Occasionally water is ejected from the mantle cavity to liquefy the sand (especially if the bivalve is digging at low tide), allowing a faster burrowing job.

One of the more mobile of the shelled mollusks is the scallop in which various species have the ability to control their swimming by clapping their valves together and by directing water streams past the margins of the mantle.

Students of comparative locomotion have been greatly impressed with the diversity in locomotion of the gastropods (snails or slugs) which never impresses the average man, since he thinks of a gastropod only as a garden snail who leaves a slimy trail in his laborious crawling. Yet the gastropod class includes animals who move with undulatory peristaltic movements, who swim with the symmetrical flapping of winglike appendages to their foot, who proceed by side-to-side bending, alternate stepping, "loping," and even "galloping." In some gastropods the foot is entirely a swimming organ. In the subclass *Pteropoda* ("wing-footed") the foot has expanded its forward lobes into two broad winglike organs. In the Heteropoda the entire foot has changed into a fin and the animal swims backward by flapping it, as in sculling a boat.

It is among the cephalopods that we get into modern technology. The chief organ of locomotion of all cephalopods (including nautiloids as well as octopuses and squids) is the "funnel," which is a modified part of the less advanced mollusk foot. Behind the funnel is the mantle cavity into which the funnel opens. The cephalopod takes water into this cavity, after which he closes the entry by a special valvelike contrivance. Then, by powerful contraction of the mantle muscles, he forces water out through the funnel in a propulsive jet. This results in a jet-powered submarine which advances in jerks backward. Thus in swimming the cephalopod assumes a position in which the apex of the trunk is ahead of the rest of the body, while the arms trail out behind. Squids, unlike the more sedentary octopuses, roam the seas freely and have a more specialized, streamlined funnel. Aside from certain aquatic insects, this highly sophisticated mode of locomotion is peculiar to cephalopods, but one must note that it has certain deficiencies. Even the squid has not found a way to make the jet operate continuously, so that its jerkiness is intrinsic, and man has actually done better with the modern jet engine, both under water and in the air. The cuttlefish has a more sophisticated means, however, than a man-made submarine for controlling its buoyancy. Instead of a compressed-air pump (to ballast with sea water), it sets up an osmotic force arising from this difference in salt concentration between the cuttlebone fluid and its blood. With any change of sea pressure, the osmotic pressure changes in order to balance the sea pressure. In some squids the coelomic fluid accounts for two thirds of the animal's weight and has a density appreciably less than that of sea water. The cuttlebone is both a skeletal support and a flotation device. As the animal grows, successive independent hollow chambers in it are filled with gas and liquid. Like a submarine, the cuttlefish ascends with secretion of gas and sinks when flooded. The gas is formed at night when the animals hunt. If they are kept in a darkened tank for two days they become so buoyant they cannot stay on the bottom.

To Swim Like a Fish

ONE CAN truly say that the greatest invention in marine locomotion was made by a creature so primitive that it had neither skull, brain, heart, jaws nor true fins. This was the lancelet (amphioxus), who discovered how to get around by side-to-side undulation, which remained through evolution's experiments the most efficient means of aquatic propulsion until the screw propeller. Even advanced mammals, like whales or dolphins, use this method. There is a good reason why the lancelet was able to learn to undulate. For this to be an effective maneuver, there must be some degree of both stiffness and of flexibility, and the lancelet was the first animal to develop a gristly interior rod—the notochord—which gave the paired antagonistic swimming muscles something to pull themselves against so they did not cancel out each other's action. (Two muscles without an unyielding central attachment cannot undulate any more than can a piece of muscularized gelatin.) The lancelet was thus not only the first undulatory swimmer but the ancestor of all of us vertebrates, from the bony fish onward.

Fishes with true bone instead of gristle in the central chord increased the strength of the wriggle in the fresh, streaming water of rivers. In the course of hundreds of millions of years various fishes for various reasons substituted other actions for the immemorial wriggle. *Propulsive* swimming, in which the pectoral fins are used much as crude propellers, became popular. Some fishes learned to walk and some even to glide in the air. From an evolutionary standpoint, the sea horse and pipefish are probably the most sophisticated, but in gaining this sophistication they have given up all claim to streamlining and to speed. They use their paired median fins as one sculls a boat. The dorsal fins vibrate ten times a second. Yet it takes one of these tiny creatures five minutes to cross a bathtub.

Flying fishes (*Cypselurus*) do not flap their wings in the air —they glide like flying squirrels. When ready to emerge from the sea for a flight, they swim at highest speed, preparing to taxi. As they reach the surface they spread their paired fins, membranes taut between the fin rays. The tail is enlarged to give the boost necessary to get up to taxiing speed. They rarely take off with the wind but prefer to head into it at an angle. The glide in the air rarely lasts over twenty seconds. Presumably it was developed by evolution as an emergency tactic to get away from insistent predators.

The ray has developed a propulsive method that can only be described as flying under water. This fish has no dorsal or anal or caudal fins at all, or only in atrophied form. The pectoral fins have grown into wings. Although one has an instinctive dislike of rays because of the concealed dagger that many of them carry, it is impossible not to be dazzled by the sheer loveliness of their undulations. When the ray moves, the fleshy wings themselves undulate. A sinuous movement takes place from back to front, with most grace at the edges, creating a movement like the waving of a silk handkerchief.

Among the great fishes who have amazed men by the speed and strength of their majestic wriggles are the swordfish and its closest relative, the sailfish. The swordfish's top speed is estimated at fifty knots, based on calculations of the minimum velocity required to penetrate, with both beaks, an oak ship's hull one foot thick and sheathed with copper. (The Kensington Museum in London has this exhibit.) Swordfishes lose their tempers easily, especially when annoyed by the nautical devices of man, and in 1967 one attacked the small experimental,

three-man submarine *Alvin,* wedging its beak between upper
and lower sections of the Fiberglas external hull. The sailfish
is estimated to have a top speed of seventy knots, although
this is not confirmed by any very scientific methodology. Since
man has not been able to make a torpedo that will go over
thirty knots, the U. S. Navy has been interested in finding out
how these great fishes do it. Investigators of the Naval Ordnance
Test Station have reviewed the stages of a fast fish's swimming
process. They find that when the fish is stationary in the water
he still moves his fins. He compensates for gill propulsion
(the jet effect of water being ejected through the gills at
higher speed than it is swallowed) and for the tendency to
overturn by gently waving the pectoral and side fins. Quick
darts or acceleration to cruising speed are achieved by violent
body undulation (large amplitude) with the head moving from
side to side. Moderate cruising speeds are maintained with most
of the fins folded close to the body and the body undulating
like a traveling sine wave.[2] At maximum speed (as when the
animal intends to spear a submarine), rapid ripples pass aft
along the body, with the motion approaching a *multiple* traveling sine wave. The amplitude and wave length are decreased
but the frequency is greatly stepped up. Most fins are completely folded. Naval Ordnance now believes that the secret
of the fast, quiet locomotion of such fishes is "body participation." Only a living animal can do this. The fish body
creates what is known in hydrodynamics as a "propeller race"
in the same location as the "hull wake," thus wiping the wake
away and eliminating the main cause of turbulent drag. Some
approaches to the body-participation technique have been made
by engineering design, which we shall discuss when we come
to look at the dolphin's swimming skills. Heinrich Hertel, the
German engineer, has pointed out that, using the body shape
of a tuna as a model, the air resistance of airplane fuselages
could be vastly reduced. According to him, the trend of design

[2] A sine wave is the simplest symmetrical periodic movement of undulation. The pressure wave made in the air or water by a pure sound tone is
described by the same equation.

has been grossly contrary to nature in such unsatisfactory embodiments as the teardrop shape or the circular cylinder with bow and stern caps. If the tuna shape were used, for example, in the Boeing 747, the fuselage could accommodate three times as many passengers and fly faster. Hertel is recommending the tuna-type laminar fuselage for the new generation of vertical take-off airplanes.

The Pacific salmon is not a speed specialist but it deserves awards for the incredible endurance feats that both sexes perform in swimming up fierce, sometimes torrential, rivers in order to assure that their young will have a chance to be born in relative serenity to enjoy the quiet of the ancestral pools before they venture downstream and take their now dead parents' place in the never-ending cycle between fresh and salt water. In going home from the sea to the pool in which they were born, the Pacific salmon swim steadily day and night without rest and without food. The effort required for swimming at top speed in the warmer waters of the rivers is much higher than it is in the cold sea, hence the ascent of the Fraser River in Canada, for example, is a costly business. The studies of J. R. Brett have shown that salmon have the unexpected ability of increasing their energy output by a factor of more than twenty in attaining top sustained speed at the now unfavorable temperature. This puts the salmon actually in the class with a race horse. Study of salmon confirms the obvious fact that a large fish can swim faster than a small one, but the performance does not increase in direct proportion to increase in size. If we describe the speed in terms of *fish lengths per second*, the smaller fish does better. When a salmon breasts the three-mile-per-hour Fraser River, he or she covers 640 miles in twenty days. Since this indicated sustained speed is physically impossible, it must be deduced that the salmon have some hydro-dynamic short cuts, choosing water paths where the downstream flow offers less resistance. By the end of the journey, after laying her eggs, the female sockeye salmon has consumed 96 per cent of her body fat and 53 per cent of her protein reserves. She is hardly more than an ovary supported by skinny tissue. In fact a considerable part of her energy has been spent in the development of this large ovary, and a parallel situation exists in the emaciated male. Their daily output of energy in swimming up the Fraser has been 80 per cent of the maximum steady rate they could possibly maintain for any length of time, leaving little margin for emergency demands, such as a leaping up the spillovers from a dam. Brett also finds that the salmon's hydrodynamic efficiency depends on body participation. The drag on a live salmon is much less than that on a dead model, except at very low speed. The difference increases up to the maximum sustained speed, at which the power required for the live fish to overcome drag is less than one half that required for a dead model. It is obvious that, in order for the Pacific salmon to perform its suicidal procreative mission, evolution has endowed this animal with magnificent muscles as well as steely purpose.

Some fishes decided to learn to walk. For people who were not aware of walking fishes, the sight (in Florida, for example) of certain catfish jumping out of the aquarium and appearing in the living room, like little men walking on their elbows, has been demoralizing. (The Florida scare was apparently caused by the escape from import packages of members of the Claridae family, originally African or Asian. With dual breathing equipment, they move around if left alone, eating snails, frogs and the like, and some of them have been reported by excited Floridians as capable of leaping as high as four feet in the air.) The red gurnet, which belongs to the same family—Triglidae— as the "true" (Mediterranean) flying fish, has armor-plated cheeks. It is a gullet-breather. The gullet and floor of the mouth dilate instead of the gills. A striking elaboration of the pectoral fins, which have three separately moving extensions like fingers, allows them to walk along the bottom of the sea bed as spiders walk. The champion walker is the so-called "climbing perch" of Southeast Asia and the Philippines. The body lies within a thick coat covered with rugged scales, overlapping like roof shingles. Each gill cover has a spine projecting backward. This fish is so versatile that it has *aerial* vision (unlike normal fish it can see acutely when out of the water). A special lunglike apparatus in the cavity above the gills enables it to breathe air. Its ordinary gills are not adequate for a total aquatic life and it has to rise to the surface now and then. When the walking perch leaves the water for a visit on land, it steps along on its pectoral fins, waving its tail to get added motive power. Its thick skin retards the loss of moisture and is thus as important to this animal as its skin is to a frog. Of all such fishes, the mudskipper (*Periophthalmus*) is perhaps the weirdest. He climbs trees with his fins and pursues insects. He is as agile on the tide flats in snapping worms as a robin on the front lawn. He too has aerial vision and his behavior is somehow foreign to that of a creature of the sea as he dodges and evades with a certain bug-eyed insolence, suggestive of some land animal, perhaps a mongoose.

First Flight on Earth

IT IS a shameful admission, but neither aerodynamicists nor entomologists have decided how it is possible for many insects to fly. By the technology of slow cinematography we can describe in great detail the motions but we cannot understand clearly why the motions result in sustained flight. In the case of insects with very frail bodies, who weigh very little, the wing-loading is so small that the so-called "lift coefficient" need not be very great. But in beetlelike insects, such as the June bug (*Melolontha vulgaris*) of the British Isles, which weighs almost a gram, the mathematics of standard aerodynamics would predict the necessity of a lift coefficient of from at least two to four to get off the ground. However, Leon Bennett of New York University, who has built a mechanical replica of the June bug's wings, estimates a lift coefficient of less than one, whereas the most effective man-made, unflapped, low-camber airfoils produce a maximum of one and a half. Obviously there is something about the June bug's wings or a subtle unnoticed trick about their use that has eluded the most expert scrutiny. The dilemma is not unlike the question of how, by body participation, the live sailfish can go faster than a rhythmically wriggling dummy, and the answer may be of the same character: The live insect's body has less drag or more lift than any mechanical model. Obviously the discovery of the nature of this mystical ability of living things to exceed the set boundaries of aerodynamic law would be of incalculable practical and theoretical value to man as an aeronaut. If we yearn to be angels, we must learn to fly like beetles. Let us consider some of the things that are known.

The first insects on earth undoubtedly crawled. It was only when terrestrial vegetation, the insect's first sole source of food, took to growing out of reach, that the insects had to learn to fly, which they did in a most revolutionary act of evolution, not by modifying limbs or hands (as birds and bats later learned to do) but by a quantum jump in anatomy—by growing wings out of their breathing organs—more specifically, from the thoracic vanes or, one might say "louvers" of the tracheal system. This is nearly as imaginative a way to grow wings as from the upper back, as angels are said to do, although, as we shall see later, the seraphim and even the cupids portrayed by Renaissance artists are (as Leonardo realized) veritable aerodynamic monstrosities, a million times as aerodynamically improbable as the June bug, and thus in such creatures one must presume not only mysterious body participation but a special super-whammy of grace to get them into the air.

An insect very like a mayfly over 150 million years ago was probably the ancestor of all arthropod aeronauts. With the discovery of flight, insects became truly oriented to land. The ocean is peculiarly deficient in adult insect life, although it is by no means uncommon for insects in the larval stage to develop in fresh water. A number of small aquatic animals, such as copepods (crustaceans), shifting up and down in a daily rhythm in many lakes and ponds, are eaten by the larvae of the phantom midge fly that rise and sink with their food supply by the skillful compression or expansion of two pairs of gas bubbles each. The larvae of dragonflies, damsel flies, mayflies and caddis flies are equipped with gills—closed tra-

cheal systems—and do not have to surface to breathe. Dragonfly nymphs (one stage further in development) are peculiar
in having gills within the rectum. The water is sucked in
and out, is used in respiration and also, in exhaling, serves as
a jet to propel the nymph through the water. For those few
insects that prefer water to land, the high surface tension can
be useful. The tiny water springtail can hop about over the
water as if it were solid. When insects are serious about making
water a permanent residence, they develop propelling organs
that usually consist of legs modified into oars. This is true of
the water boatmen, the back swimmers and the diving beetles.
The fairy fly (actually a minute wasp) can *fly* under water
and uses this mode of locomotion to locate dragonfly eggs
in which it deposits its own microscopic eggs.

If one looks again with a critical anatomist's eye at the
wings of a prototype insect, one sees that they are attached
to the upper corners of the boxlike thorax. But the box is by
no means rigid. Large muscles extend from top to bottom,
the contraction of which pulls the thorax down, causing the
wings to rise because of the way they are attached. Their
other muscles extend lengthwise and their contraction causes
the wings to beat downward because they cause the roof of
the box to bend upward. All these muscles are indirect in
action, since they move the box, which in turn moves the
wings. However, there are also direct muscles attached to
the bases of the wings for other motions than simply flapping,
and now we begin to see what a subtle flyer the insect is.
On the downstroke, these direct muscles cause the wing to
move *forward* and on the upstroke to move *backward*. Furthermore, as the wings move up and down they also rotate on
their axes. As the wing rises, its hind part is deflected downward and when the wings descend the hind part is deflected
upward. We begin to see that the wing of an insect is more
nearly like the rotating blade of a propeller than like the fixed
wings of an airplane. Merely flapping four artificial wings
would never simulate insect flight. The wing tips in fact describe a figure eight, not up-and-down arcs, and the form of

the eight is not vertical but downward and *forward*. This seems unnatural to us, since one would naïvely think that progress would better be made if the movement were downward and backward, but this is simply because most of us do not understand how a propeller works. In fact, the latter kind of pattern (downward and backward) is described by insects when they want to stand still in the air—hover—as do syrphid flies, hummingbird moths or bees pausing to take the nectar or pollen from flowers.

Since insects evolved as four-winged creatures, the question immediately arises as to how they solved the problem of avoiding the turbulent effect of the front wings on the hind wings. The Diptera (flies, mosquitoes, etc.) had a simple if drastic answer. They simply eliminated the hind wings which became little knobs called "halteres," whose cryptic functions we shall describe later. Many advanced four-winged insects, such as bees, butterflies and moths, evolved contrivances for hooking the two pairs of wings together so they function as a unit. The dragonflies, which are the most prodigious flyers of all, learned many millions of years ago when they were as big as eagles to alternate the beats of the two pairs of wings, the front pair beating downward as the hind pair rises. This alternation is so exquisitely timed that the hind wings meet undisturbed air before it is made turbulent by the front wings.[3]

The flight control system of the locust has been recently studied in all its peculiar complexities by Donald M. Wilson of Stanford University and his conclusions are important in a

[3] Since aerodynamics involves the terribly complicated mechanics of a compressible fluid, I am sparing the reader some rather formidable quotations from the vast and recondite literature. However, some of Leon Bennett's conclusions from his study of the simulated June bug may be presented as exemplary. He finds that the flight of this animal, especially in the hovering condition, simply cannot be explained by steady-state aerodynamics. In fact, *unsteady* effects (which in classical aerodynamics are commonly neglected for the sake of mathematical simplicity) evidently dominate the flight regime of this insect. The possibility exists that the June bug uses an extremely sophisticated procedure, being used experimentally in advanced airplanes—the forced circulation of air along the upper surfaces of the wings to avoid stalling.

general way for distinguishing the proprioceptive imperative—which, as we have seen, may demonstrate itself in a piece of a bristle worm—from the non-reflex actions controlled by the central nervous system. The locust is an ancient, man-abominated insect that combines individual behavior with periodic, enormously destructive socialism. Even in the nymph form the locust shares a tendency to massed army movement. When the blood potassium is low, the nymphs will march in company with each other. The stupendous migrations of adult locusts curiously enough have nothing to do with the search for food. Rather, temperature and weather conditions seem to govern their mass whims. They may even fly *away* from food. One swarm of Rocky Mountain locusts was estimated to consist of 124 *billion* creatures, sounding as they passed overhead like a distant waterfall. During the great locust plagues of the last century, Nebraska was so badly swarmed under that the original state constitution had to be rewritten to take care of the economic exigencies. The new document was known as "The Grasshopper Constitution."

How was Professor Wilson able to study the individual flight behavior of such a neurotic small animal? He accomplished this by having the locusts fly in front of a wind tunnel while suspended on a pendulum that served as the arms of a very sensitive double-throw switch. The switch operated relays that controlled the blower in the tunnel, so whenever the locust flew forward the wind velocity increased and vice versa. This made it possible for the insect to choose its preferred wind speed, but nevertheless to stand still in space. Devices automatically measured the lift and the positions of body and wing. Tiny wires that terminated in the muscles or on nerves conducted electrical impulses to amplifying and recording instruments.

What Wilson was trying to decide was whether the locust's flight movements are the result of a patterned reflex response to the nerves that carry the proprioceptive information from the stretching or hinge receptors of the wings or whether there is some built-in central control system that dictates what the locust does. He found that when he cut the sensory nerves carrying information about lift forces, the locust continued to fly undisturbed, although he had trouble with certain tricky maneuvers. Cutting out or burning the stretch receptors that measure wing position and angular velocity resulted merely in reduction in wing-beat frequency. Even when *all* the nervous feedback was eliminated, the locust could be made to fly by giving a small electric shock to its brain. The co-ordinated action of the locust's flight muscles therefore seems to depend on a built-in motor system that responds to any central stimulus whatsoever. Why then does the locust even *have* a stretch reflex that controls the wing beat frequency? Why not code the frequency also in the brain? There is a good answer to this question, and it involves the compromise of the locust as a genetically coded animal and the locust as an individual—as a distinct person, so to speak. The wings, muscles and skeleton of an animal in flight form a mechanically resonant system with a preferred frequency at which the conversion of muscular work into aerodynamic power is most efficient. This preferred frequency is a function of size. Even insects with the same mothers may reach different sizes because of different special environmental conditions during egg production and development. Hence each adult insect must take into account, as it were, its own size to find the best frequency of beating its wings. This account taking is provided by the stretch reflex which automatically adjusts the wing-beat frequency to the mechanically resonant one.

If one continues to look upon the locust as flying by the seat of its internal tapes, so to speak, what would happen to a locust with damaged wings? Much to his surprise, Wilson found that even if a pair of the locust's four wings is removed, the insect still does a respectable job of flying. Now for a crippled locust to fly it must change its whole pattern of nervous motor output. At this point we must remark that the free-flying locust has at least two extra sources of proprioceptive feedback about its flying progress. It has signals from its eyes and signals from directionally sensitive hairs on its head that respond to the flow of air. These signals tend to keep the locust flying straight in spite of anatomical error or deficiency. The locust flight-control system thus consists only in part of a built-in motor pattern (what electronics people call a "score"). It also shows the adaptability expected of the type of control that is expected of a system that depends on sensory reaction to a model or template. It can be concluded in general that there may be no such thing as a pure internal motor-tape or a pure sensory-template type of control. Locomotive systems of the invertebrates and even of the higher animals combine internal tape and automatic sensory adjustment.[4]

Getting back to aerodynamics, the locust wings have a constant average lift force in normal flight. When the inclination to the wind is artificially changed by about 15 degrees, the wing twists itself, under nervous control, so that average lift remains unchanged. Pitch and roll are probably controlled by feedback from the eyes. The mechanisms for control of yaw (the side-to-side waving motion) are unknown.

The speeds of flight of various insects have, in the past, been argued in the hot-stove league of amateur entomologists with great bombast and fervor but with little data. With the advent of radar tracking, such absurdities as C. H. T. Townsend's claim that the deer botfly careens through the air at 820 miles per hour have been exploded. Insects often are the cause of the so-called "angel" radar echoes observed from an otherwise apparently clear atmosphere, and the flight of specific species, such as hawk moths, tobacco budworm moths, honeybees and dragonflies has been studied with radar techniques.

[4] Some other locomotive systems in invertebrates are quite massively influenced by reflex rather than by tapes in the brain. The walking pattern of a tarantula shows diagonal rhythm in that the diagonal pairs of legs are in step. Yet tarantulas can lose one or more legs and still manage to walk. The spider adjusts the relations between the remaining legs to maintain the diagonal rhythm. The real nature of the oscillating reflex nervous loop involved in this adjustment is unknown, but obviously it must be of a kind so plastic that the organism can recover from unpredictable accidents without a period of learning. Wilson advances the interesting suggestion that this is what reflexes are really for—to equip the animal for anatomical catastrophe.

The fastest insect known is the *Austrophlebia* genus of dragon-fly who gets up to 36 miles per hour with a wing-beat rate of only about 30 per second. Honeybees, depending on whether they are carrying a load or not, can fly at from 5 to 14 miles per hour at a wing-beat rate of some 250 per second. The housefly can go only at about the speed that a man can jog, although when we try to swat him we are under the impression that he is much faster—an optical illusion based on the scale of his surroundings. Since insects are cold-blooded, they are often unable to fly on a cold morning and have to warm up by cautiously vibrating their wings in a ground stall.

The flight ranges of insects depend on how well they utilize their fuel and what the fuel is. Fats are three times as efficient as nectar, which is why a horsefly can fly 60 miles while the honeybee (a sugar burner) can get only about half of that. Desert locusts can fly over 200 miles without refueling. Some butterflies are known to fly at 20,000 feet, and the monarch butterfly, which takes part in great mass migrations, is an extraordinary exception to the fat-sugar rule, since it can evidently get 600 miles on one tankful of nectar. Such butterflies have for over 100 years made the town of Pacific Grove, California, a special wintering resort where they cluster on their favorite eucalyptus trees and where City Ordinance No. 352 makes it a misdemeanor to kill or threaten any of these gorgeous creatures. The painted ladies, the most widely distributed butterfly in the world, like to winter in Mexico and have been seen flying over Pakistan at 17,000 feet. The noctuid moths, whose larvae are the cotton worms, are even more neurotic than locusts in their migratory habits, since they will often set off en masse northward to assured suicide by freezing.[5]

Most of us are of necessity students of houseflies. Did you ever think of how, if you were a fly, you would land on the ceiling? In slow motion it is made clear that the fly brings

---

[5] This should offer one approach to the elimination of pest insects that has not been exploited—to turn their tendencies toward mass neurosis against them. All colonial or swarming insects have sociological weaknesses —witness the fratricidal wars of colonies of ants of the same species.

the front end upward so that the forefeet can come in contact with the overhead surface, after which the other feet are attached by an exuded glue. The fly has, in other words, gone through half the cycle of an aviator's simple backward loop, but with such effortless ease that one has to pause and consider that this is a rather complicated trick. The fly and all other diptera are well equipped for such maneuvers by means of their flight-control systems which are somewhat more subtle than that of the locust. The halteres (the knobs that replaced the missing pair of hind wings) are actually little vibrating bodies that act as gyroscopes. If moved from their plane of motion, like a gyroscope they will exert a force couple (or torque) at the point of attachment, so that each haltere gives the brain information about rotations on vertical and horizontal axes through its plane of vibration. J. W. S. Pringle, who has made the study of insect flight his life work, suggests that in the fly a distinction between pitching and rolling movements is made possible because the torques on the two halteres act together during pitch but are out of phase with each other during a roll. The removal of one haltere has little effect on a steadily flying fly but a large effect on responses to rotation of a fly with its eyes covered, showing that the eye reflexes are tied in with the haltere reflexes. Unlike the honeybee, who uses the weight of her trucker's abdomen to measure gravity, the fly does not respond to gravity alone and a housefly would never have invented or have understood Newton's laws. The fact that the haltere is an evolutionary adaptation in a rather advanced insect is made probable by experiments in which artificially induced mutation in fruit flies often gives rise to individuals in which the halteres have disappeared and been replaced by a pair of hind wings. The halteres are of variable cruciality to different species. In the fly *Sarcophaga* the loss of its six legs does not stop flight, but the loss of the halteres does. After removal of one haltere in *Tipula*, the posture of this insect is still normal but if both are eliminated, the poor animal can only drag its body, resting on the ground. The fly *Philonicus* is unable even to walk after removal of wings and halteres. There are various flight-initiating mechanisms, an important one being the tarsal reflex, when contact is lost with the ground. Wind or air current is frequently necessary, the antennae on flies being especially sensitive. Predator insects that carry their prey (such as wasps) will fly, although their tarsi (feet) are firmly on the ground before take-off. Suspended insects stop flying when tired but are set going again by a sudden falling movement. One automatic flight stimulus allows an insect to crawl up to the tip of a blade of grass. In the housefly, nerve excitation (probably from Johnston's organ) influences the wing movements in relation to air speed and the hairs of the little sensory organs (sensilla) of the head must be excited if the fly is to continue in flight. After loss of the head, the tarsal reflex alone causes a clumsy kind of flight (no more edifying than the reflex running of a headless chicken) but the flight does not continue for long. The antenna of the fly serves as a flight-speed indicator, as shown by the fact that flies without antennae crash clumsily because they land too quickly.

In that very ancient and great flyer, the dragonfly, the movements of the head relative to the thorax excite hair plates on the head. The head, so to speak, tends to get left behind in sudden rolls and registers its distress. The beautiful flexibility of the juncture of this head to the body allows a big "darner" to drop his head and look underneath and behind and thus to fly with exceptional precision. He may fly backward and forward with equal poise and speed.

For almost incredible speed and precision in dive-bombing maneuvers, however, the parasitic *Pyrgota* fly is a maestro. It attacks May beetles, but only when they are in flight, since it is only in this posture that the beetle's tender back membrane is exposed. The fly singles out a female beetle, darts in and thrusts an egg into this soft spot before the beetle realizes that she has been had.

The sexual swarming of small insects, such as mosquitoes, has often been a cause of amazement and sometimes of fright, since the dense swarms are easily mistaken for smoke—in the

Netherlands fire brigades have turned out because a church tower was reported to be burning. The mosquitoes seek warm and moist places to put on their flight orgies. In the early evening the entire crown of a tree is a reservoir of warm air and moisture and is thus a good place to dance above. A TV aerial, conducting warmth from the roof, may also be a place for a mass mosquito rendezvous. Such swarms have indeed been included among the causes of UFO rumors.

Before proceeding to consider the locomotion of land vertebrates, we should say a word or two about spiders, millipedes and the non-flying insects. In many-legged, brisk walkers, we come back again to the problem of central control versus peripheral reflex control. How to explain how the many legs walk at all by the same precise pattern to the point that they walk precisely in the same set of tracks? Removal of the brain or the protocerebrum alone simply leads to increased activity, probably because the animal has its optic nerve center here and it is only active in the dark. Removal of the whole head stops co-ordinated walking in some species but in others the locomotive pattern is little changed, even in pieces of the body. Some pieces even retain the righting reflex, for turning right side up. Nervous waves between nerve centers evidently play a greater part in myriopod walking than in insects and crustaceans.

That fierce and versatile insect the mantis has a wide range of gaits associated with a specialization of the powerful prothoracic legs which can be used for climbing, running as well as capture of prey. A cockroach when scuttling about is found to have a nervous discharge in the leg muscles when the leg is not touching the ground. The most likely leg to step is one which bears the least weight. If the act of putting a leg down relieves some other legs of the load, the sequence will be alternate. The co-ordination of the sequence is thus due to exterior forces and is in part necessarily caused by the movements of the other legs. No leg is lifted until the leg behind it is in a supporting position. The least loaded leg is the next one to be raised. It is thus clear that walking insects of sensible weight are quite dependent upon gravity and, unlike the house-fly, should be on communicating terms with Isaac Newton.

The climbing instinct of young female spiders should not be overlooked, since without it the spider would not be distributed widely enough to survive as an animal type. When, finding a wide space beneath her after climbing to the top of a bush, she sends up her thread and sails with it, she has come to childhood's end. Thereafter she will be interested only in climbing as it involves her webs. Spiders are remarkable in that the end joints of their legs have no extensor muscles. The flexor muscles, instead of pulling against muscle antagonists, act against blood pressure. In the jumping spiders, a valve controls the flow of blood into each leg, and before a jump the leg may have a blood pressure of five times the resting pressure. Orb-weaving spiders, such as *Agalena*, learn their way around the web (although no one knows how they have been able to design and build it) by a combination of visual and kinesthetic (proprioceptive) sense. It takes her about half an hour of exploration to make herself at home. This spider can then make a beeline from any part of the web to the lowest point. In *Agalena* the strange proprioceptive homing sense is as well developed as it is in ants. If taught an obstacle-strewn indirect route home from a food site, *Agalena* will, upon removal of the obstacles, immediately take the direct route.

How to Slither

BEFORE there were snakes (a relative newcomer on the vertebrate scene) there were lizards, and it would seem that a large proportion of lizards would prefer to be snakelike. Half of all the families of lizards include species either lacking legs or with legs too small and weak for walking. This evolutionary tendency to lose legs is not connected with a desire so much to slither as to burrow. The fossil record plainly indicates that the poor excuses for legs seen on some lizards does not mean that the burrowing animals are acquiring legs but they are losing them by the usual process of degeneration. Both snakes and lizards at one time or another in the pageant of biological history made feeble attempts to fly, and in recent times the lizard (the flying dragon of Asia) accomplished a sort of volplane flight somewhat along the order of the performance of the flying squirrel. In ancient epochs, of course, the reptiles achieved flight, but later forgot how it was done. Whereas bats fly with their hands and birds with their forearms, the pteradactyl flew with monstrously developed "little" fingers.

In the obscure whim of divesting themselves of legs, there is among lizards little generic regularity. We may see two species of a single genus, one with strong legs, the other with useless appendages. We may even find differences in the number of toes between normal individuals of a single species. The locomotive transition (or perhaps one should say ambiguity) is especially noticeable in the tiny teiid lizards of South America. They may walk leisurely like a respectable quadruped.[6] If excited, however, they will change to serpentine slithering, with legs uselessly fanning the air. Sometimes, as in the sand skink of Florida, the legs have become recognized as superfluous and even embarrassing, so evolution has contrived grooves into which these pieces of excess baggage fit. What many lizards would evidently like to do is to lose at least their front legs, so that, like the fringe-toed lizard, they could dive into the sand and literally "swim" under it. In this animal the little front legs are held against the body and the swimmy burrowing is achieved by pushing movements of the hind feet together with slithering of the body and tail. It is rather surprising that no modern lizard has become two-legged, or bipedal, like so many of the gigantic early reptiles. However, some lizards resort to bipedalism when a burst of speed is required. Basilisks are famous for two-legged running and can even make short dashes across the surface of water, like petrels. (The term "petrel," incidentally, is derived

[6] Quadruped walking is a much more complex operation than one would suspect and will be discussed at greater lengths when we come to mammals.

from Saint Peter who found that in an emergency and with moral support he could walk on the water.)

Some lizards have mysterious and poorly understood gifts of locomotion. The toe of the gecko has been described in matter-of-fact zoology texts as a "suction disk," but actually it is composed of thousands of tiny hooks too small to be seen with the naked eye, these hooks in turn having still tinier suction spots. The hooks do not explain how the gecko can climb up a glass wall or walk across a ceiling. The hairbrush feet do not cling by the exuding of an adhesive fluid, like. flies, because the gecko has no secretion glands. It cannot create a vacuum under its foot, as the limpet can. That no vacuum device is involved is proved by the fact that the gecko can cling to a vertical glass surface in a vacuum jar. Supposedly the tiny hairs could penetrate fine cracks in the glass, but the gecko is not an insubstantial creature like a fly, and his weight should simply pull the hairs out.

Until quite recently the gecko's thumbing his nose at the science of human dynamics has been as intimate an insult as the bite of a snake. Luckily the human race has rebuffed this particular challenge by one of its rare and brilliant inventions—the so-called "electron microscope scanning." Although this technique is much newer than television scanning, and there are unsolved problems of the type that are much more serious than those of the Milton Berle era of TV entertainment, the technology is more important to the human race in the long run than the present gross TV war on the nervous stomachs of two or three billion human beings.

As described so charmingly by Joseph F. Gennaro and others, this three-dimensional use of electron-microscope principles has opened up a new world of insight at an especially crucial time in biologic history. Biochemistry and biophysics have not been previously so concerned as now with the little wavelets of membranes that seem as vital to the scenario of the living cell as the DNA molecule, which is itself a rather majestic wavelet rather than a molecular statue.

What one does in order to *see* rather than merely to deduce very small dynamic adventures is to coat the membrane, i.e., the surface structure, very thickly with gold (evaporated under vacuum and condensed onto the crucial surface). The gold is a trick to get the little membranes, the little pieces of fierce life, to reveal themselves to instruments that scientists can in turn use to translate things seen into established physics as old as Newton.

In this case, with an incisiveness that Galileo would have relished, the scanning electron microscope reveals the cunning-ness behind the gecko's ability to cling to a smooth glass ceiling, not with the mystical grip of an angel but with a submicroscopic trick that characterizes the gecko as a remarkably subtle student of surface chemistry. What actually does the scanning electron microscope show?

It makes known the fact that hitherto imperceived rows of setae (submicroscopic hairlets) comprise the brushlike lamellae (little plates which we *can* see) and present what are indeed powerful suction cups to a surface. We learn the practical lesson that a really enormous number of infinitesimally small suction cups has almost horribly unexpected force. As Gennaro has so poetically maintained, in this powerful surface system, each seta is seen mounted individually on a small bristly knob—an arrangement providing nevertheless socialistic co-operation between the setae "like shocks of ripe wheat in a field." Under magnification with the scanning electron microscope one can see that each division of a bristle has at its tip a cuplike structure about eight millionths of an inch in diameter (just beyond the resolution capability of the best light microscope). When one scrutinizes these extraordinary cups one can see that they each possess a membrane so thin and active that it can easily conform to the irregularities of any surface—even plate glass or polished steel. The gecko has simply discovered that what we regard as smooth is only so to an engineering degree, which evolution with arrogant ease has been able to cope with. (Indeed, I have suggested that a gecko be added to the laboratory equipment of people who specialize, for example, in the manufacture of precision bearings for rocket gyroscopes. The difficulty, as in all suggestions to government or industry, is one of categorization—is the gecko an inanimate instrument or a potential member of a labor union, deserving twenty dollars per hour?)

It is also important to know how this incomparably tenacious lizard can let loose if it wants to: Its adhesiveness to a polished ceiling is not a politically indefinite posture. When the gecko rolls its toes back the release is immediate. Rolling the toes back flattens the rows of setae and curls them up. Each seta pulls its stubborn cups so as to raise them from the surface.

This is a more extraordinary co-operative exercise than would appear at first glance. If you were an animal composed essentially of millions of suction cups, like those on the end of a toy arrow, how would you assure that the command "Okay, let's all let loose" be immediately obeyed? One would expect a few hundreds of thousands of clinging membranes to be asleep at the switch, like soldiers dazed by pot or simply by the usual sleepiness of armies at rest, and one would therefore expect a gecko release from a surface to be as clumsy as a military retreat. However, the gecko is a remarkably nimble fly-catcher and not one who waits, attached, for events to drift toward him. He is himself an event-maker. As far as we can deduce with the scanning electron microscope, the two thousand or more membranous cups of each of the gecko's setae are *not* attached like toy suction arrows, and this is the secret of quick release. Each of the thousands of cups on each seta sits at the end of its bristle *at a jaunty angle*. When the command for release comes, it is not so much like standing up as like *sliding away*. Sliding is always easier than standing and marching.

We see, as in all life we have examined, that evolution has outguessed us, even in processes we regard as having been invented by Archimedes or Galileo or Newton or Edison.

If a modern lizard wants to evolve into a snake, he probably can, since his ancestors did. But what is so good about being a snake? How does he get around? The answer to this is quite complicated and agreement among herpetologists has been reached only after many decades of bitter controversy. In the order of importance to the average snake there are four types of locomotion. (None of them involves the fantastic maneuver seen in old books on natural history or in the comic pages in which the snake crawls with its body curving up and down, like a mythical sea serpent on dry land.) Most important is the horizontal undulation or slither. The snake's body is kept in a series of curves just as in swimming snakes. This supple bending is easy for snakes because they have so many bones in the vertebra, not because they are loosely jointed. The snake's body pushes at the rear of each curve and this push piles up dirt or sand as the snake moves forward. This requires a viscous medium (such as water) or a rough surface. If the surface is smooth, like glass, the snake is in a silly predicament, since he simply remains "swimming" in his tracks. Many heavy snakes use a caterpillar or straight-line crawl. The belly is covered with narrow scales that are overlapped and this overlapping permits expansion and contraction in a forward and backward direction. Whole sections of the belly scales are raised slightly and are moved forward before being laid down again. As a result one sees waves along the body like those that appear to flow down the body of a caterpillar. Contrary to popular misconception, the ribs do *not* take part in this maneuver. The skin and the muscles attached to the skin move independently of the ribs. The free edges of the scales do not actually cut into the surface, since they are quite delicate. In crawling caterpillar-style over a smooth surface, the snake relies entirely on friction between the scales and the surface. He can crawl across glass, but not across glass with a film of oil on it.

There is also what is known as "concertina" locomotion in some snakes. The snake throws his body into a series of curves, alternately straightening out his forward part and then bringing up the rear. This is a rather slap-happy way to get around and is neither efficient nor speedy. Finally, there is sidewinding, or crotaline crawling, used chiefly by desert snakes over loose sand. When a sidewinder moves, it seems literally to *flow* sidewise or obliquely. The track is a series of nearly straight, disconnected but parallel depressions, proving that the snake has actually been off the ground a good deal of the time as it rolled or, one might say, *bounded*. This is a very tricky way of getting around and has always fascinated students of locomotion. It is in keeping with the fantastic sensory gifts of the crotaline snakes like all pit vipers, such as the incredibly exact temperature-detection devices in the pits at the sides of the head.

In order to climb up a slender pole or tree (which is not too smooth) those snakes that are addicted to such adventures use a modified concertina technique, consisting of a series of alternate hitches and releases, the hind part gripping while the forward part reaches up to get hold. Like the telephone wire repairman with spikes on his feet, the snake that knows how to climb well has specially designed scales that form an angle extending along either side of the belly.

A forgivable error on the part of the great Sherlock Holmes, whom many middle-aged people at one time regarded as a sort of eccentric nineteenth-century Apollo (and perhaps still do), occurred in *The Adventure of the Speckled Band*. In this story Holmes determined in his usual inscrutable and debonair fashion that the victim had been killed by a Russell's viper that had been encouraged to climb up a bell rope (with which every Victorian Englishman affluent enough to afford a butler was as familiar as with a flushing chain for a toilet). What Holmes (or his alter ego Conan Doyle) had not realized was that the Russell's viper is not a constrictor. The snake is therefore incapable of concertina movement and could not have climbed the rope. If attached to the rope by a villain, it would have fallen off and most likely ended up coiled around inside the toilet bowl—certainly a most un-Victorian place to commit a murder—but a very likely place for a wild snake to wind up in a house.

There is a widespread superstition about the speed of snakes. When I was a boy, I used to hear stories of the fearsome "red racer" that could catch up with a running man. Tests show that probably the fastest of all snakes, the coachwhip

(*Masticophis flagellum*), proceeds at the dizzying maximum velocity of three miles per hour. As in our illusions about the housefly's speed, the snake seems to be going faster because we see him slithering by things of small scale, such as bushes and rocks. Furthermore, a fast crawling snake (using the slither) quickly tires because of the slow rate of oxygenation of the blood. Snakes would be poor Olympic racers at the altitude of Mexico City. We have mentioned before that tens of thousands of country people claim to see hoop snakes rolling about like hoops, but these creatures stop rolling and adopt a modest crawl or slither when a herpetologist shows up.

To Fly Like a Bird

In order for birds to fly, evolution had to brush up on its aerodynamics again and teach in a different mode the lessons that had been learned long ages before by the flying insects. There were, of course, variations in both scale and organic design. Evolution waved its wand and lo, four wings sprouted from the thoracic box of the insect, still leaving him with his original six legs; but making a flying machine of a four-legged reptile took a longer magic. Evolution decided that the extremities of the front legs should sprout aerodynamic feathers and become flapping members, leaving a two-legged creature who could still walk about when grounded.[7]

There were certain grave problems in designing a relatively large flying animal. We come back to our old geometric dilemma in which the volume (or weight) increases as the cube of some linear dimension (say, the size of a rib), while the

[7] Paleontologists are now disposed to believe, however, that the invention of body feathers, to provide a new sort of insulation much more effective than reptilian scales, came about before birds began to fly. It is noteworthy that the warm-bloodedness of birds, which they share with the mammals, demands good insulation to be at all practical in cold regions. The mammal's hair or fur and the bird's feathers were revolutionary inventions in the art of insulation that came about at approximately the same time geologically.

surface area (including the wing) increases only as the square. What this means is that a large bird must have disproportionately large wings. Because of the high moment of inertia of big wings, it is hard to make them strong enough for flight without making them too heavy. Heavier birds thus have higher wing-loading and a bird the size of a condor probably represents the limit of physical possibility and, in fact, this bird is only able to fly with a small margin of safety because of his skilled use of vertical air currents. (The roc of the *Arabian Nights* is as unlikely as the winged heads of the cherubim.) The body weight of a flying bird is limited to about thirty-five pounds. Birds, such as the ostrich, the rhea and the cassowary, when they exerted a preference for eating like pigs, found themselves permanently grounded. The kiwi weighs only four pounds, but in the insular ease of New Zealand its wings never became more than puny. The penguin, instead of flying, returned to the ocean and learned to swim with unexampled swiftness and purpose. There are no flightless fresh-water birds except in ice-free climates.

The size limitation cuts both ways. As size is reduced, the surface-to-volume ratio goes up so fast that heat loss becomes critical. Thus we see the hummingbird panting on the very verge of life's boundary, resorting to nightly hibernations in which his blood temperature falls to that of the surroundings, in order to recuperate from the day's frantic work as a tiny living helicopter.

An average bird is a marvel of aeronautical engineering. Compare bird and man in flight as regards fuel economy. The golden plover flies 2,400 miles on two ounces of body fat, which is equivalent to flying a small airplane 160 miles on a gallon of gasoline rather than the usual 20 miles actually achieved. Yet the bird has the handicap of greater heat loss and greater friction, because his design has necessarily involved providing him with auxiliary devices to feed, to protect and to reproduce himself. We do not design an airplane to feed at a trough or to conceive little airplanes. Some of them *are* designed to avoid predators in times of war.

To inform ourselves of the brilliance of bird design, let us consider first the structural details of a feather. Light and springy, the thin walls of supports are built around a solid foam structure and the structure is as strong as an alloy-steel strut. Yet the feather is at the same time as flexible as a rubber tube. In the "remiges," or flight feathers, of the swan and pheasant, the wall thickness varies around the cross section of the shaft, which is an ellipse at the root and a rectangle at the tip. The corners and upper walls are thickened, with the upper wall holding toothlike projections that increase the resistance of the shaft wall to sudden bending and also help bond the shaft to the core of foam. A bird's feathers are stronger, weight for weight, than any man-made substitute. Once formed, any feather is a dead horny structure without living cells. The feathers grow from the base and not at the tip. There is naturally a good deal of teamwork between the parts of a feather. The outmost barbules on a barb have little hooks, and since the barbules overlap at right angles the smooth inner barbules of a neighboring barb, they cling stubbornly to hold all the barbs of a feather vane parallel and together to face the moving air. In some birds, such as the owl, the barbules' hooking system is so cunningly designed that the wings make no sound at all in flapping so that silent flight is assured to this predator of the night.

The *primary* feathers are those that extend from what would have been the bird's hand, if he had developed into a primate. They are anchored, in fact, to three bones of the third "finger." The *secondaries* are the feathers which extend from the bird's "forearm." The number of big flight feathers on the wings and tail are extremely constant. It is as hard to find a pigeon or a chicken with an unconventional number of tail feathers as it is to find a man with six fingers.

The wing feathers overlap each other, so that the leading edge of one feather lies above the more flexible trailing edge of the feather in front. The wing surface formed is quite impermeable to air on the down stroke but may open like a venetian blind on the upstroke to let the air slip through. In order to understand both insect and bird flight one must constantly bear in mind that the wing of flapping flyers is both wing and propeller. The bird's hand with the large primary feathers does most of the propelling, while the forearm with the secondaries gives most of the lift. During flight the hand moves through a slanting oval or figure eight, while the upper arm and forearm move very little. The removal of a small part of the tips of the primary feathers of a dove prevents it from flying, yet shearing the secondaries to cut the surface by 55 per cent hardly embarrasses the bird at all. His gliding is hampered, but doves are not much on gliding anyway. The wings of birds are in fact designed for the kind of business the bird is in.

In addition to the primary feathers, the bird's hand has a few small feathers in the "thumb." This so-called "bastard wing," or alula, is actually a wing slot, just as we see on the leading edges of airplane wings, and is located about half the way to the wing tip. One should by no means overlook the bird's tail as a part of its flight equipment. When the tail is lowered it is acted upon by the horizontal air stream and tends to lift the body. Various clever tail movements help the wings in balancing, steering and braking during flight. Birds with miserably short tails, such as ducks, cannot make sudden turns. Some aquatic birds have such short tails that they substitute their webbed feet for steering themselves.

The easiest flight plan to understand is that of soaring birds who rarely flap and, in taking off or landing, are notably clumsy. Most of their active life is spent in riding the air currents and the winds. The best soarers have very long, narrow wings like those of the shearwaters and albatrosses. In hawks and eagles, when a heavy prey must be carried, the wings are wide as well as long. Aerodynamically speaking, there are three kinds of soaring. Two depend on upward currents of air, either thermal or deflective. The third method (*dynamic* soaring) depends on knowing how to manipulate oneself with or against a horizontal wind. Thermal soaring birds, such as hawks and vultures, make use of the warm air rising from sun-baked fields or rocks, a kind of updraft that produces cumulus clouds. The bird that uses such thermals usually climbs them in great circles. Deflective updrafts are formed by mountains which simply deflect a steady wind upward. The convenience of this to certain soaring birds can be seen in the masses of migratory hawks that follow the deflective updrafts along the eastern edge of the Appalachian Mountains. At Hawk Mountain near Dreherville in eastern Pennsylvania, the ridges funnel migrating hawks into a narrow flightway. A bird census taken there registered every known kind of hawk and eagle in eastern North America, often in very large numbers during the southward migration in the fall. This is practically automatic transportation for a hawk because he can travel along ·this corridor for many miles at speeds up to forty miles per hour without flapping a wing. A bird that soars on thermals must often choose the right country for nesting. Thus the range of the more buoyant turkey vulture extends into southern Canada, but the slender wings of the black vulture restrict him to the southern United States and the tropics, where the warm sun more richly generates thermal updrafts. For such maneuvering the wing must be well furnished with slots, to avoid stalling. In that famous soarer, the California condor, 40 per cent of the wing span is in fact occupied by slots. This would not do for oceanic flying, because wet feathers cannot be easily manipulated into the slotting configuration.

Dynamic soaring is the method used by ocean birds like the albatross and the frigate bird. The bird moves against the wind in a series of cyclic maneuvers. It first rides up at an angle of about 40 degrees to the wind until it stalls; then it turns and falls rapidly until it nearly hits the water. At this point it executes a remarkable maneuver: it banks sharply and coasts up into the wind until it stalls at another crest in the cycle, repeating the dive to pick up momentum, and so on. This mode of wind exploitation is very clever. The effect is like a man hopping off a moving bus to run up a slope at the edge of the road. Birds that use this technique spend their lives in the great oceanic wind belts. The wandering albatross is aerodynamically perfect for such locomotion since its wings have an "aspect ratio" (ratio of length to width) of 18 to 1, and a lift over drag ratio of 40 to 1, and it has the greatest of all known wing spreads—about twelve feet.

Contrary to soaring, flapping flight is very difficult to understand, although most but not all birds, like insects, are born with the capability of carrying out this excruciatingly complex operation. One must distinguish between this kind of flight in small birds and large birds. When a small bird decides to take off from a twig, his wing moves downward and *forward* on the downstroke (as we emphasized with insects). The trailing edge of the wing bends upward and molds the whole wing into a propellerlike shape which *pulls* (it does not *push*) the bird forward through the air, the feathers of the wing biting the air with their under surfaces like propeller blades. On the return stroke, upward and *backward*, the wings do little or no propelling. In *large* birds, the upward stroke cannot be wasted, since the bird has a higher wing-loading and must take advantage of every instant to get going fast enough to avoid stalling. Thus propulsion takes place also on the upstroke. It was a long time before anybody could figure out how this was done, but the mechanical pattern is now clear. In rising, the wing bends slightly at the "wrist" and "elbow" and the whole arm (humerus) rotates backward at the shoulder joint to such an extent that the mighty primary feathers now push against the air with their *upper* surfaces and drive the bird forward, again like a propeller. The downstroke is the same as that of small birds.

The hummingbird is an extreme case. He is not so much a propeller-using job as a helicopter. A hummingbird can fly backwards a small distance and *hover*. The wing is practically all hand (no secondary feathers) and there is no slotting. The entire wing may be looked at as a variable pitch propeller. During hovering the wing oscillates at seventy-five times per second at a steep "angle of attack" (angle at which the wing hits the air or vice versa), forcing the air downward with *both* up and down strokes of the wings. Evolution actually did not do as well as man has done in developing this operation. Compared to a rotating helicopter blade (remember that evolution never invented a wheel) the twisting, vibrating wings of the hummingbird are sadly inefficient and draw an exhausting amount of power from this poor little creature. The breast muscles make up 40 per cent of a hummingbird's total weight. The breast keel, which anchors every bird's flying muscles, is relatively enormous.

Birds that fly in formation show an instinctive knowledge of aerodynamic tricks, much after the fashion of automobile racers. In long files each bird is so spaced that he beats his wings against the rising wake of the bird in front. Usually the wings beat in unison, and if one bird is out of step, he is either sick or silly and in either case is encouraged to leave the flock. In the V-formation of ducks and geese, each bird touches only the inner wing tip on the rising vortex of air from the bird in front.

Some birds practice an aeronautical technique known as "gliding flight." They jump into the air, flap their wings violently and often very noisily, then glide on for some distance. This is typical of quail, pheasant and other gallinaceous birds.

Wings can be "cambered" (curved so that the surface is concave below and convex above, to obtain more lift). It is the upper surface that provides about 75 per cent of the lift, hence the flow of air should be as smooth and as fast as possible over the upper wing. (Pressure is lower, when the velocity of air is higher, hence a bird obtains lift by being, so to speak, *sucked* upward by lower pressure rather than being pushed upward by higher pressure. The lift process is essentially the same effect that makes a fast rotating baseball curve. The air speed is faster at the surface of the ball that is rotating in the direction that the air is striking it; hence the pressure is lower on that side, and the ball curves in that direction.) For a given wing the angle at which the lift vanishes is a stalling angle. This angle can be increased (hence the stalling speed lowered) if the air over the upper surface can be prevented from separating and creating eddies. Wing slots achieve this smoothing of air.

The shape of the wing is adapted to the way the bird makes a living. Elliptical wings are best for a forested or shrubby habitat. The bird has to maneuver in close quarters, and this calls for a low aspect ratio, reduced wing tip vortex and a high degree of wing slotting, especially in the form of separated primary feathers. One sees this design in the dove, woodpeckers, most perching birds and the gallinaceous species.

High-speed wings are good for birds that feed in flight or make long migrations. A high-speed wing has a low camber, a high aspect ratio, a taper to a slender wing tip and no slots, while the body is "faired" and given "sweep-back" contours to get low air resistance. One sees this kind of configuration of wing and body in shore birds, swifts, falcons and swallows. The peregrine falcon dives at 180 miles per hour. Some rapid flyers have baffles in the nostrils to prevent excessive pressure from building up at high speed in the lungs and air sacs. Sandpipers have been timed at 110 miles per hour while ducks can fly steadily at about 50 miles per hour. The specialized, highly slotted, high-lift wing of moderate aspect ratio and deep camber is seen in terrestrial soarers such as vultures, hawks, owls and predator birds that carry heavy loads in their business.

All of a flying bird's anatomy and even his diet are highly specialized and he must adopt a constant flight maintenance program. For example, he preens with oil from the uropygial gland or with dust—in fact, the preening operation occupies a good share of a bird's waking time. A bird's bones are light because they are hollow. (Darwin smoked a pipe whose stem was made from the hollow wing bone of an albatross.) They are also very strong. The internal bone struts of the metacarpal bone of a vulture wing is very like those of a Warren truss used in aircraft and bridge design. Teeth are too heavy for a bird to carry so the grinding of food is taken over by the muscular gizzard. In dispensing with teeth, the bird has also gotten rid of heavy jawbones and muscles. The ribs of flying birds are long, flat, thin, jointed and overlaid. While saving in weight (most of which has to go into the keel) this provides the same strength found in a woven splint basket. A flying bird cannot be burdened with a urinary bladder and has no urethra; uric acid passes directly into the cloaca whose walls absorb water. Muscles are "dark meat" and are built of finer fibers than white meat, such as one gets from the breasts of many gallinaceous birds (grouse, quail, pheasant, chicken, turkeys). Birds with white breast muscles cannot take long flights, although the dark meat of their legs shows that they run well. If the ruffed grouse is flushed three or four times, his breast muscles become so tired that he can be picked up by hand. The breeding season is sharply limited so that the bird for only a fraction of the year is burdened with heavy sex organs.[8]

Since the keel is the chief anchorage for flight muscles, its size is a good index of a bird's capacity for flapping flight. Reduction of the weight of muscles on the back of a bird is made possible by the rigidity of the synsacrum and the dorsal bone. These eliminate the need of strong dorsal muscles (such as the loin muscle of mammals) to hold the flexible backbone against the stresses imposed by flight or running. The large pectoral muscle and its antagonist, the supracoracoideus, lower and raise the wings. The arrangement is similar to a rope and pulley, the supracoracoideus exerting an upward force on the wing by a downward pull and keeping its center of weight in the body. These two paired muscles make up to one half of the total weight of a strong flying bird's weight (e.g., a pigeon).

Since flight entails high temperature of the blood, the temperatures of flying birds may run to what in a mammal would be deathly high —107° in some sparrows, 110.5° in some thrushes.

---

[8] Many water birds lose all their wing primaries at once so that the birds are flightless for several weeks after the breeding season. This would be fatal for land birds. The early adoption of breeding plumage encourages the winter pairing of ducks long before the spring breeding. The sex organs swell up only *after* the northward migration.

The red corpuscles (erythrocytes) are smaller and more numerous in good flyers, once again illustrating the importance of surface-to-volume ratio, since the total oxygen-transferring capacity of a lot of small corpuscles is higher than that of the same weight of large ones.

With all this power generation, the bird must have a much better cooling system than a man and indeed he does. A pigeon flying 40 miles an hour produces twenty-seven times as much heat as he does when perching on General Sherman's statue. This very serious cooling problem is solved much better in birds than it is in mammals by the system of air sacs through the body which act primarily to evaporate moisture as the air whistles through them and thus constitute a built-in air-conditioning system. The high-speed air entering this system of sacs also acts in a supercharging fashion to burn the body's fuel faster.

Although we have admitted the decisive superiority in mileage per unit of fuel in birds compared with airplanes, when the natural and man-made flying machines get in each other's way it is always disastrous for the bird and not infrequently for the passengers of the airplane. In 1962 the collision of two whistling swans, whose remains were found lodged in a horizontal stabilizer, caused the fatal crash of a United Air Lines Viscount. Ducks, geese, seagulls and starlings have caused at least a dozen airline accidents in the past ten years. The starlings did their damage not by collision but by being gulped into the intake of jet engines. So fearful of the disastrous effect of ingestion or of collisions of jet aircraft with seagulls, rooks, plovers, etc. have the Pakistani become that old-time falconry is being resorted to for keeping the nuisance birds off the air strips. Yet mankind can immobilize birds by means other than killing them. The leashed goose with the swollen liver, the swan who tries piteously to fly at migration time but who has been "pinioned" by amputation of the wing bone at the metacarpal joint, the bird in the gilded cage are easy to bring to mind. In the winter of 1968 thirty wild ducks were thought to be frozen in Lake Aracataw in Michigan. Actually they were too fat to take off. They had been fed too much by lakeside residents. Thus even in our clumsy attempts at fraternization with this great and naïve class of animals, we seem always to manage to defeat them or to bring them harm.

The Versatile Mammals

THE ANCESTOR of all of us mammals (including the seal and the whale as well as the Harvard professor) got around like a lizard on four legs and this is still the mode of the great proportion of mammalian species. It is a fantastic example of how poor an observer man is that the act of walking (not running or hopping) on four legs has been misunderstood for thousands of years—in fact, ever since man took up painting, sculpturing or animal description. As has been pointed out by such modern experts on quadrupedal locomotion as Edward Muggeridge, Samuel Chubb and Lewis S. Brown (all Americans), practically all paintings and sculptures throughout history that portray even such a familiar companion as a horse, show him walking in a manner that would cause him to fall over if he tried it. (The paintings of Frederic Remington are notable exceptions, since his horses and buffalo are seen to walk in a scientifically correct manner.)

Man's usual failure to depict accurately the walking of an animal must involve some peculiar evolutionary deficiency, and it may be significant that, while nearly all four-legged animals truly walk in a universal patterned manner, there is one and only one notable exception—the four-legged primates (such as lemurs), and it is only when they grow up that they choose what Brown calls the "false walk." As babies, the lemurs walk (or crawl) in the immemorial sequence that is shared by human babies, the horse, elephant, cat, dog, camel, giraffe, lizard, amphibian, even the sloth as he "walks" upside down on the branch of a tree.

What is the "true walk" that must have been decided upon by evolution for the first mammal?[9] The starting sequence is *right hind foot—right front foot—left hind foot—left front foot,* in which the front foot begins advancing only after the hind foot of the same side has done so. If one examines this sequence from the standpoint of mechanical support, one notices that this is the only manner in which the feet and legs, as they move, form a series of good sound tripods to hold the animal's weight. In none of the other five obvious sequences are the tripods as supportive. They would all either throw the animal off balance or the animal would likely tangle his feet up. This is an exceedingly important sequence to remember since undoubtedly at some point in evolution walking was the way to achieve maximum speed. Running and trotting and hopping came later. The original idea was to find a way for so-called "planagrade" locomotion to thwart gravity without falling down.

A big dictionary will say that, in walking, two of the quadruped's four feet are always on the ground, but it does not specify *which* two feet. Actually it should say one of each pair of feet, front or back. This actually amounts to two bipeds, one walking behind the other, each having one foot on the ground. The walk is, of course, one of several symmetrical gaits. Yet in all gaits in four-legged animals, the second half of the stride is a mirror image of the first half.

Now if the feet form triangles that are small and do not lie under the center of gravity, the animal is in walking trouble. In what Brown calls the "false walk," so popular among pictorial artists and sculptures from the Egyptians to the present

[9] One must note that four-legged walking is more complex than the walking of spiders, insects or centipedes, in spite of the greater multiplicity of legs in this other phylum. A simple diagonal symmetry is involved which in centipedes amounts to a constant marching plan of all legs. But there are mathematically six ways in which a quadruped can start to walk. One scientist proposed 21 varieties of walking gait and another suggested 108 different gaits for quadrupeds. Any gait has four factors: foot sequence, foot support, velocity and the rhythm produced by the feet striking the ground.

day, the sequence is *right hind foot—left hind foot—left front foot—right front foot*. Superficially this looks practical as well as graceful, but it is mechanically unsound, giving bad triangles and poor support. A heavy animal, like an elephant or a horse, would never think of risking its torso with such a performance, nor even would a cat. Most animals never use the false walk. It must be admitted that animals sometimes, though very seldom, use another gait that Brown calls the "thinker's walk," in which the movements of the legs on one side are synchronized, so that the locomotion somewhat resembles the trot. This presumably is resorted to only when the animal is absent-minded and more attentive to the digestion of his dinner or preoccupied by some inner mystery of the soul—a rare mood in a walking animal—but this too is a configuration happily reproduced by medieval and modern artists, none of whom probably ever saw a quadruped in this unusual configuration.

If one wants to see the true walk at its most classical, note a hunting dog frozen alert in the act of walking. The good tripods of body support are at once apparent. A hunting dog trying to progress by the false walk or the thinker's walk would be a disgrace to his breed, sneered at by his master, his companions and even by the game that he scents.

The axis on the lemur's false walk may show the effect of his confusion between walking with four legs and tree-climbing (in one case) and with two legs on the other. Most monkeys run along on the top of branches on all four limbs and leap from one branch to another much like a squirrel. Among the platyrrhines, only the spider monkey uses brachiation (swinging by his arms underneath branches). The first move to get into the trees and make a life there probably occurred about 50 million years ago. Fossils of lemurlike animals show the "vertical clinging" posture, which encouraged long hind legs and short front legs. Getting around in the trees became a master art in the case of the gibbon, which of all the anthropoids is the farthest removed from man. Gibbons are as specialized for swinging in trees as is man for walking on two feet. It is all the more curious that gibbons are the only anthropoid apes that do not make nests in trees, although they sleep aloft. This habit on the part of gorillas, chimpanzees and orangutans perhaps betrays an ancient memory of the security of living in trees, so for the night they make a temporary house there, while the gibbon never comes out of the trees, night or day, if he can help it. Some adult orangutans weigh over 200 pounds and they have learned to climb trees very cautiously, like an old acrobat who has had a tough life. Their caution is justified since examinations of orangutan skeletons in the forests show that over one third had suffered broken legs during their active youth. Chimpanzees, in spite of their show-off acrobatic stunts, prefer to spend their active life on the ground. In walking, the gorilla places its long foot solidly and flatly on the ground. He begins to look like a man learning to walk after an illness and the resemblance is strengthened by the beginning of a heel—a human trait.

Before the great adventure of bipedalism (which was unquestionably the most important invention that any primate ever made, before or since), certain climatic changes had to take place. When Proconsul (the nearest thing to a "missing link" connecting apes and man) was living, the theatrical Miocene period got under way—an age of the birth of mountains. The Alps, the Himalayas, the Andes and the Rockies were thrusting up their titanic shoulders and great climatic changes were freeing a new kind of living space—the grassy savanna. This was the domain of new forms of vegetation that in many parts of the world (especially in Africa where man was born) took the place of the interminable rain forests of the Eocene and Oligocene. The grassy savanna, however, is a dangerous place to learn a new way of getting around. There are too many big cats behind the bushes. A better gymnasium to try out new locomotion techniques is in the *woodland*-savanna, where the safe old trees are nearby and can be reached by a sudden scramble on all fours. (Chimpanzees and vervet monkeys occupy these places today.) The australopithecines probably learned to get around on two legs in these loosely wooded arenas, but they did not learn the true walk or stride there.

During the Pleistocene, this first manlike creature was bipedal but he probably got around in a sort of jog trot. One can strongly infer this from the australopithecine skeletons. The degree of extension of the legs required in true striding can only be achieved if the ischium of the pelvis is short and the muscles of hip and thigh (the gluteus maximus and minimus) are well developed. But the ischium of *Australopithecus* is almost as long as that of an ape and the muscles that stabilize the pelvis during each stride were poorly formed. This nervous jogging is a most inefficient kind of locomotion and it requires a lot of power output. It may therefore have caused a revolutionary change in australopithecine diet. The best high-energy foodstuffs available were the bodies of other animals. Pre-man thus became a hunter and probably learned to stride when he moved into the open savannas in search of more animal flesh.

What is involved in the stride? In order to get around at all on two legs (and not just fitfully, as a bear does) some crucial anatomical novelties must be bought from evolution's store. Upright posture requires a lumbar curve in the backbone to pull the trunk back and over the legs. If the body were not pulled back by a reverse curve in the lumbar region, the twisting of the pelvis during striding would throw the trunk completely out of balance and we would fall flat on our faces. Biologically the human foot is a wild and improbable thing —as noted even by such Greeks as Anaxagoras. The foot is our secret of success and came before the ballooning of the brain, which caused hunting tools and fire to be developments of so early a pre-man as *Australopithecus prometheus*. Note, for example, that by using the heel (a human novelty), the outer border and the ball of the foot as a tripod basis of support, man can even stand on one leg and often does. The natives of the Nilotic Sudan rest in that way. But it is the big toe that is the secret of true walking. We know for sure that *Homo habilis* walked with a striding gait, since his fossil big toe is both tilted and twisted with respect to its shaft— an anatomical feature found otherwise only in modern man.

When we look carefully at the act of human striding we realize that step by step the body teeters on the edge of catastrophe. It is only the rhythmic forward movement of first one leg, then the other, that keeps us from falling forward, although this is not true of the early australopithecine trot. We begin the strange exercise when the muscles of the calf relax from the tension of standing still and the body sways automatically forward, acted upon by gravity. The sway places the center of body weight in front of us so one leg must swing forward in order to widen the pedestal and ensure that the center of body weight again rests within the pedestal. The amount by which the pelvis can rotate decides the distance the swinging leg can move forward. We do not paw our way forward. The "stance" or rear leg provides the propulsive force. It pushes against the ground first with the ball of the foot, then the all-important big toe achieves the push-off. Once the stance foot leaves the ground, the leg enters the swing phase. As the leg swings forward it can clear the ground because it is bent at the hip, knee and ankle. At the same time that the pelvis is stabilized with respect to the stance leg, it also rotates to the unsupported side. This small rotation has the effect of increasing the length of the stride. One must note a sexual difference here. A woman generally straggles behind, not because of high heels, but because the proportionately larger size of her pelvis has the effect of lessening the range through which her hip can move forward and back. This is why for a given length of stride women must rotate the pelvis through a greater angle than men, a bone movement which involves a certain swing of the buttocks which men have always found peculiarly charming and provocative.

During normal striding, the stance phase takes up about 60 per cent of the cycle, the swing phase 40 per cent. Not all walking is striding, which is especially characterized by striking of the heel at the start of the stance and the push-off at the end. On a slippery surface such as ice, short steps are used in which the push-off and heel strike are omitted, or if they are not, the walker finds himself skidding to a crash landing.

There remains the question in incentive. Why did the australopithecines *want* to walk on two feet? Probably the answer is in order to hunt better, since walking is a good way to cover long distances with an economy of energy. Bipedality also gives the creature the freedom of his hands to carry food from one place to another for later eating. The development of the powerful thigh muscles, peculiar to man, actually was not necessary for walking on the level in most of the African savannas. Such muscles are needed for running or walking up slopes and probably occurred later in evolution than the other changes—the lumbar curve and the marvelous human foot.[10]

Let us return to the progress of the four-footed mammal. As we have mentioned, the "true" quadrupedal walk is a locomotive pattern that we see everywhere non-human mammals are present, but of course the life of mammals also involves a lot of running, hopping and leaping. Animals that are used to a life of constant locomotion, such as foxes and wolves, are the most pitiable of all caged animals. The coyote has been timed at forty-three miles per hour in a straight line, which puts him in nearly the class with the greyhound. The wolf cannot sprint faster than about twenty miles per hour, but he can get along for many hours at an implacable lope, eventually to wear down the fastest deer. Coyotes and wolves, by running in relays, often are able to pull down that dazzlingly fleet animal, the antelope, who can travel up to sixty miles per hour for several miles. Most hoofed animals have four toes on each foot, but the antelope has only two.[11] He has lost even the bony remnants of the lateral toes (called "dew

[10] Although walking was a good way to move armies around through several thousand years, it no longer is efficient enough, even for "armies of protest." It is interesting to recall that in the depression year of 1893 there was unemployment and rioting in many American cities and in 1894 "General" Jacob Coxey started from Massillon, Ohio, to march on Washington. By the time he got there, he had about 400 people left from the tens of thousands who had started from all over the country. Yet in 1963 Martin Luther King called for a march on Washington and 250,000 people poured in—a triumph of modern transportation over the human foot.
[11] From an evolutionary standpoint, the modern horse walks elegantly on the nails of its middle fingers.

claws") of his ancestors. Antelopes are not only fast but also incredibly nimble. They can flash through a space no more than a foot high between the ground and the lower strand of a fence.

The fastest mammal in the forest country is the varying hare who can go at thirty miles per hour and may leap twelve feet. As it speeds up, its hind feet swing farther forward and at full run the hind feet hit the earth several feet ahead of the front paws. To a less exaggerated degree, this is common practice in all four-legged running. The jack rabbit, living as it does in open country, is still faster. In times of real stress, as when hunted by a coyote, he may reach forty-five miles per hour with leaps of from fifteen to twenty feet and can be pursued and caught only by the still faster greyhound. Some animals, such as the mountain goat, put their trust in nimbleness rather than speed. The bottom of each cloven hoof is hollowed out and the edge is sharp, enabling this shy animal to stick to rocks with what amount to suction cups. His greatest hazard actually is not predators but winter avalanches. Snow slides are believed to kill more mountain goats than any other single cause.

Some quadrupeds never walk. The legs of the guinea pig, for example, are adapted for running and nothing else. It does most of its living at night, and its wild ancestors probably escaped by running in the dark.

Although an opossum walks (and with notable absent-mindedness—I have had one approach me with an abstracted expression and walk right between my legs), its favorite locomotion is climbing. Its hind feet are even better "hands" than the front feet because they have very long flexible front toes. Like the thumb of a man, this big toe can meet any of the other four toes of the same foot. Thus the opossum goes around grabbing things with its hind feet the way people use their hands. (Indeed, the extraordinary handiness of this ancient creature would seem to prove that simply having hands and even opposable thumbs is not enough to pull oneself out of the animal abyss. One must probably, as in man, combine handiness with "footiness.")

Let us consider the mammals who prefer swimming. But first of all, why do so many people drown because they never learned to swim, while any dog (an animal who is not normally fond of water sports) can swim? A dog does a most remarkable and wise thing when he finds himself in deep water. First he paddles furiously, gasping in air as fast as he can. Then he relaxes, because he has *swallowed* enough air to inflate his intestinal tract—he has turned his bowels into a kind of swim bladder that keeps him afloat. He is able to swim without panic and with purpose. (I don't know whether this could be made to work with a human being, but the ease with which even babies can be taught to swim indicates that man, although far from an aquatic animal, can readily adapt. The recent discovery that the human lung can actually obtain oxygen when submerged in aerated water emphasizes still further this innate adaptability. The trouble is that a drowning person needs more oxygen than he can get from breathing water, because he burns up energy so fast in hollering and flouncing around.)

Ocean mammals, such as seals, who decided to return to water long after the cetaceans (whales, porpoises) made their historical move, had to make some fundamental adjustments in their blood circulating systems. When a seal dives, certain arteries in the body automatically constrict. This blocks the blood supply to the outer tissues and preserves the oxygen supply for organs that have to have it continually, such as the heart and the brain. The air that the seal has taken into his lungs before diving must be parsimoniously spent. The constriction of small arterial branches is so intense that the blood flow is completely cut off to the muscles, the skin, the kidney, the liver, the spleen—all organs except the brain and heart. How necessary this automatic reaction is may be seen by preventing it. If you drug a trained seal with atropine, which blocks the arterial diving response, the seal will drown within four minutes.

There are some people that have, in effect, made themselves into seals by rigorous training. The famous diving women of Korea and Japan, who harvest shellfish by diving as a profession, have been studied in detail by Suk Ki Hong of Yonsei University (Korea) and Herman Rahn of the State University of New York at Buffalo. Theirs is an ancient art and in South Korea was probably practiced before the fourth century. Up until the seventeenth century, the profession included men, but it is now confined to some 30,000 women. For physiological reasons the female is better able to stand the cold water, since she is more richly endowed with subcutaneous fat as insulation. The women (called *ama*) sometimes dive as deep as eighty feet, holding their breath for two minutes. Pregnant women may continue this work up to the day of delivery.

One of the problems is the obvious one of needing goggles, since the human eye does not see clearly under water; yet at eighty-foot depths the goggles create a hazard because the blood pressure increases to an amount that is so much greater than the air pressure in the goggles that the blood vessels in the eyelid lining may burst. Nowadays, in place of goggles, most of these oriental diving ladies use a face mask covering the nose, so air from the lungs can boost the air pressure in front of the eyes. It is traditional but not particularly scientific for the *amas* during a hyperventilating stage before diving to purse their lips and whistle. The hyperventilation removes a goodly amount of carbon dioxide from the blood. By the time the *ama* has dived to a depth of forty feet, the oxygen concentration in the lungs is reduced because the blood has been taking it up, but this is compensated for by the fact that water pressure has compressed her lungs to one half. So the oxygen *pressure* is greater than before the dive. For the same reason, the blood also takes up carbon dioxide during the dive, since compression of the lungs raises the pressure of this gas to a point greater than it is in the veins. When the diver comes back to the surface, carbon dioxide flows out of the blood, the concentration of the lung oxygen drops suddenly and the blood may lose instead of gain oxygen. This is a dangerous moment. For this reason, many unwise sports divers faint and even die after long, deep dives.[12]

By what bodily mechanism does the professional woman diver accustom herself to long summer and winter diving days in a professional career which may last thirty or forty years? Her body does not have the automatic reflexes of the seal that channel the blood entirely to the heart and brain. (She would not be very useful with bloodless hands.) Her most important acquisition, by training rather than heredity, is "vital capacity" —the volume of air that she can draw into the lungs in a single breath after a complete exhalation. Her heart also is unusual. During hyperventilation before the dive, the heart rate reaches 100 beats per minute. Twenty seconds after submersion, it has dropped to seventy and after thirty seconds to sixty. The deep body temperature goes down to 95° Fahrenheit or less. There is a total heat loss of about a thousand kilocalories per day. To compensate for this, the Korean *ama* eats 50 per cent more high-energy food than the average Korean woman. Nevertheless these extraordinary females subject themselves daily to a greater cold stress than any other group of human beings on earth, including the Eskimos. The Eskimos show almost as high a basal metabolic rate, but this is probably on account of their very high protein diet. It is possible that severe and habitual exposure to cold water stimulates the thyroid gland to jazz up the body's chemical machinery.

Although, by virtue simply of being women, these divers lose less heat than they would if all their fat were turned to muscle (which conducts heat twice as fast as fatty tissue), the divers lose heat more slowly than non-divers with the same amount of fat. There is evidently some kind of vascular adaptation that restricts the loss of heat from the blood vessels to

[12] This syndrome has nothing to do with the "bends," which used to be frequent among male pearl divers in the Tuamotu Archipelago of the South Pacific, whose repeated dives to 120 feet or more resulted in accumulation of nitrogen in the blood, which burst out of solution in quick ascents to the surface, causing vascular hemorrhage.

the skin, especially in the arms and legs. In the winter the *ama* loses half of her fat, probably because the food intake does not compensate for the greater heat loss. But her body has learned one amazing trick. She does not shiver. Shivering, which was a device invented in order that our ancestors could make their luxuriant body hair stand up and encompass more insulating air pockets, is a disadvantage for hairless bodies since it increases the skin surface and therefore boosts the rate of heat loss. It would be better if we shivered when it is hot. The *ama*'s victory over shivering is an impressive demonstration of human adaptability and gives us hope that many of the bad habits of our ancient forebears that evolution has not had time to erase may yield to training or skilled biological sculpture.

When it is a question of getting around better in water, we tend to pay more attention to the dolphin than the fish, primarily because it is a fellow mammal in the range of our weight and size and obviously in possession of a sophisticated brain and of some emotions that we can share. He also gets the point. For example, if we want to find out how fast he can swim, we blow an underwater whistle and he starts over a measured water course, receiving three fish as a reward but six fish for a fast run. This encourages fast dolphins. In their careful study of the Pacific bottlenose dolphin (*Tursiops gilli*), Professor Kenneth S. Norris of UCLA in Hawaii and Thomas G. Lang of the U. S. Naval Ordnance Test Station at Point Mugu, California, have recorded a well-documented maximum speed of 16.1 knots, which may disappoint some dolphin enthusiasts who imagined speeds in the 30-knot range. During a fast run the dolphin will swim partly on his side less than one yard under water, while the tail never breaks the surface, each tail beat making itself known, however, by separate little boils in a smooth surface of sea. The tail beats averaged out at two and a half per second. When accompanied by a boat, a dolphin tends to horse around, attracted much like a dog chasing an automobile. He may spend a good deal of his time swimming in the bow wave of a speed-boat or aft in one of the spilling waves of the wake, probably obtaining some artificial thrust from the pressure field of the boat or from the wake. Norris and Lang concluded that no mysterious body-participation or water-smoothing apparatus in the skin was necessary to explain the hydrodynamics of this kind of dolphin.

Other students of dolphin swimming do not agree. Perhaps other species show more astonishing feats. In fact Lang himself, in collaboration with Karen Pryor of the Oceanic Institute of Oahu, Hawaii, later found that the smaller dolphin (*Stenella attenuata*) could attain a speed of twenty knots over a period of seven seconds. Calculations showed that either the water drag (resistance) was several times lower or the power output was several times greater than that expected of a torpedo with power equivalent to that of a human being. They seem inclined to give the credit to the greater ability of the dolphin to put out bursts of power to explain what has become known as "Gray's Paradox"—the fact of the unexplained high speeds of fishes and porpoises, compared to mechanical water vehicles. They also find a pronounced difference in the performance between species, the pelagic (oceanic) dolphins being faster than the coastal dolphins.

Short-term high-speed bursts of activity of any animal can usually be explained by the fact that the muscles use up more oxygen than is replaced; they go into the "oxygen debt" that has become such a well-known phrase since the 1968 Olympic Games in Mexico City. Human athletes can produce 6 horsepower in a single movement of the arms and legs, but at six seconds this goes down to 0.32 horsepower and to 0.03 horsepower for one day. At the same time that Gray's Paradox becomes less paradoxical, the intensity of research into activities (such as speed swimming) became enhanced. The 21-knot pelagic porpoise *Phocoenoides dulli* is credited with three times the total blood-sugar content of the beloved Florida dolphin *Tursiops trunctatus*, and the top speeds of these two species lie in the same order. For a period of a second and a half at least the power output of any dolphin is about two and a half times greater than a human athlete of the same weight. The dolphin is advantaged by a greater ratio of muscle weight to body weight, a better muscle distribution and greater oxygen content in the blood. Lang and Pryor still find no evidence that the dolphin's water resistance is any less when swimming than when coasting or any less than an equivalent rigid body.

In spite of these rather disillusioning measurements, the fact remains that the dolphin and all cetaceans have very unusual skin structure, and some engineers, by imitating it, have designed faster torpedoes. The dolphin's skin consists of a pressure-sensitive diaphragm on the surface of a multichanneled, fluid-filled, three-layer hide. The diaphragm can transmit pressure oscillations caused by turbulent water to the fluid-filled ducts below the surface where a kind of damping takes place, just as your tossings and turnings are damped on a well-designed bed. The fluid, which is water, absorbs part of the turbulent energy from outside the skin. Because the fluid is water (a dolphin's entire outer layer of skin is waterlogged) and water is not as good a damping fluid as, say, molasses, the underskin ducts are also filled with soft spongy material like foam rubber. Max Kramer, a German engineer who has been studying the dolphin's skin structure since 1955, designed a coating to simulate it, consisting of a rubber diaphragm supported by parallel ribs, between which an oily damping fluid is stored. When tested as a covering on torpedo models towed at speeds up to forty knots, this was claimed to give a 50 per cent reduction in drag. Somewhat similar artificial dolphin skins have been experimentally applied to reduce the drag of surface ships and to cut down the pressure loss in large water pipes. A summary of all experimental developments to date seems to show that such skins work best at the top speed for which the dolphin was designed by evolution—at about twenty-two knots, which seems reasonable. If we are after much higher speeds, we should imitate water animals that are intrinsically faster than the dolphin.

As for flying, the mammals can boast of a splendidly skilled aviator, the bat, who is a much more accomplished night-flier than the owl. And we have the endearing flying squirrel, who is a million or so years from attaining full aeronautical capability but is nonetheless a cuddly and nimble little friend. For thousands of centuries he has been trying to fly and has learned only to glide. Perhaps sixty feet above the ground in a tree he will gather his feet together and with a great spring will leap off into space, cheeping "Geronimo!" Immediately he spreads out all four legs at right angles to the body. This stretches the "wings" which actually are folds of skin covered with fine, closely knit fur. Extending from the sides and lower flanks as far as the wrist and ankle, they connect the fore and hind legs on each side. By varying the slack in his wings, he can control the angle, speed and course of his glide. Mostly he will steer with his tail and may in midair make an abrupt turn of 90 degrees or more. For people who know how to make friends with squirrels it is great fun (for the animal too) to play catch with a flying squirrel. No matter how hard you throw him, he will check himself and reach the catcher with the momentum of a dove's feather. They are very gregarious and practice group living. When a multiapartment martin house in Idaho was taken down for the annual fall cleaning, it was found to be occupied by six screech owls, twenty bats and twenty flying squirrels.

If the squirrels were trying to learn better flying from their nocturnal neighbors, they were out of their class. The Mexican free-tailed bats, who make a sort of capital home city out of the Carlsbad Caverns in New Mexico, have been studied in modern detail by Harold E. Edgerton of MIT and his associates. Every evening, about 250,000 bats leave the cavern for the Pecos River feeding area, some fifty miles away. The air traffic is naturally congested and the bats must usually circle many times to clear the cave entrance, but their foolproof sonar instrumentation avoids any collision incidents. (The crowded air over our airports and our inability to do anything about it would astonish a bat.) The wing membrane between legs (or actually between "hands") plays the crucial role in flight for climbing, diving, turning and braking. The tail membrane of the free-tailed bat also could give greater maneuverability, but there is a catch in this. All the naked skin of wings and tail, when fully extended, loses heat and water at a tremendous rate. The bat is thus at a disadvantage compared with a bird, since a bird's feathers contain no circulating blood and the bird's problem while flying is to lose heat rather than to conserve it. It goes without saying that a bat does not need and would be embarrassed and probably frozen to death by the air sacs that birds are equipped with.

High-speed photographs show that the bat does not flutter its wings in a birdlike manner but uses them mostly in the half-folded position as air brakes to control the velocity of a dive. As in a bird, the sternum bears a keel to which the large pectoral muscles are attached. The shoulder girdle strangely resembles that of a brachiating (tree-swinging) primate, such as a spider monkey. By radar tracking, it has been found that certain semitropical species of bats can easily find their way home when released ten miles or more from the home roost. When the bats are blindfolded, however, they fly any which way, hence there is nothing more mysterious involved than a birdlike eye-mindedness.

In the course of man's sudden lurch into the air and beyond the air, he has come up against the stern biological fact that he was not designed to be in several wide longitudes of the earth within a few hours (his own circadian clock, that governs his appetite and his sleeping habits, was not wound up for such world-hopping) and certainly evolution did not sculpture his body with the idea of popping up to the moon or visiting around the solar system. In trying to find out what happens to terrestrial life under violent and peculiar circumstances, he has experimented with many organisms, including himself, subjecting them to super-acceleration (high-G) of take-off from the earth and to prolonged weightlessness.

Three generations of mice, for example, were made by NASA to live, make love and bear their young in an animal centrifuge simulating three times the gravity of the earth. All appeared healthy but were a little on the overweight side, possibly from underexercise. Although pregnant mice centrifuged for their lifetime never lost their ground-level agility, their offspring raised from birth at two Gs were never fully as lively as ground-level mice. On the other hand, Professor A. H. Smith spun generation after generation of chicks for six years in a similar centrifuge. This animal is more like man in one sense: It walks upright on two feet and its organs are vertically arranged, unlike mice and guinea pigs. One of the significant changes was dwarfing. The heart became smaller in size and there was a delay in reaching sexual maturity. Yet the most hopeful sign was that the chickens can develop resistance to these high-G forces and *this resistance is heritable*. Soviet scientists have concentrated on an unusual animal which shows remarkable tolerance toward superacceleration—the giraffe. Probably because of the long pumping distance to the brain, the giraffe's heart is a very powerful machine and the Russians think that further study may help them in either the selection of astronauts with stout hearts or in training the human heart muscle to withstand the jolting accelerations of space flight.

The problems of weightlessness (of what happens to organisms in zero G) have been even more closely studied, and of course a fairly large amount of experience with live astronauts has been collected, although we still do not know what would happen during a long voyage, since a moon flight or two weeks in orbit represents, so to speak, merely suburbanite astronauting. Plants, who are conservatives and have been completely satisfied with living for eons in the one-G environment of our good blue little world, show a loss of cool when they try to grow in an outer-space rocket. A pepper plant, for example, has a kind of nervous breakdown. Its leaves fail to grow in the normal horizontal position and the stems do not stay vertical but bend in weird distortions. The individual cells of plant tissues in zero G, in fact, show an abnormal mitosis (cell division), so that in the process of growth it is evident that the plant has been perturbed in its profoundest fundamental comforts.

What little research (mostly Russian) that has been done on insects shows that houseflies tend to develop very curious and specific mutations when they breed in zero G. One half of the body of the space-born fly tends to be shortened and one wing is poorly wired with nerves. One half of the thorax may be missing and one eye may be smaller and roughened—probably useless. Although it is a long time before we face any problem such as human parturition or even conception in deep space, some studies are being carried out on opossums because they are born in the embryonic state only twelve days after being conceived and one can therefore get a lot of data on a mammal, even if it is only a marsupial.

As far as humans are concerned, man shows his usual brilliant, perhaps even silly plasticity. The problem is actually not that man cannot adapt to a weightless state, but that he adapts too well. Being precisely the other end of evolution from a pepper plant, his body becomes addicted to zero G. One can simulate long space voyages by simply keeping a man immersed in water for days or weeks, and invariably it takes a lot of will power to leave the tank even for routine tests. Just by keeping the body erect on earth against the pull of gravity, as we have seen, results in the distribution of calcium in the bones. Without the stimulus of gravity, the bones do not yell out for calcium and because, just as in the case of amino acids, the body cannot *store* calcium, it is excreted in the urine. Not only is 5 to 7 per cent of the body's bone content lost after from seven to eight weeks of weightlessness, but there is a strong possibility that kidney stones will form. This points to the necessity of some regular exercise during a trip to Mars, where the muscles instead of pushing or pulling against gravity must exert themselves against inertia. A fist fight between astronauts (an eventuality by no means impossible to imagine in a very long voyage) would be quite spectacular, and the first knockout would undoubtedly be received by the man who missed with his Sunday punch and catapulted himself with a jarring crash against the capsule wall.

However, the exercise schedule must be mild because of another, perhaps even more serious effect of weightlessness. The body loses blood during space flight, both in plasma volume and red cell mass. Exercise with friction devices, isometrics, etc., can cause a further decrease in red blood cells, because the bone marrow output of the blood cells is reduced by the lower demands in general on the circulation system during weightlessness.

The psychiatric factors of deep space have undoubtedly been exaggerated, since it is man's mind that is his most resilient possession and even when he is in a crazy situation, he is less likely than other animals to die of craziness.

CHAPTER 6

The Unknown and
Forgotten Senses

Look Homeward, Angel

IN THE COURSE of this chapter we shall be confronting
kinds of animal behavior that escape analysis and in some
cases even classification. For the "practical" scientist such con-
frontations are nearly as traumatic as the experience of seeing
a ghost. Aside from the risk of a nervous breakdown, there
is another reason for scientific distaste of the unexplainable
that involves the process of getting to be an accredited scholar.
Behavior that eludes systematic applications of textbook neurology is not likely to be good material for a Ph.D. thesis. In
order to proceed in an orderly way up the stately stairs of
Academe, one should start with a modest, *soluble* problem,
even though it adds up to no more than a footnote to one's
professor's textbook. The work need not involve actually any
new experiment. One can get by in biology by the application
of awesome statistical abracadabra to data accumulated by great
numbers of separate biologists. It is thus for very human reasons
that the field of the "homing" of birds and other animals, once
the focus of enthusiastic bionics research, has suddenly dropped
almost out of the picture or, as Robert Ardrey suggests, has
been swept under the rug. The answers did not come—or at

least answers *within* the domain of established scientific principles did not come, so biologists, young and old, abandoned the area as if it were plague-ridden.

It is not plague-ridden; it is simply haunted by unknown signals. It is as if an eighteenth-century naturalist were suddenly handed a transistor set and could hear the transcribed sounds of the electromagnetic waves of the future. In a sense this is not an adequate simile because the theory of electromagnetic waves was already inherent in the concept of "forces at a distance" assumed by Newton. Radio and television were immense but nevertheless reasonable extrapolations. In exploring unexplained happenings one needs to draw a line between explanations that are supernatural and those that are merely *superhuman*. The original experiments on the "sun compass" of ants showed that they could face themselves toward their home colony even when enclosed in a box so that the sky was visible but the sun was not. The people who became discouraged over this finding rather feebly assumed that the ants were in some way perceiving the stars during daylight and thus using them as points of orientation. This is a silly, *supernatural* explanation, since there is nothing about insect eyes which would allow them to filter out all the interfering light from the sky and still leave that of the stars. A *superhuman* explanation would be that ants have an unforgettable memory of directionality that man does not possess but that is the natural heritage of a large number of animals that have been in the universe a good deal longer than man. (Or, said in another way, these animals have neural capabilities that have in man been buried under the complex weight of a brain preoccupied by *symbolic* rather than *natural* signals.)

In this book I have emphasized and shall continue to emphasize the pragmatic usefulness of metaphysics, especially for animals of a low degree of cortical complexity. To posit the existence of transcendental memory is a much more practical way to explain otherwise inexplicable animal behavior than other answers, for example, the incredible notion that a bird is able within a few seconds to decide infallibly how to use a phantom sextant, how to measure and correct precisely for time changes due to longitude changes and how to correct such data continuously while changing longitude or latitude at the speed of an early airplane. In the case of the green turtles and other island finders, we have no adequate explanation at all, although such gifted naturalists as Archie Carr have not yet quite given up.

The pragmatism of the metaphysical approach to animals and even to plants divorces naturalism from the almost ritualistic attempts to explain everything in a computerized mechanistic manner. Before we are able to make a computer as good as a homing pigeon or a pregnant female green turtle determined to lay her eggs on Ascension Island, we shall ourselves need to have changed the human mind to such an extent that it will no longer be sensible to call it human. We shall have realized that infrahuman life has secrets we can never learn until we are superhuman. In the meanwhile, contemplating the greater familiarity with this planet of lower species, we tend toward hoary rituals as predictable as other rituals of human life.[1] Finding them unsuccessful, petulantly we throw our marbles in the gutter and go home to find some more tangible task such as plotting the complications of the DNA molecule. (Yet here, precisely, we butt our heads against chemically incorrigible, inexplicable behavior. We find ourselves asking ultimate questions as frightening as how fishes and cephalopods can predict earthquakes. For there is no weak salient in the wonderfully massive fact of life. If we abandon the homing of birds, we will abandon the far more impenetrable mysteries of "what" tells the DNA molecule "when" to do "what.")

Before we get to the birds, it is noteworthy that homing

[1] Some of the rituals have been engraved in patterns of intellectual games. For example, the "mystery story" and the "spy story" are based on fictions that the reader readily accepts as ordinances in a never-never land of gamesmanship. There was never in the history of the world any murderer one tenth as clever as those in the mystery novels of Agatha Christie. Even science fiction of the "adventurous" type (e.g., *Star Trek* on TV) may be based on absolutely unacceptable assumptions, for example, that men have learned how to travel faster than light.

instincts are unmistakable in forms of much lower organization. Eugene Marais contends that the directional influence that the king and queen of a termitarium exert on worker or soldier castes cannot be explained in full by chemical signals, particularly in the case of the queen, who can summon or control her sexless offspring as if they were still attached by invisible threads to her swollen body. A worker termite can be encased in chemical insulation in a steel box buried a good distance from the royal chamber. Yet even amidst succulent food, it will respond to an unheard, unseen, unsmelled influence that tells it to get home. It will desperately try to pierce the unpierceable walls of its artificial prison, always in the direction of the unhearable call. What is it sensing? If the queen is killed, the worker subsides into apathy. We can say "This is a *psi* phenomenon. The termite has extrasensory perception." But let us make it clear that such a statement has no mystical significance; in fact, it has very little significance at all. When we say "extrasensory," we should imply simply that the termite has senses that we do not know about, since we do not normally have such senses ourselves. Lacking any better information, it would be better for us to say that the signal between queen and termite worker involves *superhuman means of communication*.

As we have discussed previously, ants, bees and, in fact, all the colonial hymenoptera have not only a vivid sense of home and how to get there, but when things are to be "taken home," there is an exquisitely accurate estimate of how to go about doing it. For example, an ant wandering far from the hill may come upon a dying dragonfly. This is, for an ant, a huge creature, as big as a whale is to a man, but it is valuable food. What does the ant do? It races home by the most direct route and returns with several comrade workers. They begin, like skilled butchers, to dismember the corpse. Nothing is wasted. The legs, wings, head and thorax are separated into slices of portable size; and, with each ant carrying its precisely maximum engineered load, the group files back with its communal booty to the distant mound. There have been exactly enough ants to do the job. There is not an ant left with a skimpy load or with time on its hand to get a drink or smoke a cigarette, as would be the case in a similar human project employing labor union workers. The communication has been as exact to the home colony as is the language of bees.

In Chapters 1 and 2 we dipped into the much-disputed bee language, but we did not mention a remarkable instinctive visual sense concerned with the mating time and place. The females of a colony mate with the drones at a specific place, far from the hive, year after year. This rendezvous conceivably could be recalled by the long-lived queens, but the poor drones are born for one exquisite hot-weather honeymoon and never survive a winter. Yet every drone, spoiled rotten as he has been since birth by his infertile worker sisters, must find his way to the mating area without guides. Entomologists in Germany discovered that the mating area invariably lies on a straight line from the hive to the *lowest* point on the horizon. The drones are born with an instinct to select this line of flight, year after year, generation after generation. Since the lowest contour point that he can see would be, from the standpoint of a human surveyor, practically indistinguishable from another contour point perhaps in an entirely different direction, it is evident that the compound eyes of the drone have incredible sensitivity to perhaps a few minutes or even seconds of an arc. His whole life's mission (the only purpose of his eyes) is to find this precious direction rapidly and, having flown it, to locate the object of his affections, again with rapidity, for the female is imperious and impatient and there are a lot of other suitors buzzing around. The drone, as a sort of seeing baggage of spermatozoa, may not make it. He may die in vain. Yet he has tried—he has always flown in the right direction.

We have already considered under Chapter 3, "Signaling with Molecules," the probability that the Pacific salmon finds its native brook by a search after a home stream smell or taste. But this is only the last lap. First he has to locate the right river. And in many cases the reverse process (by which the yearling salmon, or smolts, find the right outlet from a lake to an ocean-bound river) is equally mysterious. The Dutch zoologist C. Groot investigated this behavior in some lakes of British Columbia. All around the shores of the lake front he observed that the smolts began moving toward the outlet at the same time. Their lake trip was far from exploratory; it was as direct as a rifle shot. In holding the precise heading, the converging schools of little fishes were not confused by wind or by thermal currents in the lake. Since they were fresh out of the nest and had never been anywhere at all, it is clear that this "reverse homing" behavior, which enables some of them eventually to reach the Pacific Ocean, is an inherited virtue of the particular race of salmon involved. The geography of the lake (the compass direction of the outlet stream) is something that has been born into them and is as old as the lake. (Of course, a lake is not ageless. It can dry or silt up or be cut off by geological chance. Yet the homing instinct persists in fish species that have been landlocked for ages. The lake red salmon returns to spawn, as do trout, in streams where they were born; a lake has taken the place of the sea.) Professor Groot's experiments convinced him that the migration of little salmon from a nursery area to the lake outlet could be governed geographically by more than one sensory system. On clear days the fishes could instinctively use the sun as a compass and perhaps the pattern of polarized light in the sky.[2] Of course, guidance by light polarization is just a form of orientation by the sun serving as a compass. The distribution of differently polarized patches of light in the sky can indicate where the sun is, even when it is not directly visible. This could be quite important to smolts because most of their migrations start at dusk when, although the sun cannot be seen, the polarization patterns are the most pronounced. Groot found no "bico-ordinate" sense in smolts (i.e., the ability to locate oneself not only by latitude but by longitude), but that is not needed until the young salmon swim

[2] As we have previously explained, light that is reflected from water is polarized; that is, the electromagnetic waves that constitute light vibrate only in one plane, the other planes of vibration having been cancelled out by the act of reflection from the water surface.

in the great ocean. All they need as nestlings is to find the river outlet. Years later, in finding their way home to spawn, they will need a more sophisticated navigation system and a tremendous growth in bodily strength and valor.

In truth the story of the Pacific salmon as a navigator is not only dramatic but it means money in the bank. It is a case where the prudent, hard-working, hard-drinking salmon fishermen find themselves up against ghosts. None of the theories work.

For, note that although scientists from Canada, Japan and the United States have co-operated (rather warily) for over a decade in tagging hundreds of thousands of salmon, the co-operative group still has not the faintest idea how the salmon operates as a navigational animal—it only knows its general route. Anthony Netboy of Oregon State University has quite recently summed up the dilemma, but it has been summed up many times before. It is a perfect case (even beyond that of the homing birds) of ancient animals knowing instinctively more about the world than we do.

When the smolts find their way to the ocean from their fresh-water nurseries, they first of all have to establish a reasonable eating schedule. After starting on plankton, when they reach the estuaries, their jaws become powerful enough to eat crustaceans, then small fish such as anchovies, pilchards and herring. The young salmon from northwestern America enter a gigantic counterclockwise movement, not as true schooling fish but as "bands" (brigades rather than hosts), facing toward Alaskan waters, then circling southward then northeastward again. Salmon bands are not comparable to the astronomically sized schools or shoals of fish like herring. Salmon may congregate in numbers equivalent to the human population of a city the size of Baltimore or Seattle.

Note now the international element. A given species of salmon (say, the pinks) will be simultaneously coming from the great Asian rivers of Kamchatka, following a similar revolution throughout the Pacific. They will mingle with their kissing cousins from North America somewhere during these vast sweeps of the Pacific. They will mingle with absolute peaceful-ness (unlike the men who are after them), but when the biological bell starts sounding, the Asian bands and the North American bands will begin swimming for home and at prodi-gious speed and with incredible accuracy. No Kamchatka pink has ever been known to arrive in a North American river and the converse is true. The pinks from both continents make an elliptical 2,000-mile circuit during their salt-water lives, but the chum and the sockeye, which stay longer in the ocean, may make two to three circuits and travel 10,000 miles before re-turning to spawn in Alaska, Canada, Washington or Asia.

The scientific controversy about how the American Pacific salmon and their Asian counterparts carry out this tremendously fast spawning navigational return to their native rivers is much more complicated than the question of how, once in the proper river, they can locate the home stream—the place where they were born. The theory that the fish uses the sun as a compass does not seem to stand up in the face of meteorological data. Along the Pacific routes there are few clear days from one end of the year to the other. Around the Aleutians the skies are almost always overcast, with winds blowing continuously and storms roiling the seas. Even in the milder summer periods the sun is persistently hidden by fog, mist or clouds. If the salmon are sun navigators, they have discovered a technique of sun navigation impossible for a mariner to imagine. A rather ingenious but completely unproven theory of Professor William F. Royce and his associates at the University of Washington would have it that salmon navigate in the open sea—on their fatal dash toward their home rivers—with the help of almost infinitely small voltages generated by ocean currents as they travel through the earth's magnetic field. The sum and substance of our knowledge is that we have none. If we did know, we would be in possession of priceless insights, not only into life but perhaps into the total nature of the earth.

The end of the brilliant return is pathetic and possibly we have a clue to why this is. Geologists have pointed out that most of the incredible up-river runs of the salmon for spawning developed long ago behind the retreating ice of the Pleistocene. The difference of runs between various species represents differences in the reserves of energy of the fish themselves on leaving salt water, those stocks with the greatest reserves pushing on to more and more remote spawning areas as the ice withdrew.

In other words the tragedy of the Pacific salmon in his mass spawning death may be simply a matter of geologic memory. Yet the end is singularly touching. Each female, upon arriving at the native burn or pool, pushes the male (who may indeed be her brother) aside and commences to dig the "redd," the nest for the eggs. After spawning and after the male has released his fertilizing milt, the gaunt female continues in a rather drunken way to dig at the gravel with ever-weakening efforts until she dies. The eggs have been laid, they have been fertilized, and her husband is dead. But this postspawning digging, which may continue for ten days, becomes shallow, off-center, ineffective. The poor mother is in a haze of impending death, and the fact that her fainting, excavating nuzzlings do more harm than good would seem to indicate that the whole cycle is indeed a mistake in geologic time. She is remembering, but without purpose, the cycles of her remotest ancestors.

Consider this splendid animal who, as it enters the sea, is too oily to can, but at the end of its life contains only enough oil barely to provide food for dogs or bears. Yet if it doesn't know how to survive more than its poor cycle, consider also that it knows something about the seas, the rivers, the burns, the universe, in effect, that man with all the elaboration of mathematics and physics available to him has never been able to understand. In another book I shall try to show that man's intricate equipment of scientific thinking—despite his seeming engineering and technical triumphs—has been on the wrong track in trying to elucidate the mysteries of life's ways and life's sojourn on earth.[3]

---

[3] Perhaps the most perceptive hint so far in the last eighty years was that of H. G. Wells in *The War of the Worlds* in which he told how his hypothetical Martians, enormously superior to us in every technical

Note that there are two kinds of migrating fish. The *anadromous* (salmon, shad) migrate from salt water to fresh water to spawn. The *catadromous* (fresh-water eels and gobies) reverse the process. Under the International Council for Study of the Sea, the Danish government appointed Johann Schmidt to spend all his time on the eel problem, which he did from 1905 until his death in 1933.

All eels in rivers of countries that touch the Atlantic Ocean originate in the central mating grounds of the Sargasso Sea. The larval European eels, or *leptocepheli*, except for the Sargasso Sea nursery, are found no deeper than about 150 feet in the waters of the Gulf Stream. Many seem to have no directional urge and, feeding on plankton in a leisurely way, gradually drift toward Europe. However, there *is* a general directional trend, since they would be most embarrassed to find themselves in North American waters, where their cousins go. The European and North American eels are distinguished mainly by a difference in the number of spinal vertebrae (107 for those that wind up in America and 115 for the Europe-bound); yet one would not be found dead in the other's hemisphere although all are born in that mysterious biological magnet—the Sargasso Sea. In the autumn of the third year of life, the drifting, grazing leptocepheli become "elvers," which can swim. The European elvers move into fresh-water rivers and at this point the sexes say good-by to each other for a long time. The males stay near the river mouths and the estuaries, while the females swim far upstream into headwaters. Both eat ravenously, but the females grow bigger. They may sojourn without any sex life for five or even twenty years. (In a Paris aquarium a female eel lived comfortably for thirty-seven years.) When the urge to mate descends upon them, both sexes find their way back to the Sargasso Sea where they breed in the springtime and

---

sense, *had never used the principle of the wheel*. This seemed at the time and still seems to all right-thinking engineers of our world absolutely incredible. Yet the wheel is a simplistic notion. Although it has made our present kind of civilization possible, the wheel is never used by evolution in any of her various creatures. It is as alien to total life as an advertisement for cigarettes.

die. How they guide themselves in making this mass rendezvous (which is nearly equivalent to the green turtle finding Ascension Island) is completely unknown. It should be pointed out, however, that the eel is a creature even more ancient than the marine turtle and has had a long time to become familiar with the geography of the seas, the ways of currents, the smell of seaweed, the signals of the earth as a watery planet.

Curiously there are no fresh-water eels in the Pacific rivers of North or South America but there are several species in the Western Pacific and the Indian Ocean. A. W. Herre of Stanford University saw an "eel fair" (a sexual migration of millions) in the Sepik River of New Guinea. These Pacific eels don't go to the Sargasso Sea and it is simply not known *where* they go or how long it takes them to develop from leptocephali into elvers or how they behave as elvers. (Dr. Schmidt's duties, as he saw them, were to solve the problem of the *Atlantic* eels.) The problem of eel navigation, even to the Sargasso Sea, from all the oceanward flowing rivers of Europe and America, is a dead issue. Nobody has any ideas or feels sufficient incentive to do any more work. This problem has indeed been swept under the rug. In effect, we say, "This is how eels behave. Don't ask us any more please."

We know that the much more modern goby fishes carry out similar movements—to fresh water to mature and enjoy life and back to a salt-water rendezvous to mate; but, aside from the fact that the goby is likelier to have a more personal home than a mere territorial river, we know little or nothing about the goby's navigational techniques. In cases like this we are indeed like Newton's somewhat insincere picture of himself as a witless searcher playing with pebbles on the shore of an illimitable ocean of undiscovered truth.

Even such a humble mollusk as the limpet knows its way home. E. S. Russell, the English ethologist, marked limpets for individual recognition and found that they always returned to the same place at low tide. The limpet in fact becomes branded by his home. As its shell grows, it takes on the shape of the · particular piece of rock it regards as its home rock.

Since man is more compatible with the air than with the water, it is natural that the homing feats of birds have fascinated him ever since he became a bird watcher and bird hunter. The seasonally migrating bird has solved a population problem which should be edifying to man in a time of population and food tensions. By alternately exploiting two different habitats for food, more birds are able to make a living. (Before man became a farmer with fixed property, he too possessed some of this logistic advantage. It is now proposed in fact that, in order to maintain extremely large future populations it will be necessary to move the bulk of the human race to the arctic or antarctic regions—honeycomb them in ice—so that the rest of the planet, including the oceans, can be used merely to grow food. A romantic extension of this is the proposal to colonize other planets of ours or other solar systems. This is essentially a birdlike idea.)

The technique of massive bird movements varies. In so-called "molt migrations" some ducks leave their cool summer breeding areas for sheltered marshes where they molt their old flight feathers and grow new ones; then they fly to their winter headquarters. The migratory urge is not symmetrical over the planet. Thus very few birds native to the Southern Hemisphere are very resolute migrants. In South Africa some twenty species migrate up to the equator for the winter but not one of these gets as far north as Europe. There is a topographical reason for a difference in migratory habits of birds of the New and Old Worlds. In the Americas the great mountain barriers run north and south, while in the Old World they run east and west. In relation to the vast Eurasian breeding ranges, the southern land masses attractive for wintering are displaced toward the west (Africa) and toward the east (the East Indies and Australia). Storks and other soaring birds must remain over land in order to use the thermal currents for long flights. There are zigs and zags and east–west diversions in order to reach the lands of warmth and food. There is nothing as simple as the great duck and geese flyways in North America (the Mississippi, the Pacific, the Atlantic, the Central) or for hawks and other soaring migrants the luxurious up-draft corridors down the Appalachians. While at the famous sanctuary at Hawk Mountain, Pennsylvania, one will see the soaring birds pause on north–south flights, on Kurische Nehrung, the long off-shore island near the southeast shore of the Baltic, one will see as many as half a million birds a day fly by but not necessarily northward or southward.

Some migration paths of birds are, in fact, crooked for no apparent reason but nevertheless constant year after year. It is thought that this is a matter not of biological compulsion but of tradition. Birds are slaves of tradition. Probably the change in the northern landscapes brought about by the recent ice ages and the subsequent recession of the glaciers has affected the migratory flight patterns of birds of older lineage.[4]

The arctic warbler makes its winter quarters in southeast China, Indonesia, the Philippines and Malaysia. One would expect the warblers in Alaska to fly south to equatorial America, but instead of that they take their winter route the hard way, first flying west across the Bering Strait, then migrating south along with the Siberian birds. Warblers in Norway or Finland first fly east about 3,000 miles across Siberia, then go south with their relatives.

It should be emphasized that the migrations always occur long before the late summer or early autumn food supplies grow sparse. The birds are, in fact, usually fat before migrating, because they have to store body fuel. In some species, a sort of training schedule for the big flight is in order, practically the reverse, however, of a prize fighter's training. The wheatear, for example, needs a week of steady, ravenous eating to fatten itself from its very lean condition at the end of molting, just in time to be plumped up for migration. There are some unexplained facts. In the Northern Hemisphere migrations north

---

[4] The strange and pointless maneuvers made by swarms of monarch butterflies flying over Lake Superior on their way south may have some similar origin. At one point over the great lake they all turn east for a while before continuing south. Each successive swarm repeats this pattern year after year.

in the spring always take place at greater speeds than migrations southward in the autumn. This may be connected with sexual phenomena. Sometimes the males and females fly north separately. This may postpone the maturing of the female's sex organs, keep her in better flying trim and ensure a better synchronized honeymoon when the rites of spring take place.

In addition to building up fat for fuel, the birds, days before taking off, start to sleep restlessly at night. This unease is called *Zugunruhe* and in captive migrant birds is especially noticed during warm weather in the spring and by cold weather in the fall.

The homing feats of the migrants have, of course, entered the language of common legend. Banded long-distance migrants have returned to the same pinpoint nesting sites and to the same restricted wintering area. Swallows are reputed in both tale and song to return to the mission of San Juan Capistrano in Southern California precisely on St. Joseph's Day (March 19) every year, come rain, fire or earthquake. Their cousins, the purple martins, show spring migrations at about the same time—arriving, for example, around March 20 in their national capital at Griggsville, Illinois. (This once mosquito-ridden town was one of the first to create vast martin "apartment houses" and, since each martin is supposed to eat up to at least 2,000 mosquitoes a day, Griggsville is regarded as a place singularly free of both mosquitoes and flies. The St. Louis Veterinary Medicine Association recently participated in a big drive to erect more martin houses to help prevent heartworm infestation in dogs, a serious disease carried by mosquitoes.) Also according to local legend, turkey vultures return to Hinckley, Ohio, on March 15 of each year—where they spend spring and summer in the cliffs and caverns of Old Whipp's Ledges.

Actually, there is a somewhat more complicated process involved in such migratory homing than simple mass descent. The swallows, for example, send out scouts, to see how things are in Capistrano (and probably in Glocca Morra) before the true mass migration. The purple martins have similar advance agents who check the condition of the houses and apartments, and report back to the flocks who may have made a half-way stop.

Not all birds migrate, of course, and some, such as wrens, English sparrows and doves, do not even seem to have much homing sense. Experiments with the migratory California sparrow, however, have shown an unexpected mastery of strange geography. It can find its way home to San Jose, California, for example, if carried in a box by airplane to Baton Rouge, Louisiana, and even to Laurel, Maryland—a distance of over 3,500 miles and over country it has never seen before. This is a much greater homing feat than migrating in a flock northward or southward along traditional flightways. The Manx shearwater, a sea bird, has been shown to be capable of an analogous stunt. One was carried by airplane from England to Boston, Massachusetts, about 5,000 miles from its breeding island off the coast of Wales. After banding and release in Boston, it decided at once to escape its barbarous surroundings and was found twelve and a half days later back on its home island. Transoceanic flights of this sort (westward or eastward) are thoroughly unnatural, even to sea birds, and usually happen only by accident, usually on account of storms. Because of prevailing winds it is more unnatural for land birds to fly westward across the North Atlantic than eastward. Fewer than twelve species of European land birds have been known to cross the Atlantic to North America, although forty-eight species of native North American birds are recorded in Europe. The cattle egret and the fieldfare are the only Old World species known historically to have established themselves in the New World as breeding birds without human help. The egret (originally from Europe but now more common in South Africa) has also expanded its activities—which include debugging cattle—to Australia. Much to the consternation of present bird lovers and lovers of peace and quiet, men and women deliberately established the European starling in North America, where it has become one of the most boisterous successes of history. The house sparrow and the Chinese ring-necked pheasant have been perhaps even more successfully introduced here by forcible invitation. The presence in America of these sometimes undesirable aliens is due to a wave of nuttiness in the late nineteenth century among dewy-eyed but reckless bird romanticizers, one sect of which insisted that every bird ever mentioned in the works of Shakespeare should be made to live here. There were also "acclimatization societies" in the United States dedicated to the importation and release of all exotic bird species, regardless of whether they had been known to the great bard or not. A group in Cincinnati liberated 3,000 birds of twenty species, but had no luck. None survived. In the Hawaiian Islands, however (a more bland and hospitable environment) some fifty species have been introduced but at the expense of about two thirds of the original native birds. (It has thus proved possible for man to extinguish animal species, not only through minding his own business, which is usually at odds with the business of other living creatures, but by *failing* to mind his own business. The gentle and attractive bluebird, for instance, has in this country been harassed in the direction of extinction by that ubiquitous and aggressive hoodlum, the starling.)

One must not overlook, however, the great help that the wide interest in birds among people everywhere has been to scientific studies. The bird-banding program, which the U. S. Fish and Wildlife Service took over in 1920, includes the banding with little pieces of aluminum of about 15 million birds in North America alone. Many spectacular facts have come out of this program. It has been found, for instance, that the yellowleg can migrate 1,900 miles in six days. The arctic tern has been crowned the champion of all. It nests in the far north, then sweeps down the Atlantic and Pacific flyways for a second polar summer in Antarctica. The round trip is over 23,000 miles. By banding, such mysteries as the wintering area of the chimney swift, long an exasperating problem to ornithologists, was solved when some Peruvian Indians turned in thirteen banded birds in the upper Amazon basin.

In sea birds of enormous feeding range, such as the albatross, the homing instinct for nesting is nevertheless infallible. Albatrosses (gooney birds) mate for life and the pairs invariably build each year's new nest not only on the same island but within a few feet of last year's nest. On the island of Guam this insistence on a pinpoint "home" was a sad problem for bull-dozing crews during and after World War II. In order to build landing strips the crews had to move about 100 nests with live chicks up to 100 yards from the original sites, a job they thought they had performed with the utmost of care and even tenderness. But the chicks' parents ignored them in the new location. As far as the mother and father albatross were concerned, their offspring had disappeared from the world. Bringing food back from the sea the adult birds returned to where their homes *had* been and dumped the fish. All the chicks starved to death. The ferocious bird, the skua, also marries for life and returns to the same breeding colony where he was hatched. This is usually either next door to a penguin colony, on which the skuas prey, or near where the Weddell seals have their young, since the skua has developed a perverse appetite for seal placenta. (It is also one of the few cannibals known among non-human animal species.) The skua's navigational instincts are superb. When released from an airplane at the South Pole, it will un-erringly find its way home over an immense continent as unfamiliar to it as the mountains of the moon.

For land and even sea birds one might conclude that whole continents and oceans are maps remembered in the genes. Before considering any such heritage, it is useful to remind oneself that birds have better eyes than we have. A bird has colored eye droplets and may discern things invisible to us. From up in the farther air, birds may recognize a terrestrial physiognomy as a person recognizes a face in a crowd or the photograph of an old friend.[5] Since we have mentioned the penguin, consider the homing abilities of such a bird *who cannot even fly*. He has not even man's standing height to make his surveys from. John T. Emler of the University of Wisconsin and Richard L. Penney of the Institute of Animal Behavior (a New York

[5] We have noted in Chapter 1 that pigeons can distinguish between photographs that contain images of man or man-relevant objects and pictures free of human taint.

facility sponsored jointly by Rockefeller University and the New York Zoological Society) carried out a most difficult field study on the Adelie penguins who form migratory societies in the Antarctic. Each spring and fall the Adelies travel hundreds of miles between the outer fringes of the antarctic pack ice and their rookeries on the coast of the continent. The penguin is, of course, a splendid swimmer, but otherwise it walks and tobog-gans its way and fasts completely for weeks during the nesting season. Since its range is along the coast, it has no more reason to be familiar with the vast inland areas of this continent than did Robert Scott in his tragic venture toward the pole. Individual birds were released far inland from man-made underground burrows, one by one, so that they could not follow one another. Most of them had been taken from Cape Crozier where about 300,000 birds gather each nesting season. The season of these experiments was polar summer, during which the sun never rises nor sets but moves around above the horizon. The sun's movements are therefore mainly azimuthal (that is, it seems to cover a lot of ground from one direction on the horizon to another, but is never overhead). To navigate with the use of a sun-compass that is behaving this way is much more of a job than with a sun that properly rises, attains a prominent position at high noon and proceeds regularly toward its setting. Never-theless it was apparent that the penguins, when released, used the sun to point themselves north toward the sea. When freed the bird would make a few excited waddles in various directions, then stand and peer at the experimenters' transit tripods, the human shelter buildings and finally see the sun. Then they would set off, infallibly northward. On a clear day their waddles and tobagganings were in amazingly straight-line distances. When the sun was veiled by thin clouds, the performance of the penguins became uncertain and when heavy clouds prevailed, the pen-guins would zig and zag in clownish frenzy and at random.

From a technical standpoint, in order to hold a constant course while one's sun-compass is swinging around the horizon calls for a continuous knowledge of the passing of time—not only a continuous but a very accurate internal clock. Yet the penguins did not care what time of day they were released; always they turned northward. In the morning this meant heading about 90 degrees to the left of the sun; at noon, straight toward the sun; and in the afternoon 90 degrees to the *right* of the sun.

The fact that all the Cape Crozier birds, wherever released, went along parallel courses, regardless of the direction of their rookery, shows that they were primarily trying to *escape*, to reach the good cold water and to elude the desert of snow and massive mountains of ice. Birds taken from Mirnyy, a coastal colony in the Russian-controlled area far removed from Cape Crozier, took the same direction as the American-colony birds. Note that this involved a resetting of internal clocks since the time zone of Mirnyy is 88 degrees to the east of Cape Crozier, equivalent to the six-hour time difference between London and Chicago. With reset clocks, the Mirnyy birds chose also the straight-line route to the sea.

All of the penguins, both from Cape Crozier and Mirnyy, having come in sight of the Antarctic Ocean, then appropriately changed course to get home. Thus, back in their respective rookeries once more, they had performed two sequential tasks: they had gone north to reach the sea (which is explainable if one assumes the penguin is a much more skilled navigator-walker than is man and combines a knowledge of geographical directions with a clock that is not only infallible but can also be reset accurately to the time zone from which he was taken) and they had an additional sense of finding home after having reached the coastal ice pack. We do not know what this additional sense is.

Some of the most earnest experimental attempts to understand how birds accomplish their navigational feats were done by Gustav Kramer in Germany after World War II. He studied pigeons, starlings and a variety of birds and, in general, found that birds can be released in a strange place and, with only a few seconds for reconnaissance during daylight, will take off immediately homeward. Kramer recognized the importance of the sun's angle, combined with a good clock, in keeping the bird on the right course. Yet he remained puzzled until his death by the bird's ability always to *start* in the right direction.

G. V. T. Matthews of Cambridge University believed that a bird first determines its geographic location in an unfamiliar area by measuring the arc the sun travels. The bird is using an inborn sextant; but note how many corners he is cutting. A human sailor, in trying to find out where he is, obtains his latitude in the following way: If he has a good chronometer he waits until local noon, when the sun is at zenith (highest in the sky). Then with a sextant he measures the angle of the sun with the horizon. Then he compares this angle (in tables that he carries with him) with the angle at some known latitude which he may call "home." The tables then tell him what latitude he is in. According to Matthews, the bird supposedly can, first of all, compute the zenith without waiting until noon by merely observing the sun "for a few minutes." By measuring the tiny arc traveled in that short space of time, the *future zenith* position of the sun is estimated by the bird. The bird then compares this estimate with the sun's zenith back home and can therefore tell if he has to fly north or south. The height of the sun can also be used to compute longitude. If a traveler has an accurate clock marking New York time, the homeward-looking angel can obtain his position west or east of that celestial city. Thus a bird with a chronometer running on home time can determine if it is east or west of home, depending on the sun's position.

This seems completely incredible. Some pigeons need only a few seconds to set their homeward flight, a time in which the sun has scarcely moved, even as recorded by sophisticated astronomical devices. It has been shown, in fact, that pigeons do not need *any* time to circle for taking solar observations, reading their biological clocks, etc. Theories of navigating by means of the earth's magnetic field have been proposed as substitutes for the sun-compass notion. Bar magnets were attached to the wings of homing pigeons and had no effect at all save to encumber the bird as one encumbers a race horse by a weight disadvantage. Kramer carried out a number of experiments in the homing of starlings near an East Baltic station near which occurred deposits of magnetic iron ore that made man-made

compasses totally unreliable. He reported, "The compass behaves wildly, the starlings do not."

Although the magnetic field of the earth may not be a critical
factor in influencing the behavior of most animals, the *absence*
of the earth's field (of about 0.5 gauss), as might be expected
on planets such as the moon and probably Mars, gives astronautical scientists something to worry about. At the Franklin
Institute in Philadelphia mice were exposed for a year, mating,
bearing young and going about their business in a magnetic
field of essentially zero. There were an unusual number of pre-
mature deaths and a lot of alopecia (loss of hair). The hair
fell out in both white and brown mice and was caused by the
plugging of hair follicles by the overgrowth of skin cells. Internal
organs and tissues showed abnormal cell growths—not quite
cancerous but on the verge of being so. In experiments with
men at the Indiana University Medical Center, the only effects
noticeable were a slight loss of dim-light vision and brightness
discrimination. On the other hand, plants seem to thrive when
the magnetic field is cut off. Seeds of white clover and wheat
germinated faster and in the wheat cells the roots of the seeds
were more robust.

The experiments of E. G. Franz Sauer in Bremen, West
Germany, showed that birds flying at night can apparently
substitute the fixed stars for the sun as a navigational aid. In
planetarium experiments he took the European lesser whitethroat
warbler (*Sylvia corucca*) on an imaginary trip to Africa without
leaving the cage. When a replica of the night sky of autumn
over Germany was projected on the planetarium dome, the bird
faced southeast, the direction of migration. The positions of
the stars and constellations were continually changed so that the
bird was apparently making progress. As the sky became a
replica of that over North Africa, the bird turned exactly south,
acting as if it were near the end of a migration. A trick was then
played on the warbler: Instead of the night sky of Germany, he
was presented at migration time with the stars over Siberia. With
such a drastic shift in longitude the bird became visibly confused for a minute, then he turned as if to fly westward—to

Germany—in his own cage—trying to get back to where he was so that he could start from true scratch.

When all the stories of celestial navigation by birds have been told, it always turns out that there are verified and unexplainable exceptions that do not fit in. Sauer himself pointed out, for example, that a flock of murres, flying in dense fog, overtook a ship heading by compass and chart to the same little island in the Bering Sea—their spring mating grounds. A female purple martin removed from her nest containing young in northern Michigan and transported 350 miles south to Ann Arbor was released at 10:40 P.M. The next morning at 7:28 A.M. she was back at her nest feeding the babies. She had made the trip through a night in which the sky was completely overcast with a double layer of clouds.

The homing instinct for the most part is more accurate than can be taught by constant experience. When the bird is old enough to fly, it is old enough to carry out prodigious feats of navigation—often better, as a matter of fact, than older birds of the same species. Experience often seems to confuse rather than magnify the innate gift.[6] Birds differ in this. Young geese are dependent during migration on the leadership of older geese. Young crows, released in Alberta, Canada, long after their parents had taken flight to wintering grounds in Kansas or Oklahoma, made a beeline for the same grounds, flying for the first time over the prairies. The New Zealand bronzed cuckoo, although brought up in a strange mother's nest, has an irresistible cuckoo clock in him that tells him to follow, by a month, the migratory flight of his true parents (whom he has never seen before). Thus he will suddenly migrate about 1,800 miles north over water to the Solomon and Bismarck islands where he will join his peculiar family. In the young cuckoo, the compass and clock of his genes are far more powerful than the nurture of his long-suffering foster parents, whatever species they happen to be.

[6] We observe here a remarkable affinity with human experiments with "extrasensory perception." It is normally on the first trials of a series of tests on ESP cards that the largest percentage of correct guesses is made.

Perhaps the most magnificent navigator known is the great marine green turtle, whose capacities Professor Archie Carr of the University of Florida has studied with such devotion and reported with such charm. Here we are face to face with a very ancient animal—much older than the birds.

Once every two or three years the female green turtles swim from the west coast of Brazil all the way to Ascension Island— a target five miles wide and 1,400 miles away in the South Atlantic, where they lay their eggs. As we have discussed in Chapter 1, on hatching and emerging from the nest the young green turtles set off on a direct course for the sea, even when the water itself is completely hidden by dunes. But the hatchlings on Ascension Island have the further job of swimming 1,400 miles to Brazil. Although the original instinctive sense that impels them to scramble toward water probably has nothing directly to do with the compass sense of directional swimming, the latter may grow out of it. At any rate, not long after reaching the water, they are engaged in finding the continent of South America—certainly a much plainer assignment than their mothers had in making landfall on the little dot of their native island.

Even human navigators, with their ability to measure the position of the sun and stars, were unable to calculate their location exactly until the development of precise chronometers in the eighteenth century. Our discussion of homing in bird flight has indicated the necessity at least of a clock sense, a map sense and a compass sense and in many cases (perhaps in *all* cases) these have not turned out to explain the facts. In the open sea, where the features are only those of terror and loneliness, some kind of guidance beyond a simple compass sense is required if the turtles are going to be able to correct for current drift and wind drift. The smell or taste of water may be of some help but certainly not across a stretch of 1,400 miles of deep ocean.

It is possible that the green turtles use an old island-finding technique that was used by human navigators before it was known accurately how to calculate longitude. Knowing the *lati-*

tude of the target, the navigator would sail north or south until the sun's position at noon showed he had reached the right latitude. Then he would toss a coin and decide to sail either due west or due east until he bumped into the island. In an analogous way, possibly the green turtles swim north or south along the Brazilian coast until they reach the vicinity of their first landfall as hatchlings. Perhaps something about the look or the smell of this place is remembered from their youth. Assuming this is also the latitude of Ascension Island, the female turtles may then simply swim due east.

But it is not "simple" just to swim due east across and against currents. (The turtles have to buck the equatorial current for at least 1,200 miles of open sea. There is a 3,000-foot mountain on Ascension and clouds often pile up high above it, but this is by no means a 1,400 mile beacon for an animal wallowing in the troughs of waves.) During World War II Ascension used to be a way-stop for airplanes of the Air Transport Command flying from Miami to the Burma Road. Airplanes that left Recife on the coast of Brazil had to make the Ascension landfall or go almost 1,000 miles farther on to Dakar, Africa. A very large number of planes had to try for Dakar because they lost the island. (The sooty tern, however, gets there without any difficulty. In fact, Archie Carr has pointed out the rather mystical affinity between the green turtle and this sea bird. Wherever there are islands where green turtles nest, there are sooty terns nesting too.)

Possibly the westward pull of the equatorial current is more of an advantage than a handicap. The lines of contact between different kinds of water undoubtedly are sensed by homing fish who are equipped with delicate organs on their sides that measure some quality (not a smell or a taste) of water which, for lack of a better word, we might call the water's "dynamics," and possibly the reptile has some ability that tells him "This is water coming away from near where I want to be; I will follow it back and find my secret island." The varying speeds, or dynamics, of the successive parallels of latitude may be marks, and so may be the lines of force of the earth's magnetic field. Used together, perhaps the two could furnish the green turtle with a map. Another faint possibility is the Coriolis force, which is a result of the fact that the earth is a rotating sphere and the forces due to rotation change with the distance from the equator. This is an extremely minute phenomenon. Neurophysiologists have found no anatomical instruments in the turtle for measuring either the earth's magnetism or its Coriolis force. But neurophysiologists are far from infallible, and in many creatures they have found organs that evidently sense something, but what it is they have been unable to guess.

Another nervous capability, well advanced in ants, may work on the principle of the modern inertial guidance systems for guided missiles, although it is probably much subtler in animals since in man's machines it requires rather massive gyroscopic and computing devices. Reduced to its simplest terms, such a guidance system works by very accurately recording where the missile has been. In an animal the inertial sense would indelibly implant on the nervous system all changes in speed or direction throughout any journey or movement, however long, crooked or interrupted, however slow, however fast. We have seen something remotely approaching this even in human beings with a "good sense of direction," who rarely get confused even at night or when gradual turns are made, as in a railroad journey. This gift is probably dependent on teamwork between the semicircular canals of the inner ear and the cerebellum.[7] In birds, ants, turtles and all other homing animals the inertial sense may be developed to an extent that is unimaginable to us.

When we were discussing Groot's experiments with young salmon and his conclusions that they were able to find their way out of a lake by polarized sunlight, we did not include a significant additional experiment that Groot performed. He put smolts, ready for leave-taking of their home lake, in a circular

[7] That the cerebellum has something important to do with directional movements is obvious from its peculiar geometrical structure. When the brains of migratory and non-migratory pigeons are examined, after whirling the birds in a centrifuge, neurologists find the cerebellum of the migratory pigeon continues to show electrical discharges, which are absent in the home-body bird.

tank whose top was covered with an opaque sheet. Even under these conditions the little fishes turned in a preferred position— the one that would, if they were free, take them out of the lake. Although Groot, not knowing the mechanism of this behavior, called it "X-orientation,"[8] he tried manfully to find out more about it. Could it be inertial guidance? Could the little salmon have automatically memorized all the twists and turns and splashings made during their transportation to the experimental sunless tank? He tried deep anesthesia on the smolts before taking them to the tank, but when they woke up they faced the same direction; they still knew where the outlet river was. The possibility that all the devious angular accelerations of their enforced trip to the tank could be remembered in a state of complete unconsciousness seems quite a faint one, and perhaps this is the most crushing knockout blow that this general theory on animal directionality and homing has received.

For such reasons as this the inertia-guidance idea has fallen into disfavor. The magnetic field and the Coriolis force hypotheses depend on such exquisitely small effects that few will take them seriously, at least until sensory organs are located that might account for them. We are left with guidance by sun and stars and moon. If birds use such celestial navigation, they use it in methods too deft and instant for us to comprehend. Archie Carr finds it impossible for him to visualize the sextant process being carried out by a turtle, whose horizon bobs incessantly in front of his wet eyes in air an inch or so above the surface of the crest or trough or sloping side of an oceanic wave. Carr resorts to his conviction that the pregnant green turtle needs none of the complexities that a human navigator must resort to. He feels that the problem may be reduced to the simpler one of

[8] The algebraic instinct to call the unknown "X" is reflected with typical medical pomposity in the use of the absurd term "idiopathic" for a symptom or syndrome the cause of which is not known. The medical profession compounds this pomposity by referring to "etiology" when they mean "cause." Some of the most important, now familiar effects in science started out as "Xs." It is pleasant to reflect on the admittedly remote possibility that Groot's "X-orientation" may someday be as well understood as X-rays are today.

keeping on the same latitude that it starts on, from Recife east to Ascension. But to prove this he must have a way of following the turtle's itinerary. Simply sticking a radio sending device on a turtle's back was not good enough because of poor reception at sea level (polarization of radio waves over water and the obstinate curvature of the earth). He plans—with the co-operation of NASA and the Office of Naval Research—to try to follow the ponderous female's course by earth satellite. All good luck to him.[9] In the meantime, Carr remains one of the most eloquent deplorers of the general loss of interest (or perhaps gain in entropy of scholarship) in the whole problem of animal guidance —especially of birds. He points out that it has been theorized that birds may even see stars by day. This he rather doubts, but if it were so, it would sharply tilt the direction of research to explain their navigation. The work that Sauer began in the Bremen planetarium ought then to be repeated and exhaustively extended, beginning where he left off with warblers and going on to test all the important migrants.

There is one fact—a geological one—that needs to be added to the story of the turtles of Ascension Island. Turtles are older animals than birds; fishes are still older. It is possible that many of the migrational habits of the ancient marine animal families were started when the continents were not located as they are today. The Atlantic Ocean grew as the continents of South America and Africa moved gradually apart, perhaps leaving Ascension Island between them. Possibly the original commuting of the green turtles was done between an early Brazil and Africa—when that was a relatively short swim. Thus in the beginning the target may have been either less distant or less tiring. As the eons passed, evolution taught the turtles, in some way not yet comprehensible to us, how still to hit the target when it was both distant and tiring.

[9] As of the spring of 1969 the migratory habits of sea turtles and polar bears were to be studied by the use of the satellite Nimbus B2. On its first launch on April 10, 1969, however, the space craft was given the more modest task of following around a placid male elk named Moe whose home territory was the Yellowstone National Park.

Some attention is owed to the homing feats of animals closer in nature to us, such as mammals. Karl Kenyon's studies of the Alaskan fur seal prove not only the seal's sense of "home" but an infallible way of reaching home after traveling for thousands of miles. Nothing could induce a cow seal to choose a birth-place for her calf other than the ancestral home. A critical ex-amination of the Polovina rookery in Saint Paul Island in 1954 showed that man's improvements and dredging operations nearly sixty years before had changed the topography to the extent that no harems had been re-formed on the ravaged beaches in the meantime. The seals were as fussy as the gooney birds. The fur seals on the high seas lead an exciting and risky life. Although in captivity they can live longer than a horse, in nature 50 per cent of male pups and 40 per cent of females die before the age of three years. This difference in life expectation is probably because the sexes winter apart. The cows go to California, and how they are later able to find their way across the trackless ocean wastes between that sweet coast and up through the dour misty passes to the Pribilof Islands is one of the unexplainable feats in the record book of mammal migra-tion. In the meantime, the old bulls have stayed in the north, wintering just south of the Aleutians where there is more fish to build up their strength for another sexual summer. The younger bulls go just a little farther south. All the males are thus feeding in the favorite domain of the killer whale, which for a seal is an imprudent way to enjoy a winter vacation.

Unlike the male fur seal, the harp seal hasn't learned to make breathing holes in the ice. Thus the herds, both male and female, must move southward in the autumn. On the northeast coast of North America the hooded seal suddenly becomes friendly with the harp seal and both travel south together.

No one knows the migrating habits of dolphins. They are found over all the seas, and the ones that are friendly with men seem to have only a peculiar form of periodic seaward and landward rhythms. Recently fishermen have noticed that on the Pacific Coast the dolphins move offshore at sunset and return at sunrise. It is seriously considered that this may be connected with their growing preoccupation with people-watching. As the beaches become more populated with humans, the dolphins tend at night to go seaward to eat and sleep and spend the day flirting with and ogling men and women and boys and girls.

One should not overlook the skills of very small mammals in finding their way home. Deer mice, although their ranging territory is only fifty yards in diameter, can manage to get back quickly to the home burrow if moved in a closed box to a spot a mile away. Some white spotted mice, with even more limited back yards, have been known to return home across two miles of country.

There are many dog and cat stories of almost miraculous returns but most of them share the tender dubiety of pet lore. The savants of ESP are more than willing to accommodate these legendary feats in their files, demonstrating, as they believe, a mental field (as in the case of Eugene Marais' termites) attaching the minds of animal and master. What usually happens to an abandoned dog is that, instead of trying to get home, he joins a pack of other waifs. Conceivably it depends on whether the dog has been simply thrown away out of a car or has been accidentally lost by grieving owners. In the latter circumstance there are some well-authenticated cases of incredible home-comings. A collie named Bobbie made his way home to Silverton, Oregon, six months after having been lost in Indiana. Tony, a mongrel dog, rather promptly followed the automobile carrying the Doolen family from Aurora, Illinois, to Lansing, Michigan, a distance of 250 miles. In the terminology of parapsychology this is known as "*psi* trailing." (We shall later ask the embarrassing question as to why this is essentially any more weird than the theory of the Coriolis force guiding an equatorial turtle.)

One might close this section by examining how some of our own species, the ninth-century Vikings, made their muscular way by boat to North America and other far places, *before the magnetic compass was invented* and before there were any good clocks. They navigated by the sun and by the stars, but it now appears that they had a little help that we did not realize before. Even on a cloudy day they could locate the sun by the use of "magical sun stones." In 1967, the Danish archeologist Thorkild Ramskou, enlisting the aid of Denmark's royal jeweler, found that in Scandinavia minerals can be located in which the molecules are aligned parallel to each other, just as crystals in a Polaroid filter. One in particular—cordierite—turns from yellow to dark blue whenever its natural axis is held at right angles to the plane of polarized light from the sun. Thus, by use of the "magic stones" referred to in runic inscriptions, a Viking skipper could locate the sun even on a misty day by rotating a chunk of cordierite until it turned dark blue. Ramskou proved the magical stone out by taking it on a flight to Greenland, keeping track of the sun with his stone while the pilot used the twilight compass. The cordierite observations were always correct to within two and one half degrees of the sun's position and had the virtue (common to all sensors of polarized sunlight) of being able to track the sun even when it had dipped seven degrees below the horizon. Thus man, even at the dawn of marine technology, was beginning to exploit tools to make up for the lost senses that he had sacrificed in becoming human.

Time Machines

In exploring the navigational genius of animals that are able to find their way to their homes or to traditional nesting places or breeding grounds, we have referred many times to inner clocks. It is evident that this notion of a biological clock is fundamental in all life—in fact, in all living cells and even in the crucial chemical systems that make the cells work. A circadian (daily) rhythm, for example, can be detected in those enzymes of the cells of the mammalian liver that are responsible for digesting amino acids. The enormous question is whether such rhythms depend on certain external rhythms of the surroundings (the rotation of the earth, for instance, and the periodic changes in the magnetic fields of the earth) or whether time itself is sensed within the living molecules as sensitively as pressure or temperature or radiation.[10]

There are two schools of thought on this question, which verges at once upon metaphysics if the implications are pursued to the dark caves of the mind where we realize the ambiguity of time as a concept. One group of scholars believes that clocks in each animal species are inherited characteristics, just as a kidney or a gill or a color. Thus the eel inherits biological clocks that developed in all eels over the eons of the evolution of eels. These clocks direct not only the eel's circadian doings— its feeding and sleeping—but the rhythm of its irresistible urge to go home to the Sargasso Sea for breeding. This group believes that the inherited clocks are wound up at birth or perhaps even at conception and are free-running and immutable, although some of them are reset every day, throughout the life of the organism.

The other school, most prominently led by the great experimental biologist Frank Brown of Northwestern University, thinks that all living clocks simply measure the rhythm of the environment. Brown compares a biological clock to an electric clock which actually does not measure time at all but measures the oscillations of an electric current and adds them up. Thus an organism, in Brown's conception, is literally plugged into its environment and receives a continuous flow of information which regulates its activities. The nature of this "plugging in," however, and the nature of the information may be much more sizable than we have imagined. A number of extraordinary experiments convinced Brown that there are superhuman senses in many animals that detect things of which we are able to become aware only through the design of supersensitive machines and probably some things of which we have not become aware at all or have only guessed at. Many living creatures are capable

[10] Some exception to the universality of rhythm may have to be made in the case of bacteria and blue-green algae and possibly viruses. It is perhaps significant that these particular single-celled creatures possess no membraned nucleus.

of picking up minute changes in the world by signals obtained through the walls of a box sealed from any variation in light, temperature, humidity or sound. Brown sealed a rat in a laboratory tomb of this sort and found that it ran about three times as much when the moon was below the horizon as when it was above. What is this "moon sense"? Are the rat's moods affected by lunar tidal pulls? If so, the rat has a sense as old in life as the oyster. On the east coast the oysters open their shells twice a day when the moon's tidal pull is highest. When Brown shipped the same oysters to Evanston, Illinois, after a short period of acclimatization, they adapted to the longitudinal change and their shells opened twice daily when the moon's gravity was a maximum in Evanston rather than on the east coast.

Brown proved that certain creatures of low estate, such as snails, can apparently sense the subtle rhythmic change in the earth's magnetic field caused by the rise and fall of the ionosphere. (Your transistor radio can readily respond to the gross lowering of the ionosphere at night, which is why you get so many stations on it after the sun has long disappeared but this is because more radio waves are bounding back to earth.) In thousands of experiments, Brown released mud snails straight down a track and recorded which direction they veered. At certain times of the day or night they preferred to turn in one direction, twelve hours later in the other. Using a weak magnet that corresponded to the faint changes that occur in the earth's field of magnetism, he could make the snails turn against their habit.

Those that contend that magnetic pole reversal in the earth, which has occurred many times, could not possibly result in the unloading of enough strong radiation to cause a burst of biological mutations must still face up to the fact that paleontology nevertheless traces a faunal and floral map of discontinuities that coincide with geologic evidence of pole reversal. The more the radiologists argue that pole reversal could have had no radiation effect, the more support they add to the still stranger suggestion that magnetic field changes by themselves must have affected life on earth.

Brown believes that some organisms similarly sense incredibly small changes in the electrostatic field, the background radiation and even to a shift in radio frequencies. All such changes occur in our earth environment in regular twenty-four-hour rhythms. When the moon goes around the earth it not only affects the tides in the oceans but the tides in the atmosphere. These air tides rise and fall very slightly not only in a lunar-day rhythm but also in a superimposed rhythm corresponding to the phases of the moon. These tides in turn cause extremely weak but measurable periodic changes in the electrostatic and radiation fields of the earth.

The tiny sand flea *Talitrus* navigates not only during the day by shooting the sun but also at night by shooting the moon. It is able to correct continuously for the passage of the moon across the sky. A computer capable of this automatic correction would weigh about five pounds.

(I do not perceive any essential difference between the two schools of thought mentioned above. Time is, after all, only *what happens*. The reason that circadian rhythms are so common in life is that the earth has been rotating on its axis throughout life's history, the moon has been circling the earth for a similar time and the earth has been revolving about the sun from the time of the first living cell. The really critical changes in life's rhythms would occur if one exposed a race of organisms to a sufficiently long space trip through the solar system or the galaxy where the inherited rhythms of life on earth would be gradually erased through probably a thousand generations or so and possibly be replaced either by an inconceivably complex set of new rhythms or with complete rhythmlessness—an interesting evolution to contemplate.)

Frank Brown also found that one does not have to be an animal to perceive the tenuous, fairylike changes in the world. Brown sealed potatoes, as he had done the rats, in boxes under constant conditions of light and temperature. The rate of "breathing" of the potato depended on air tides, but was more influenced by the tidal pull of the sun than of the moon. Because solar heating occurs on only one side of the earth each day, the air tide cycle caused by the sun is definitely circadian and can be recorded by sensitive barometers. This tide rises in the morning, reaches its maximum about 10 A.M. and drops to a low point in the afternoon. The potato plugs (containing "eyes") responded to these changes in air tide and behaved like living barometers, taking in more oxygen as the minichanges of barometric pressure occurred. At one point in the breathing pattern, the potatoes seemed actually to be weather prophets by predicting barometric changes two days in advance. (We shall see that the sense of time, as the sense of something happening, can in many other living organisms be a kind of extrapolation to what is *going* to happen.)

One wholesome thing that the remarkable experiments of Professor Brown have done is to disabuse experimental biologists of the crude idea that "constant conditions" in a laboratory experiment can truly isolate a living thing from every environmental change to which it is sensitive. It appears that many organisms have more subtle, Houdinilike tricks than we had ever dreamed possible.

Of all *normal* circadian stimuli, the simplest and most predictable is, of course, the light of the sun. World-wide, perhaps, the daily *vertical* migration of tiny animals (zooplankton) in the oceans is the most crucial to the life of the planet. We are here faced with a problem of unexpected differences in what had always been regarded as a sort of gigantic blob of oceanic porridge. The effect of light under artificial conditions may or may not change the rhythm with which these tiny animals (mainly crustaceans) tend to rise and fall in the sea. The common and expected behavior is that when the sun shines, the whole population of various species descends into deeper water and rises again at night. Yet, by a careful collection technique and laboratory tank experiments J. T. Enright of the University of California (San Diego) and W. M. Hammer of the University of California (Davis) showed that some species of zooplankton, contrary to oceanographic lore, do the precise opposite: they congregate at the surface during the daylight. Certain species insist on going up and down according to some internal rhythm regardless of the lighting.

The effect of light on the sexual rhythms of sparrows has been studied by Michael Menaker and Arnold Eakin of the University of Texas. What they showed was that the effect of a light-dark cycle (for example, the gain in weight of the male sparrow's testicles) depends on an underlying rhythm, and that the light is effective only when it is applied at certain phases of this underlying rhythm. In other words, it is the *light-sensitivity* of the basic glandular process that is rhythmic. Thus a bird's response to long days can be initiated by exposure for short times to light during the night, provided the exposure is made at the right time—at the right part of a basic rhythm that was doubtless inherited in connection with a glandular pattern in which the long day was the natural stimulus.

In birds, very dim light does not cause any stimulus of androgen hormones and green light is much less stimulating than white or red. Very dim light or darkness controls the phase and period of the light sensitivity rhythm. The sparrows were presented with a cycle of fourteen hours of very dim green light and ten hours of darkness. It was found that the fourteen hours of dim green light was no more effective in maintaining the bird's testicle size than complete darkness. The addition of white light at the time of the transition from darkness to green light or twelve hours later, just before the green to darkness transition, likewise had no effect. But at any other time the sensitivity of the glandular process to white light was enough to make seventy-five minutes the equivalent of a long day in swelling the sparrow's testes. The Japanese quail is a good animal to use in studying the effect of light because of the prominent extrusion of the male cloacal gland when stimulated with androgen. One does not have to kill the animal in order to weigh the testes, since the size of the cloacal gland as determined in the live bird is an even more accurate index.

Internal glandular clocks, regulated by the length of the day, are probably present in all animals that depend on deciduous vegetation for food and who live in temperate zones. This is especially true of plant-eating insects, such as the pink boll-worm, studied by Perry Z. Adkisson of Texas A. and M. University. Insects of this sort do not migrate south during the winter, so they must plan well ahead for a period of dormancy, analogous to hibernation, which is called in insects "diapause." The insect clock in this case has an uncanny pre-cision. The onset of diapause in a given population (for ex-ample, the first insects to go to sleep for the winter) may occur regularly each year at almost the same date within a day or so. But, most important, diapause does not hit all the insects at the same time.

During the long summer days the larva of the pink bollworms may eat its way out of the cotton boll, drop on the ground and pupate immediately. There will appear a new generation of moths with time to mate and lay eggs before cold weather. During the shortening days of fall the larva will prefer to stay inside the boll and spin itself a silken bed, or hibernaculum. All growth and development are frozen. The larva enters a state of diapause that lasts until spring.

The transition from a short- to a long-day response occurs when the number of hours of light per day increases from 13 to 13¼. Yet at 80° Fahrenheit nearly 30 per cent of a bollworm population fails to respond immediately to the short-ening or lengthening of the days. For diapause to occur in all the larvae simultaneously, they must have been raised in short days of temperatures of 68° Fahrenheit or less. This lag in photoresponse has great survival value for the population. Since both the start and end of diapause are under light control, both the going to sleep in the fall and the waking up (in the form of moths) in the spring are spread over several weeks. This is a kind of insurance against natural disaster. It promises that no single sudden catastrophe (perhaps a hail storm or a flood) will kill all the members of a population. What if you try, as in the case of the sparrows, to substitute short periods of bright light during the night for long days? You bump into the same phenomenon, which is now called the "Bunning effect," that was found in sparrows. The light, in order to have any effect (as in the inhibitor of diapause), must be introduced at a time of rhythmic light sensitivity. In the pink bollworm, light has the greatest effect on diapause when it is flashed at from eight to ten hours after dusk or from eight to ten hours before dawn. The *length* of day is not important in determining whether diapause is inhibited or whether it is prematurely induced by the artificial light. Apparently the inhibitory light interruption presented early in the night acts as the terminator of the day or as an artificial dusk. Interruptions late at night act as initiators or as artificial dawn. Thus the effect is to "reset" the dusk or the dawn. The process that induces diapause may be set in motion in the insect egg. Exposure of the eggs to twelve hours of light and twelve hours of darkness during the incubation period produced immediate diapause in nearly 50 per cent of the larvae from these eggs. They had been born to the "short day." This sort of "light memory" would be beneficial to bollworms, since diapause could be programmed by light while in the egg or early larval stage. Thus, an older larva, feeding deep inside the cotton boll where little light intrudes, would nevertheless be so sensitive as the result of the rhythm of sensitivity imparted earlier in life that it would stop chewing and start to make its winter bed at the right time.

The actual mechanism of such light-sensitized insect clocks involves a nerve-gland reciprocal action in the brain, perfectly analogous to the nerve-gland reciprocity in the pituitary of mammals. It was found that the sexual identity of aphids could be controlled by illuminating the mid-area of the brain. Later it was shown that the action of light in controlling diapause in the oak silkworm is directly through the brain. When the brain of the pupa of this insect was surgically transplanted to the tail end, the photosensitivity also went to the tail end. It is evident that evolution has assured insects that only in light periods connected with climate suitable for growth and development can the brain be activated by light and the brain hormone released. This hormone in turn stimulates the prothoracic glands, which secrete ecdysone, which then acts as a stimulant to growth and development of all the cells of the body. If the light does not synchronize with the inner rhythm of sensitivity (in other words, if it is an inappropriate light), no brain hormone is released and diapause takes the place of growth and development.

The hormone nature of the *daily* rhythm of activity of insects has been ingeniously demonstrated by the famous tandem-cockroach experiment of Janet Harker of Cambridge University. She joined the blood circulation of two cockroaches so one was riding on top of the other. The rhythm of the bottom one had been temporarily stopped after being exposed to a very long period of light. When the artificial Siamese twins were placed in perpetual "daylight," the bottom one suddenly began to follow a definite daily pattern. Thus the hormones of the top one had triggered a cycle in the lower one.

The inheritance of the rhythm is stubborn and hard to break. Bees whose parents were raised in the dark nevertheless had twenty-four-hour cycles like normal bees. Lizards raised from eggs under constant light still showed a circadian cycle of activity. Fifteen consecutive generations of fruit flies raised under constant light still maintained the same daily rhythm. When a fiddler crab is placed in a dark laboratory it continues to change color and to run about busily at the same time as its free fellow crabs back on the beach.

Yet in mammals a rather curious steady change in the arithmetic of the circadian rhythm may occur when the animal is specially protected from visible day and night. Patricia DeCoursey of the University of Wisconsin kept flying squirrels in darkness, housed in special revolving cages that turned like a treadmill each time the squirrel moved. While free squirrels capered and took off in the woods and rested, the squirrels in their dark cages also went through a cycle of work and rest. The cycles of the captive squirrels, however, varied from twenty-three hours to slightly over twenty-four hours. Squirrels with the unnatural twenty-three-hour cycle began running around one hour earlier each day. Experiments on human beings at the Naval Submarine Medical Center in Groton,

Connecticut, showed an exaggeration of this trend. Men completely shut off from the world with no clocks or sun to inform them gained from one to two hours in their normal cycle of life. Men who normally went to bed at 1 A.M. retired from one to two hours later each day. After nine days, their bedtime had shifted from 1 A.M. to 4 P.M. The circadian rhythm of the human body is, of course, subject to wild dislocations because of fast jet airplanes. So serious, in fact, are these rhythm distortions that it has been a rule of the United States State Department that its diplomats should not undertake negotiations within twelve hours of crossing various time zones. Many hospital patients seem to have symptoms that occur with clocklike regularity. As the result of observing over 500 case histories of this type, Dr. Curt P. Richter of Johns Hopkins University developed a deep-probing theory of cyclic indispositions (e.g., migraine). He believes every functioning unit of an organism has an inborn but individualistic cycle. In a normal, healthy organ these units function *out of step* (health is non-rhythmic). Shock or injury may accidentally synchronize the various cycles, resulting in illness. Therapy consists in persuading the units to stop goose-stepping and get out of phase again.

The adaptation to certain rhythms of nature has been useful to animals not only in finding their way about the world but also in increasing the efficiency of predators. Thus each day the Australian reef heron, living about thirty miles inland, arrives on the coast for his shore dinner *exactly* at low tide, although the low tide occurs fifty minutes later each day.

The well-publicized spawning of the grunion on the Southern California beaches demonstrates an exact synchronicity with the tides. The grunion always wait until the moon is either full or new before mating. At these times, with the spring tides at their highest, the females ride the waves ashore to lay their eggs on the beaches. Each time the ride comes within a few minutes of high tide. The run lasts only about one hour and because it is a good tourist gimmick, timetables have been prepared by the California State Fisheries Laboratory for public distribution. The only data needed are the height and time of each spring nightly high tide occurring the first, second, third and fourth nights after the highest tide of a series at the full of the moon and during a new moon. Evolution has allowed the grunion to synchronize the incubation of the eggs with subsequent tides. Two weeks after the eggs have been deposited comes the next series of high tides. The first has no effect but the next night waves of a still higher tide sweep up the beach just far enough to dislodge the eggs from hitherto dry sand. The eggs hatch instantaneously and the same wave carries the young back to sea.

Coyotes and wild dogs that like turtle eggs have developed an uncanny sense of anticipating the place and date of arrival of the marine turtles who are making their faithful mission to the egg-laying beaches. The ridley turtle of the Caribbean is apparently the only reptile species that prefers to lay eggs like an occupying army on the beach heads. Great convoys of pregnant ridleys (as many as 40,000) known as "arribadas" arrive somewhere on the beaches of Tamaulipas, Mexico, at no time that is predictable by man. Yet the coyotes are ready. They have come from all over the inland scrub country in armies of their own, in packs bigger than anyone ever saw before. They are hinterland coyotes and visit the beach only when the ridleys come. If they really do decide in advance the time and place to meet an arribada they are demons of cleverness because, as Archie Carr points out, that great jubilee of egg-laying can happen anywhere along ninety miles of shore on any of at least 100 days of an unspecifiable year.

There seems very little doubt that some animals can predict weather, not only a storm coming but the severity of the coming winter. In only a few cases can we guess from their behavior how they function as weather forecasters. When birds line up for no apparent reason on telephone wires during the spring and summer, a storm is probably in the offing, but this could also be predicted by a glance at a barometer. The birds are perched on the wire because the air pressure is so low that they find it suddenly harder to fly. Yet studies by research field ornithologists show that migratory birds seem to know what the weather conditions will be at their flight target twelve hours in advance and that this instinct is the chief reason for their safe arrival at the destination points. Local legends are sometimes accurate correlations. For example, in the New England backwoods, when the partridges grow feathers between their toes the winters will be hard and snowfall heavy. Some people would rather rely on chipmunks. The winter will be long or short depending on how these animals carry their tails in the fall. Straight-up or forward-cocked tails mean long cold months, while droopy tails mean mild, short winters. The tougher the winter is to be, the fatter the brown bear will become before hibernation.

In birds there appear even to be correlations between the size of the clutch of eggs laid and the probable food supply. In some species the larger clutches are already laid before the abundant food is at hand. Thus such birds seem to respond to some general sense of the amount of virtue in the coming spring. A seven-year study of British titmice (the same bird that was smart enough to learn to open milk bottles) showed that not only do the clutches increase in size in those years that caterpillars are more abundant, but the young titmice are hatched each year just as the caterpillars emerge in numbers. These two events may vary from year to year as much as a month, yet they are always in synchrony. It must be admitted that some species guess wrong. The Central European swifts may lay three eggs early in the summer, but if the weather turns rainy and cold and thus cuts down on the number of flying insects, the parent birds will remove one, two or even three eggs and drop them to the ground.

Some fishes are very sensitive to air and water pressure changes and their behavior has been used in weather forecasting in Japan. Based on the behavior of gulls, dolphins and jellyfish that take shelter long before the actual approach of a storm, scientists of Moscow University concluded that these animals were responding to sounds arising from the friction of waves against air which gives a frequency (from about eight to thirteen cycles per second), which is *lower* than the human ear can detect. The Moscow students created an instrument imitating the animal perception, which they hope will give warning of a storm at sea from at least twelve to fifteen hours in advance.

There is a further even more urgent reason to investigate devices that detect infrasound (lower than the human ear can detect). Japanese scientists have found that certain fishes and cephalopods may be able to predict earthquakes. Dr. Yasuo Suyebiro, director of the Marine Park Aquarium at Aburatsubo and son of the founder of the Tokyo University Seismological Research Institute, recounts in a book some of the strange alarums that fishes and other marine creatures try to convey preceding earthquakes. (According to ancient legend, the almost daily earthquakes in the Japanese archipelago are the result of the stirrings of a giant catfish.) Cuttlefish of great size, usually found only in remote depths, had been caught in shallow water near Aburatsubo two days before the big quake on May 15, 1968. In his book Suyebiro cites 127 instances of unusual behavior of fishes or cephalopods prior to an earthquake. For instance, a rarely caught species of deep-sea cod had been landed off Hayama, Japan, by the Belgian ambassador a few days before the earthquake of 1923 that killed over 140,000 people in Tokyo and Yokohama. It seems possible that prior to the vast mechanical slippages responsible for the *mechanical* shocks, some higher frequency sounds may be emitted—the mutters of the earth, so to speak, before it shrugs its great devastating shoulders. We cannot hear these deep-rooted mutters but maybe the fishes and cephalopods can. (Scattered over the skin of certain cephalopods are some singular structures or organs whose use is not known. They are highly pigmented and provided with nerve endings surrounded by transparent cells—they look like tiny eyes. Some think they are sensitive to temperature changes and call them "thermoscopic eyes." It may be that, instead, they are sensors for infrasound. As we saw in Chapter 2, the otherwise highly developed octopus and squid are not able to hear the sounds we do, but perhaps they can take note of the preludes to the hurricane and the earthquake.)

In the research area of infrasound, as might be expected,

the most exciting work has been done in the direction of development of weapons for killing men. As we have noted, a team of scientists under Vladimir Gavreau of the University of Aix-Marseilles made a device which would generate sound waves at less than ten cycles per second, or ten hertz. (A hertz is one cycle per second; the human ear records sound from about 16 hertz to 20,000 hertz.) Very fast air vibrations either go right through solid objects or bounce off them (the basis of ultrasonic echo-location by bats). But slow air vibration of sufficient intensity can create a sort of pendulum action, a reverberation in solid objects that quickly builds up to destructive intensity. Gavreau and his merry men built a giant whistle, hooked to a compressed-air hose. When the whistle was blown, no audible sound came out but the men barely escaped with their lives. They had to shut the whistle off quickly since all their organs—stomach, heart, lungs—were madly vibrating and they were sick for hours. The people in other laboratories of the building were sick too. Gavreau planned to build a military weapon that could kill a man five miles away. It was to be in policeman's-whistle form, eighteen feet across, which could be mounted on a truck and blown with a huge fan turned by an airplane engine. There was one problem that they apparently could not solve—at least at the date of this writing. The weapon would kill its operators as well as the enemy. The most promising idea to get around this slight difficulty seemed to be to propagate different but complementary infrasound waves backward from the machine, so the waves would cancel each other out in a backward direction, thus protecting the firing crew.

The World of Electric Senses and Weaponry

A SENSORY UNIVERSE of electrostatic fields is one that we lost when we left the water. What such a universe would be like we have no possible conception, but when evolution creates such a universe for an animal, it can be precise and violent and involves organs of great complexity and exquisitely tailored power. Usually when an animal is given senses that are not available to others, it becomes a specialist and the more usual senses disappear or decline.

It is among the fishes (some of them the most ancient order of fishes) that electric senses and electric weapons have come to be developed. Yet perhaps the oldest of all creatures, a kind of bacterium, uses one of the most modern techniques developed by human technologists—the principle of the fuel cell—in carrying out its living processes. In a fuel cell, a feed material, which can provide energy by burning (say, a petroleum hydrocarbon) is, instead of being burned, passed by an electrode of a battery where it firelessly is stripped of its hydrogen and provides electric current in the process, ending up as water and carbon dioxide but without the presence of air. These bacteriological fuel cells ("bug batteries"), if harnessed in an imaginative way, might not only provide us with gigantic and extremely efficient sources of electric power but could also be designed simultaneously into clean-up methods for polluted rivers, streams and oceans. Many of the anaerobic bacteria use garbage or other wastes rather than hydrocarbons as sources of fuel, hence essentially what is needed is the architectural cunning to place the electrodes and semipermeable membranes in the bacteria and garbage-rich waters and let the bugs go to work.[11]

Since the study of the uses of electric senses by fishes has become almost a private domain of H. W. Lissman of Cambridge University, we take a look at this unknown world with his classic studies of the Egyptian fresh-water fish, *Gymnarchus nilotica*, who hunts but does not kill by electricity. For a reason that will become obvious, *Gymnarchus* does not swim as fishes usually swim—by lashing their tails from side to side. He keeps his spine absolutely straight, down to the last joint on the tail bone. He has a beautiful undulating fin along his back by which he can propel himself forward or backward, and to see him make a turn, still with a straight back, is a dazzling exhibition of hydro-

[11] The use of specialized strains of oceanic bacteria, applied in enormous doses, might also be a practical emergency method for cleaning up oil spills, such as that at Santa Barbara.

dynamics in which complex waves ripple here and there over the back fin at one and the same time. When he dashes after smaller fish to eat, he never bumps into the walls of a tank, but dodges obstacles as gracefully as a bat or an open field runner. Yet his eyes are degenerate and can perceive only the difference between light and darkness; and he has no bat's gift of echo-location by ultrasound.

That part of the secret lies in the tail was found in dissections made as early as 1847 by Michael Pius Erdl of the University of Munich. *Gymnarchus'* tail is funny-looking (the Greek name means literally "naked tail"), being slender and finless. In this naked tail Erdl found some tissue resembling an electric eel's small electric organ, consisting of four thin spindles running up each side to somewhere beyond the middle of the body. Like all electric organs, these tissues are believed to have been muscles once. Evolution, in giving them electrical properties, took away their power to contract. (Since we know that all muscles are electrically stimulated, it is an immense but credible extrapolation to imagine the electrically activated tissues becoming electrically activated batteries, with the nerve impulse acting as a switch does in turning on an electric power system.) In fishes that paralyze their prey by big discharges, an extreme in evolutionary trend is seen, but somewhere along the line the discharge must have been weaker, as it is in *Gymnarchus*. In studying this fish in a laboratory tank, Lissmann was able to record a continuous stream of electric discharges at constant frequencies of 300 pulses per second, waxing and waning in amplitude as the fish changed its position relative to a stationary electrode in the tank. But even when *Gymnarchus* was lazy or asleep or at least motionless, the stream of discharges continued.

Lissmann found other fishes that emitted continuous streams of weak electricity. He found a mormyrid relative of *Gymnarchus* and in South America a gymnotid, a small fresh-water relative of the electric eels, belonging to a group quite unrelated in the evolutionary family tree to *Gymnarchus* and the mormyrids. (This seems to be another example of convergence. When evolution has a good idea, it may confide it independently to its pets far removed in space and time.) Lissmann had a fight on his hands with other scholars in trying to define the nature and function of these weak discharges. Some were inclined to believe that the output was of the character of an electromagnetic wave which would make *Gymnarchus'* location abilities analogous to radar tracking. But Lissmann has prevailed with an alternative theory that fits all the observed facts. During each discharge the tip of *Gymnarchus'* tail becomes electrically negative with respect to the head. The fish becomes what is known in electrostatics as a "dipole." An electric current may then be pictured as spreading out into the water in a pattern of lines that describe a dipole field. How important the field is to this fish is shown by the fact that the exact configuration of the electric field depends on the conductivity of the water and on distortions introduced into the field by objects (such as rocks or other fish) with an electrical conductivity different from that of water. (In more technical language, the *impedance* is changed.) In large free volumes of water—an empty hunting ground—the field is symmetrical. When objects of significance are present, the lines of current will converge on those that have better conductivity and will diverge from poor conductors. Such objects therefore alter the distribution of the electric potential over the surface of the fish—the living dipole—and it is these sometimes infinitesimal changes that allow *Gymnarchus* to earn a living and to elude collisions.

Lissmann found that the fish responded violently when an electrified insulator (such as a comb that had just been drawn through a person's dry hair) was moved near the aquarium. The electric effect must have been in the range of less than a millionth of a volt per centimeter. *Gymnarchus* could easily distinguish between two pots when one contained water and the other wax. This was a pushover. But he could also distinguish mixtures of a different proportion of ordinary tap water and distilled water (the latter having very slightly lower conductivity). He could tell the presence of a glass rod two millimeters in diameter inside of an earthen pot.

While the electric field emanates from the naked tail, where does it return in the head? What is the other end of the dipole? It is known that the tissues and internal fluids of fresh-water fish are good electric conductors enclosed in a skin that conducts quite poorly. The skin of *Gymnarchus* and of many mormyrids is very thick, with layers of platelike cells sometimes in curious hexagonal patterns—an insulation better than rubber. But in some places, particularly on and around the head, the skin is perforated where pores lead into tubes filled usually with a jellylike collection of cells. If this jelly is a good conductor, it must be that the lines of electric current from the water converge at these pores, as if focused by a lens. Each jelly tube widens at the base into a small, round capsule that holds groups of cells—known variously as "multicellular glands," "mormyromasts" and (more vigorously) "snout organs." This is undoubtedly where one of the most delicate senses of the entire animal kingdom picks up signals for the brain. Anatomically, the capsules send out nerve fibers that unite to form the largest of all the fish's nerves leading to the brain. The brain centers into which these nerves converge are remarkably large and complex in *Gymnarchus* and in some mormyrids they completely cover the remaining parts of the brain.

Skates also have weak electric organs in the tail. These are not bony fishes as are the mormyrids and gymnotids and are about as far removed in an evolutionary sense from *Gymnarchus* as a snail is from an octopus. Furthermore, skates live in the salty ocean which conducts electrically much better than does fresh water. Skates possess sense organs known as the "ampullae of Lorenzino" that consist of long jelly-filled tubes open to the water at one end and a sensory bulb at the other. Skates are notoriously unco-operative, being an older, more stupid creature than *Gymnarchus*, and Lissmann was unable to get them to help him in his studies.

Yet note one common feature—the indispensable feature— of all such fish. All of them swim with their spines stiff as a rail. *Gymnarchus* has his back fins, the gymnotids have propulsive fins on their bellies, the skates use pectoral "wings" to swim with. This is essential if Lissmann's theory is correct that it is the change of electric potential gradient over the surface that carries the signal. To make this work the electrode, or dipole system, must be kept in exact geometrical alignment.

Yet with *Gymnarchus*, as with all living things that perceive the external universe, we are gnawed by a central mystery. We know how sensitive the senses can be. One quantum of light can affect a good eye. A vibration of subatomic dimensions can excite a good ear. A single molecule can excite a good sense of smell. What we do not know is how such tiny signals can be extracted and pinpointed from the general noise in and around a working cell that, like an independent animal, has to do its own housework as it listens and reports on the radio. In the electrical sense of fishes, this problem of noise elimination is greatly complicated by the high frequency of discharge from the electric organ. In general any sensory stimulus grows with nerve frequency. That is the code. A small smell becomes an intolerable stink as the stimulus excites nerves to messages of higher and higher frequency. The limit of frequency may vary from one sense organ to another but 500 nerve impulses per second is a common upper limit, although 1,100 per second have been recorded over brief intervals.[12]

In fishes such as *Gymnarchus* these limitations present a very immediate conundrum. The fish's tail discharges at 300 pulses per second. A change in amplitude of the pulses recorded at the head, caused by the presence of objects in the field, is the effective stimulus at the sense organ. Assuming the reception of a single discharge of small amplitude at the head would excite one impulse in a sensory nerve, a discharge of larger amplitude (according to the code of the nerves) would excite two impulses in the same nerve. This would quickly exceed the upper limit of frequency at which nerves can send impulses to the brain, since the nerve would already be firing 600 times a second (twice the rate of discharge of the tail organ). There would be no room to convey changes in amplitude of incoming stimuli. The fish would, for example, be incompetent to estimate the

---

[12] This basic limitation in nervous frequency is the single valid reason why artificial electronic beings might be superior to living beings.

size or direction of the prey. Furthermore, the electric organs of some gymnotids discharge at rates of as high as 1,600 times per second. From the neurophysiology of the sensory nerves, it thus seems unlikely that the fish's brain is registering each pulse. What it probably is doing, according to Lissmann, is measuring the *average* value of the electric current over some unit of time. In other words the *averaging* process enables such a fish to discriminate a signal from the background of noise. Lissmann found that *Gymnarchus* is as sensitive to high-frequency pulses over a short time as he is to low-frequency pulses of identical voltage over a longer time. The fish's sensory reception thus is determined by the product of voltage times duration times frequency. Since the frequency and duration are fixed by the behavior of the generator in the tail, the critical variable for the sensory organ must be the average voltage. We have a new kind of sense not only mathematically but also, so to speak, philosophically.[13]

Gymnarchus can respond to a continuous direct-current electrical stimulus of about one ten-millionth of a volt per centimeter, which agrees with its calculated sensitivity required to recognize a glass rod two millimeters in diameter. The almost mythically small current change represented is 0.000,-000,000,000,003 amperes. If one extends this over a time of twenty-five thousandths of a second, within this time the fish can perceive the rustling of a mere segment of charged particles, while in the food it seeks there are trillions of such ions on the move. *Gymnarchus'* senses would be able to perceive the movement of a bacterium, but for him this is subjectively mere noise. He is directly aware of a universe that we can perceive only by the most expensive of equipment, but there is only a fractional part of this universe that represents a significant signal to him and to which he reacts.

[13] This averaging out of information is familiar in electronics as a technique for improving the signal-to-noise ratio. It is useful in human technology dealing with barely perceptible signals. It has been applied by special computers, for example, to clarification of the television photographs of the surface of the planet Mars.

The mystery of *Gymnarchus'* single sensory cell remains entirely unknown. If we solved it, we would be able to create an artificial electric universe as exquisitely charted as his. In structure, actually, the electric sense organs differ from species to species and in even an individual fish. Evolution has hold of a big thing, but has not decided where to go with it. Lissmann's findings strictly apply only to *Gymnarchus* and to about one half the species of gymnotids when the tail emits pulses of constant frequency. In other gymnotids and all the mormyrids, the discharge frequency *changes* with the state of mind of the fish. In this case there can be no sensory averaging process. Lissmann concludes that, as in man with many senses, the averaging process may take place in the brain itself, although this would seem to put a ghastly load on the unscrambling capability of a fishy cerebrum. Both types of sensory systems evidently evolved independently in two different fresh-water families, one in Africa and one in South America. (One should not overlook, however, the possibility that when these senses evolved Africa and South America were one continent.)

Japanese ichthyologists Akina Watanabe and Kimihisa Takeda at the University of Tokyo find that gymnotids can respond to electric oscillations close in frequency to their own by shifting their frequency away from the foreign one. Two fish might thus react to each other's presence. This would seem to be important in regard to mating behavior. How does *Gymnarchus* recognize his wife? One can only assume in this case that the electrical as well as the sexual resistivity is mysteriously changed and is apparent to both partners or that some other sense (perhaps olfactory) becomes temporarily dominant.

More recently Frank J. Mandriota and co-workers at Columbia University have found that the pulsing patterns in fourteen species of the mormyrid family can be controlled by conditioning. The frequency can be increased by conditioning the stimulus of electric shocks with light flashes. These results are novel in animal psychology, since neither secretion (as salivation in a dog) or movement are involved. Yet, if one recalls that the electrical discharge organ was once a muscle, the results are not as surprising.

The fact that nearly all the ancient cartilaginous fishes, including sharks and rays, possess the electrical sense has been confirmed by more recent findings. Some tests show that a ray can be very much affected merely by the gill movements of another fish otherwise completely stolid and motionless on the bottom of a tank. The possession of this faculty, along with his other keen senses, makes the shark a kind of superfish. He is not only the oldest kind of fish but also the most well equipped, and perhaps each fact explains the other.

Quite recently another kind of electrical organ, obviously quite different in origin, has been discovered in some bony fishes. This works on the principle of piezoelectricity—an electric force created in some crystalline solids by mechanical force. Robert Morris and L. Kittleman of the University of Oregon have come up with samples of otoliths—calcium carbonate concretions in the internal ear—that show high piezoelectric effects. The otoliths are presumed to constitute mechanisms for depth perception or frequency analysis of low-frequency sound waves or both. (Perhaps they are the earthquake-predicting organs.)

In evolution the natural advance from an organ of electric perception, derived from a muscle, was an organ designed not simply to locate the prey but to stun or to kill him. The electric eel (which is strictly not an eel at all; it belongs to the order of fresh-water fishes that includes minnows, carp and catfish), *Electrophorus electrius* of South American fresh waters, gives the most powerful shock of any known animal. It is strong enough to kill a mule. C. W. Coates of the New York Aquarium and Robert Cox of New York University made some exuberant early studies of this sinister animal. The electricity, they concluded, was generated in "glands" (actually highly converted muscles) that begin behind the head and extend along the whole length of the body. The current passes from the tail to the head but insulation protects the eel from discomfort. By using cathode-ray oscilloscopes connected to the fish, they found that the average size electric eel of four to eight feet long could deliver a discharge of about 500 volts. The impulse travels along the eel's body at speeds as high as 4,000 feet per second, which is twelve times the rate at which ordinary nervous impulses flash along human nerves. The power is ordinarily about 46 watts, but 1,000 watts could be drawn without visibly embarrassing the fish. The power pick-up (a term used with automobiles) is about 150 horsepower per second, appreciably higher than that of most motor cars. In the United States the alternating current is at 110 volts and the standard lamp is rated at around 60 watts. Coates and Cox, drawing as much as 600 volts and 1,000 watts, might have been expected to get the eel to light a good many bulbs. However, an eel cannot light an ordinary electric bulb. This is because the inertia of the ordinary lamp takes about one-fifteenth of a second to overcome, while the eel's discharge has passed its peak and gone in about two milliseconds. If the lamp, by any accident, ever did light, the filament would be burned out instantly.

The mechanism of the eel's discharge is not well understood. The individual electricity-producing cells (called "electroplaques") have been identified and pored over, but their extraordinary efficiency is puzzling. Electric eels "package" their power about 100 times more effectively than standard lead storage batteries (0.11 compared with 0.001 watts per gram). In 1967 Westinghouse Electric amused and instructed the public with an electric eel exhibit in the Aqua-Zoo in Pittsburgh. The eel's tank was wired so that the electric power generated could be used to activate equipment above the tank. The eels could be induced to attack a rod waved in front of it and, in so doing, light up a voltmeter above the tank, flash a strobe light and take a picture of himself. An eel can strike several times before pausing to recharge. His discharges have been known to kill a man standing in the water twenty-five feet away.

Electric discharges are also used, although mainly in defense, by the marine fish *Uranoscopus* (star-gazer) and a stronger one by the fresh-water catfish *Malapterurus*.

Electric rays of some species (especially along the Florida coasts and in the West Indies) use the electric organs not only for detection but also for hunting and defense. They are shaped like their close relatives, the sting rays, but substitute shock for a poisonous spear. Many rays give birth to live young, and when such infants are touched they retaliate with feeble little shocks.

The torpedo is less terrifying than the electric eel and discharges only about fifty to seventy volts. However, its anatomy has been more closely studied, perhaps because it is less dangerous. On each side of the head it has electric organs forming two kidney-shaped jellylike masses. These are made up of closely set hexagonal prisms about one and a half inches high. Each is formed of a pile of electric disks no more than about one tenth of a millimeter thick, clutched by special nerves branching out on the surface. A torpedo has about 400,000 of these disks. The comparison with a voltaic pile is obvious. In fact the electric organs of all other electric fish, catfish and electric eels function like piles. In the torpedo the resemblance to striated muscle is striking, making even more persuasive the theory that evolution can make almost anything out of a muscle, perhaps even a new kind of brain.

How to See Heat and Make Light

BECAUSE snakes are slow and rather pathetic things, evolution has given some of them a private universe which we can try to imagine with perhaps even less success than we can presumably construct the world of *Gymnarchus*, the fish that perceives faint twitches of electrical impedance. The pit vipers, which include rattlesnakes, copperheads and others, use their "pits" to distinguish between to us absolutely negligible differences in temperature in their surroundings. They can thus locate warm-blooded prey at astonishing distances and with unerring accuracy. In a sense this is perhaps the reptile's revenge on the early mammals who ate up the eggs of his enormous ancestors. The pit appears as a hole on the side of the head between the eye and nostrils but lower down. It is actually a very complex sense organ consisting of two cavities separated by a thin membrane something like an eardrum. The rattlesnake can detect differences in temperature of less than one thousandth of a degree centigrade. Copperheads will move silently through ~~the Sidewinder, which is led to its target by heat radiation.~~ see but which they trace by following the infrared heat rays from the birds' babies. The sensitivity is much greater than that of infrared photographic devices. When two balls of equal size but distinguished from each other by the merest fraction of a degree in temperature are presented to a pit viper, it will invariably and unhesitantly strike at the warmer ball.

The United States Air Force would like to know how the snake does this—quite aptly our classical air-to-air missile is the Sidewinder, which is led to its target by heat radiation. Cases are known where the missile actually entered the jet exhaust chamber of a target airplane before exploding. However, this missile can be fooled by decoys roughly the same temperature as the engine or rocket exhaust and which are launched from the target vehicle. It would presumably be impossible to fool an intelligent flying rattlesnake in this manner.

Recently it has been discovered that pit vipers are not the only snakes that have such a brilliant "thermoscopic eye." James W. Warren and Uwe Proske of Monash University, Victoria, Australia, have found that in some pythons and boas the head scales and the lip scales have depressed centers which can be looked upon as pits. These holes vary in number and depth in various species and in some they are absent. Warren and Proske prove that at least in the case of the Australian python *Morelia spilotes* they do function as delicate heat discriminating devices. If one records the electrical activity of the nerve below the pits, there is a continuous background discharge which may take place in short bursts or at random. When some object slightly warmer than the general environment is brought near, the frequency of nervous charges increases to a flutter. You may get a distinct response by waving your hand a few feet from the snake's head, even if the snake is blinded. If the radiation is filtered through water, the frequency of the discharges sharply decreases, indicating that the infrared rays, which are absorbed by water, are the ones of interest to this python.

If the balance of radiation is reversed (if an object colder than the snake is placed near him), the frequency of discharges is greatly reduced. In fact, if an object colder than a piece of ice is placed a few inches from the pits, all of the nervous discharges disappear. There no longer remains even a background of nerve chatter. Although this complete nervous silence may in itself constitute a signal, it is more likely that the snake, like the early kings of Siam, never heard of ice and has no nervous code to describe such an improbable temperature.

How the transducing parts of these extraordinary sensory devices work is completely unknown. (We do not know even how our own very crude temperature senses in the skin work.) However, since the microscopic structure of nerve endings in the pit vipers and in the pythons is entirely different, it is probable that evolution found at least two different sensory ways to compensate these snakes for poor eyesight and limblessness in a world of flying and running creatures.

In Chapter 1 we went into considerable detail about the act of seeing, but we did not emphasize that some creatures evidently go to great pains to be seen. They are able to produce cold light with a chemical reaction, a process of illumination incomparably more efficient as far as energy conversion is concerned than any electric lamps that men have been able to invent. The chemical luciferin reacts with oxygen in the presence of the enzyme luciferase, and the luciferin is regenerated by the important organic energetic compound adenosine triphosphate. The vivid point—the technical marvel—is that *all* of the energy (100 per cent) obtained from burning the luciferin is converted into light. If we knew how to do this our electric light bills would be reduced by 70 per cent since an electric light bulb wastes 70 per cent of its energy in heat, which in most cases also shortens the bulb's working life.

Luminescence occurs in nearly every kind of lower life form, including bacteria and fungi. It is especially popular (and understandably so) in ocean dwellers: sponges, corals, fishes and squids. In animals that have nerves one would like to know how the light-making process is controlled. In pursuit of this remote goal, William D. McElroy of Johns Hopkins University used to need 300,000 fireflies each year and he paid twenty-five cents per hundred to school children in the summer. It takes more than 33,000 lanterns from fireflies to produce an amount of luciferin weighing about the same as a postage stamp. In the firefly *Plotinus pyralis* the flashing lamp is located in the insect's belly. A clear outer skin forms a window for a layer of light-producing cells beneath. Another layer containing light-reflecting cells is below that.

It took many decades for biochemists to discover the basic light-producing reaction, although as early as 1887 the French physiologist Raphael Dubois found that he could create light from a substance that remained in the water that had been used to wash a certain kind of burrowing clam. During World War II Japanese soldiers made powder out of such light-creating clams. At night, when the soldiers did not want to risk revealing their positions by using a flashlight, they would add water to the powder cupped in the palm of the hand. A glow strong enough to read a map or message was produced.

Practically all deep-sea fish are luminescent, especially those who live at depths of around 1,800 feet. The light-producing organs (photophores) are fantastically varied in kind and in origin, but the most general type is composed of glandular cells in the skin. Usually they are almost as complex as an eye, being associated with some sort of lens and reflector system and being strictly under voluntary control by some mechanism completely obscure to us. The Stomiatidae, or wide-mouth family, have two rows of phosphores along each lower side of their bodies. The Myotophidae, or lantern fishes, are spotted with shining swaths like reflector road signs. One of the berycoid fish family, *Anomalops*, living in the Indian Ocean, has just one luminous organ located below the eye and attached to a movable flap or stalk. Below the eye is a small slot. When *Anomalops* wants to douse its light he tucks it into this pocket.

What are all these things for? Some are for sexual recognition, as in the case of the firefly in the meadows of the earth. Others are traps. Some deep-sea angler fish have bulblike, fleshy, luminous tentacles dangling below their chins. Others carry their bulbs at the tip of their fishing rods. This luminous lemon-colored lure has actually the function of a human fisherman's glittering Christmas-tree of hooked gadgets.

The lights can be colored and can change color. A worm found in Central and South America has two basic colors in its repertoire. It has a bright red cap and luminescent green spots on its sides. At night only the red head glows, looking exactly like the tip of a cigarette. If disturbed, the side lights are turned on. This is called the "railroad worm." In this and many other cases, the purpose of the lighting system is a little obscure, since, unlike most brightly colored but non-luminescent creatures, it is not poisonous. It simply seems to be asserting its identity—sometimes a dangerous thing to do unless your identity is feared or unless (and this is quite possible) the mere flashing of a pretty light may be in itself a fearsome thing to most of the swarming creatures of the world.

Glow worms in New Zealand caves are pretty once you know what is going on, but a stranger to such a cave could have a coronary attack upon finding himself in a place of ghosts. The worms have tiny lighted threads that are for ensnaring flies and hang like gossamer tassels from each predator worm. The general effect is like *The Lair of the White Worm* by the author of *Dracula*. If you talk loudly near the cave walls, saying, for example, "*For God's sake, get me out of here!*" the cave is instantly darkened, as if a switch had been turned off. After a while the filmy lights gradually come on again.

Ivan Sanderson, the noted explorer and amateur naturalist, discovered in a cave on the island of Trinidad probably the first luminous terrestrial vertebrate on earth, a little teiid lizard. The reptile turns on for a few seconds a series of light along its sides, suggesting the portholes of a ship at night. Since this luminescent talent is shown only by males, it is obviously as sexual as a peacock's spread of gaudy feathers.

The marine "firefly" of Japan is actually a crustacean (a kind of shelled shrimp). It gives off rich blue sparks of light when disturbed, perhaps a threat, since its luciferin system is extremely powerful. A few of these tiny individuals shaken in a tube of water give easily enough light to read by, and if alcohol is substituted, the light will persist for fifteen minutes. A proportion of one part of this crustacean's tissue in over a billion parts of water still gives a visible glow. About twelve species of ostracods of this family give off light which varies from blue to green to yellow. In higher crustacean life the light-producing organs are so complex in structure they were long considered to be eyes. In fact evolution seems to have an option here. Just as it may transform a muscle into an electric detector or into a shock distributor as lethal as the electric chair, it may turn an eye into a lantern or vice versa. One shrimp *Sergestes challenger* has 450 points of light. For some reason no true crabs have yet been found that are luminous.

Talitrus, the amphipod sand flea whose navigating abilities by moon or sun sighting we have mentioned, is often infected by luminous bacteria. These are as fatal to this creature as the bubonic plague is to rats and men. Yet the same kinds of bacteria are used for lighting purposes by certain fish and cephalopods that have special organs, or culture chambers, for carrying stores of this bacterial light without harm to themselves. This is a remarkable symbiosis comparable in ingenuity to man's discovery of a way to make fire.

Certain squids have highly developed light-producing gadgets. Too little is known of them since the most luminescent cephalopods are very confirmed dwellers in the deep sea and hard to catch. The photogenic organs may occur in almost any part of an octopus that possesses them, but they are most apt to be found in the outer integument of the arms and the mantle sac, in the eyeballs or in the mantle cavity. They are often completely internal and work as signals only because of the transparency of the body tissues in the live animal.

The fact that illumination may in some cases be a sort of "triumph ceremony" like the proud antics of graylag ganders is shown by the gaudy behavior of *Porichthys notatus*, a kind

of toadfish. Unlighted, it is dull, brownish and a nincompoop.
But if it is excited, it suddenly sports row upon row of shining
batteries—whole brigades of lights that extend from head to
tail. At the same time it makes itself heard with a humming
sound. The whole effect is of a sudden army sprung up with
banners and marching drums. Mr. Mitty transforms himself into
a tiger. Then he turns the lights off and goes back dutifully to
guard the eggs that his mate has laid and to stand watch over
the nest and the young.

The beautiful phenomenon of phosphorescence or the "burning of the sea" is a result of the sexual play of millions of
tiny copepods or microscopic shrimp. At least seven species give
off light at certain seasons of the year and conditions of the
ocean from organs scattered over their tiny bodies.

It is becoming obvious from studies made since the fateful
1940s that, in spite of the fact that the world a billion years ago
or so was bombarded by powerful rays that are now shielded
for us by the ozonosphere, most animal and plant cells show
no memory or recognition of this kind of radiation. In general
the radiation that man is able to generate that is strong enough
to split matter (so-called "ionizing" radiation) is resisted most
strongly by arthropods (insects, crustaceans, etc.). This is because of the fact that their skeletons happen to be on the
outside. This is a lucky chance, but it doesn't help if the
arthropod eats or handles radioactive material. A very odd thing
has been found out in this connection among wasps or hornets.
The common yellow-legged mud dauber will gather and use
"hot" mud (i.e., mud containing radioactive material) for constructing her nest. But the organ-pipe wasps will not. *This seems
to be the only case known where an animal has been found
capable of detecting radioactivity.* This is a sense of the utmost
value, for man himself cannot detect such dire rays without
the use of some kind of Geiger counter.

A large amount of research work has been done on special
chemicals to protect man against the ionizing radiations which
come from nuclear explosions, usually sacrificing monkeys in
this cause. It cannot be said that many foolproof compounds

have been discovered, but for people who are disposed to tipple alcoholic drinks, it may be comforting to know that a drunken monkey seems to have a better chance of surviving commonly lethal radiation than a sober one. Fatalists, expecting the nuclear holocaust, may elect to stay intoxicated, and it then becomes for them simply a question of whether the bombs arrive ahead of cirrhosis of the liver.

Since it appears that present life forms evolved in an environment of a few tenths of a roentgen per year (which represents a combination of background radiation from geological deposits of radioactive minerals in the earth and very infrequent penetrations of the atmosphere by strong cosmic rays), it has been of some interest to radiologists to study the patterns of strong artificial radiation effects on natural communities. Since a community of animals is neither practical nor humane for such a test, George M. Woodwell of the Brookhaven National Laboratory, Long Island, New York, chose instead a natural community of plants. A large source of gamma rays (about 9,500 curies of cesium 137) was suspended above the ground to provide a cone of radiation over a large area. This was enough to give several thousand roentgens per day within a few yards, alternating the normal background levels at a distance of about 300 yards. Experiments were carried out in an old field (an abandoned garden) and on a forest.

An enormous difference in sensitivity to radiation was found among the various trees and plants. The forest was much more vulnerable than had been expected. A pine tree, in fact, can stand no more radiation than a man, in spite of the fact that it was in an evolutionary sense by far the oldest organism of the group. This is apparently because it has large chromosomes compared to most of the other plants. On Long Island the normal course of things when a garden area is abandoned is that about forty species of weeds rush to take over. The first year is usually the year of the pigweed, followed by the year of the horseweed, which later gives ground to grasses such as broom sedge and to asters, followed in time by the conversion of the field first to a pine, then to an oak-hickory forest. Under radiation, the history of the field is brutally simplified. The total standing crop varied along the radiation gradient. It was 400 grams of organic growth per square meter in the control zone (no artificial radiation), *increased* surprisingly to 800 grams of growth at 1,000 roentgens per day, but in zones closer to the radiation source, it dropped off steeply to practically zero. The increase of total crop at intermediate radiation dosages is due to the fact that some low-lying kinds of vegetation are peculiarly resistant to the rays while their common competitors are not, so the resistant plant runs riot. In Long Island this turned out to be crab grass. At 200 roentgens per day it is practically all of the standing crop.

The insect population followed the food supply. Insects that can eat dead matter and decayed bacteria increased in the central zone of the forest (for example, bark lice). In the second year there was an unexplained population explosion of aphids on white oaks exposed to 5 to 10 roentgens per day. Aphids share with certain fungi, such as wheat rust, the ability to reproduce asexually very fast in order to exploit any food resource. But they do not migrate well. It seems probable that the leaves of trees exposed to 5 to 10 roentgens per day are qualitatively different from normal leaves. They produce some subtle ambrosia that is detectable by aphids but not by man, even by very elaborate chemical analysis.

The forest as a whole was much more quickly devastated than the field. Smaller plants are more resistant than trees. Mosses and lichens are the most resistant of all. This remarkably parallels the comparative resistance to climatic severity. The same species and genera that can tolerate wide swings in temperature also can best withstand abnormal radiation. Sensitivity to radiation may be a measure of sensitivity to environmentally induced mutations in general. Although the radiation within the zone of peril killed off the standing pine trees, if one continued this radiation for a few thousand years in a pine forest, one might expect to see emerge a new radiation-proof species of pine. The white oak trees obviously were at the point of some mutation of interest to aphids. In a millennium or two the oaks might have further mutated to make poison instead of attractive candy for the aphids.

Signals by Direct and Party Line

WE HAVE mentioned that for several years the zing has gone out of research into the extraordinary homing instincts of animals, and perhaps precisely because they have *proved* to be so extraordinary.[14] Nevertheless two recent expert observations on birds seem to me to have pointed the guns of theory in a new direction that may open up a whole salient in the relationship of mind and matter. One is the realization that many birds have to communicate with each other in some unknown channel in order to carry out mass migrations and mass arrivals. William J. Hamilton III of the University of California (Berkeley) finds, for example, that large flocks on the move are much better oriented than small flocks or single birds. Indeed, the V-formation in geese, he believes, is formed for the pooling of directional information. Herring gulls are creatures of such sensitive social adjustment that the arriving flock of them makes decisions of mood and readiness as if it were a single many-winged being. So dependent is one of these social birds on the community of his fellow citizens that he is unable to breed if in the spring he happens by some accident to return to the wrong gull town.

Marine turtle hatchlings come swarming and clawing their way out of the sandy bed their mother has buried them in.

[14] A somewhat similar lassitude affects research into nuclear physics, which is concerned with the phenomenon in which the artificial particles producible by giant accelerators seem to multiply in complexity beyond all reason and predictability. Nuclear physicists, such as Murray Gell-Mann and others of the Caltech group, resort to the phraseology of Hindu mysticism ("The eight-fold-way") or to extremely sophisticated literary allusions (the "quark" from James Joyces' *Finnegans Wake*), but unfortunately the language so far has proved more compelling than the experimental results.

Here there is safety in numbers and a sort of pitiful but resolute little group mind. A single turtlet would be on the open beach longer and would more likely be caught by a ghost crab or a night heron, or in the blazing sun, simply dry up. In a group there is less likelihood of the fatal lapses into lassitude that often affect single turtles, and it is positively known that a group of little turtles makes a straighter, faster walk to the ocean than single stragglers.

That permanently grounded bird the Adelie penguin goes through incredibly precise maneuvers that can only be called "drills." Thousands of them at the edge of the sea ice turn and about face in exact unison. They behave as though the horde were a single organism.

Consider also the superhuman feats of mother animals in immense breeding grounds. The harp seals produce thousands of seemingly identical babies on flat ice sheets that may circle and drift miles in a day. Thus when the mother returns from fishing she has no stable topographical home. She must locate her offspring among whole brigades of temporarily deserted offspring. But infallibly she swims and flippers herself without a moment of hesitation to her own child whimpering on his crowded ice boat. It is easy to say her child is signaling toward her with molecules, that she smells his special smell, but this would presume such an appallingly exquisite discrimination that it would exceed the olfactory powers of moths that pick up the female pheromone miles downwind, since in the moth's case it is simply the signal "female": it is not a single individual that the moth is locating. He doesn't care whether it is Florence or Mame or Dolly, just so it is not Jack. But the mother harp seal is satisfied only with her one and only child.

Another recent discovery about homing birds has been made not by ornithologists but by fanciers of racing pigeons, of which there are many. It turns out that racing pigeons, which of course are simply particularly skillful homing pigeons, are flabbergasted by powerful electromagnetic waves of long wave length. When such birds are released near a broadcasting station of sufficient power, the pigeons are completely confused. (The observation was first reported apparently by Albert Enzweiler, a pigeon-racing expert of Cincinnati.) Exposed to the long waves conveying a soap commercial or perhaps *Bonanza*, the pigeons flap about in all directions and seem to have forgotten where home is. Enzweiler points out that this has been going on for a long time and that thousands of valuable birds have been disappearing without a trace since the advent of high-powered broadcasting pylons. Assuming the validity of the observation, the phenomenon fits in with a new trend in parapsychological thinking, which we shall shortly review.[15]

If we assume a "telepathy" between animals, it could be the oldest sense of all and perhaps possessed by every living cell. The experiments of Cleve Backster of the Backster Research Foundation of New York City, if confirmed, constitute such a fantastic proof of superhuman signals between primitive forms of life that it could revolutionize not only all biology but also psychology and even philosophy. Since Backster is not an academic scientist but a technician, specializing in the use of the polygraph ("lie-detector"), his data are likely to be subjected to the most supercilious suspicions on the part of professional scientists and lumped forthwith among the sorry trash of astrological lore, dowsing and spirit mediumship. Yet Backster seems to be a straightforward young man and his story deserves attention.

As a polygraph expert, he worked for some time with the CIA in special interrogations and, at least before his fantastic discovery, he operated a school for training in the use of the polygraph. At one time he was director of the Keeler Polygraph Institute of Chicago where he introduced the so-called "Backster Zone Comparison" polygraph procedure, now used in the Army. In February 1966, idly staring at a dracaena plant that graced his office, he got the idea of using polygraph techniques to measure the rate at which water rises in a plant from the root

15 For much of the information on human ESP, which follows, I am deeply in debt to Dr. Thelma Moss of the Neuropsychiatric Institute of the UCLA Center for the Health Sciences, who has been a gracious guide in strange countries of the mind.

area into the leaves. A leaf might respond to the psychogalvanic reflex (PGR), which, in polygraphology, measures the electric condition of human skin, often affected by emotional sweating and the like. He attached a pair of PGR electrodes to each side of one of the dracaena's leaves with a rubber band and found that the plant leaf could be balanced into the PGR circuitry, since its electric resistance was in the working range of the instrumentation, including the automatic pen recorder that measured changes in resistance. Contrary to what he hoped, when he poured water into the pot nothing much happened. The plant-leaf tracing showed a general downward trend, but after a while the pattern showed the contour typical of a human being experiencing some mild emotional stimulation, such as after one's being accused of raping a nun.

Puzzled by this, Backster then decided to try some equivalent of the threat-to-well-being principle, a well-established ploy in polygraph experiments in triggering human emotionality. He tried first to arouse the plant by immersing another leaf in a cup of hot coffee. No reaction. Then he decided to do something more drastic. He would get a match and burn a leaf. (Maybe this will prove to be the most sensational decision in the history of science.) *At the instant of the decision, there was an abrupt and prolonged upward sweep of the recording pen.* Backster had not touched the plant or even moved toward it. He had not even pulled a match from his pocket. He had just thought about burning it.

Backster killed some brine shrimp by dumping them into boiling water. The polygraph needle on the dracaena leaf jumped nearly off the chart. Was this particular plant *Dracaena massangeana* a kind of spook? Hardly. With more elaborate equipment (electronic randomizers and programmer circuitry and multiple PGR monitoring devices) he found that emotional receptivity of one piece of life to another is universal. It applies to all living cells of all kinds of organisms that he has tested, and without regard to the normal function of the cell. It applies to fresh fruits and vegetables, mold cultures, yeasts, scrapings from the human mouth, blood samples, spermatozoa. Perhaps the signal is the essence of life. Parsley in the refrigerator will respond to the death cries of dying blood cells when you cut your hand on a kitchen knife. The philodendron plant on the kitchen window sill reacts when you break an egg into the frying pan.

Backster has tried to block the signals by using a Faraday screen and even lead-lined containers. But the signal is not within the spectrum of electromagnetic waves that we know how to block. It is not limited by distance. Backster's team has obtained data indicating that the signal can travel perhaps hundreds of miles. As an example of distance effects, Backster lives in New Jersey and thought about returning to his office in Manhattan. At the precise moment he had this thought, with stop-watch precision the plants in his office had registered a polygraph reaction.

A typical experience showed the reaction of plants to non-human emotionality. Backster has an electric timer hooked to a loud, pulsating alarm, located directly above the bed of his Doberman pinscher. The action of the timing mechanism is accompanied by barely audible clicks and the dog would quietly leave the room before the bell (which he disliked heartily) sounded off. Although in a different room with the plants, Backster knew exactly when the dog was leaving, even though he himself could not hear either the clicks or the dog's movements, because the plants recorded the dog's anxiety.

Until this is more firmly established as the Age of Backster,[16] we should review other less exotic evidences of mysterious signals between animals—especially between animals and their masters. Everybody is familiar with the dog or cat that anticipates that the master is about to arrive home, although too far away to smell him or to hear his car. (This may be a time sense, but there are verified observations of the same behavior, even when the returns were at unusual and unexpected hours of the day or night.) A superstition ceases to be one when it

[16] Backster's experiments have been confirmed, rather curiously, by some electrical engineers rather than by psychologists. An example is the work of Douglas Dean at the Newark College of Engineering.

is observed a statistically valid number of times. This seems to be the case in which dogs howl when their masters die, even though the death may occur in some distant hospital. A female cougar in the Washington, D.C., zoo fell in love with a mysterious woman visitor who (against the rules) scratched her under the chin and about the ears. This woman never came at regular times; yet the cougar knew when she was coming long before she appeared. From the usual cage apathy, the cougar would leap about in excited expectation for several minutes, and invariably her dear friend would appear and the fondling would appease her and make her caged life a bit more tolerable for a time. Such empathy is possible, it would seem, only when a true bond of love (love in its most Christian sense) has been established.

Professor Konrad Lorenz's Alsatian bitch Tito knew exactly which people got on his nerves and when. Against all admonitions she would gently but surely bite such people on their rear ends. The signal was received even when Tito was lying under the table. Although Lorenz hastily disavows any telepathic sense, there seems no reason for retreating so fast into standard dogmatic ethology. It is true that "counting animals" have usually been debunked, since they count only when their master is present and are supposed to receive some signal, which may be an unconscious and involuntary body movement, when the right number is reached. Thus J. B. Rhine of Duke University, practically the father of modern parapsychology, tested Lady, the famous educated horse. He found that the filly could not touch the correct numbered or lettered block when the horse's owner was not told which one the scientist had in mind. It was found that the horse had developed the habit of following the slight unguarded sway of the owner's body toward the desired block. On the other hand, the Russian psychologist Ivan Bechterev carried out a long series of more fruitful experiments with dogs trained by a professional. Bechterev eliminated the trainer and changed the already learned task from one depending on a definite number of barks to new tests, such as *silently* commanding the dog to bring a book from a table, to bark at a stuffed animal, to pick up a piece of paper, to jump on a chair and so on. He concluded that telepathy had occurred in a statistically valid number of cases. Lorenz had a gray parrot whose vocabulary consisted of *"Na, auf Wiedersehen"* ("Well, then, so long"). He only said this if the guest really departed. He would not be fooled by a false departure. Professor Wolfgang Köhler, the great psychologist, tried to teach a talented gray parrot to say "food" when he was hungry and "water" when thirsty. The attempt failed and it has always failed, becoming unquestionably a psychological mystery. Parrots are unable to symbolize. The *"Na, auf Wiedersehen"* was simply a vocal comment. Köhler's smart gray parrot in turn was probably in his mysterious way baffled that the human being could not receive such an obvious telepathic signal as hunger or thirst.

Professional psychologists are seldom willing to accept telepathy or any other phenomenon of extrasensory perception. Thus in a questionnaire sent out to Fellows of the American Psychological Association, only 16 per cent of those who deigned to reply were willing to accept the occurrence of ESP as either established or even a likely possibility. There is some reason for this reluctance. The word "telepathy" was coined by the Englishman Frederic Myers before 1900 and the supposed phenomenon was chosen as the topic of investigation of the British Society for Psychical Research. This reasonable goal quickly degenerated into a preoccupation with mediumship and messages from the dead. Furthermore, J. B. Rhine's group, not content to investigate the still untouched problem of telepathy, included clairvoyance, precognition, psychokinesis (in which one is able to move things around by mental powers—a sort of double-whammy) and even reincarnation and the gift of prophecy. Parapsychology thus became a kind of hamper for anything that would not be accepted by a reputable scientific discipline. This situation, happily, was changed during the December 1970 meetings of the American Association for the Advancement of Science, when for the first time (mainly because of the dynamic influence of that marvellous woman

Dr. Margaret Mead, who, rapping on microphones with her cane, succeeded in persuading her peers) the parapsychologists were allowed to participate in the convention.

It is useful to review what we know for sure about fields of force that surround the living human body. As far as we are aware, we possess no tangible organs, as the electric fish do, that can exert force at a distance. But there are almost gossamerlike, tiny fields of magnetism around the torso and around the cranium, because of the fact that regular movements of electric current take place in the heart and in the brain. David Cohen of the University of Illinois has studied both fields. Magnetic signals with amplitudes in the very small range of 10^{-8} and 10^{-7} gauss (in the neighborhood of less than one millionth of a gauss, the unit for measuring magnetic field strength) are detected in synchrony with the heart beat. A magnetocardiographic chest map can actually be prepared, when one plots the external magnetic field against time at various positions on the torso. This shows the general T-curve structure and other features that cardiologists look for in an electrocardiogram. It may actually have some diagnostic advantage over the latter, since it determines direction more accurately; but certainly it can hardly be regarded as a signaling device to the outer world.

Around the head, magnetic fields of even more delicate magnitude can be detected, produced evidently by the strong alpha rhythm that is seen by the electroencephalograph under conditions of repose, with eyes closed, but not asleep. Apparently under alpha rhythm conditions of the brain, there is a sufficiently regular movement of electrons in the central nervous system to evoke a magnetic field, just as any electric current in motion produces its inevitable magnetic field, which accompanies it as faithfully as a shadow accompanies a walking man on a clear day. Cohen found fluctuating values of about 7×10^{-10} gauss, which is about one billionth of the earth's average magnetic field and much less than the maximum field detected near the heart. Obviously if we are dealing simply with fluctuating magnetic fields in telepathy, it would be much easier for the earth to signal to us (as it does to mud snails) than for another human being.

Yet there is a crucial and curiously ignored experiment that indicates that this insubstantial wraith of a magnetic field or else something else that accompanies the alpha rhythm of the human brain can be communicated to another human brain. In 1965 T. D. Duane and Thomas Behrendt of the Jefferson Medical College, Philadelphia, very respectable doctors who probably are sorry they carried out the experiment, were interested in the reports that alpha rhythms in the brain that start with so-called "photic driving" (that is, with lights on and the eyes open) are not only rare, but also when they occur, the subjects become ill. They decided to add rarity to rarity and test identical twins, one having alpha rhythm in the usual way (eyes closed in a lighted room) and the other in a nearby lighted room with eyes open. One twin was being used, as they say, as a "control." They tested fifteen sets of identical twins in this way, and two of the sets showed a most remarkable and embarrassing behavior. At the precise instant that alpha rhythms (unmistakable sharp spurs in an otherwise smooth curve) were invoked as one twin closed his eyes, they occurred in the encephalogram of the other twin who had his eyes open in the separate room seven yards away. The alpha waves were exactly superimposable. This was checked and rechecked in both the two remarkable sets of twins. Nothing like it occurred in the other thirteen sets nor in any of various pairs of unrelated people.

The two sets of twins who were able to invoke each other's alpha rhythms were intelligent, educated, serene, Caucasian males twenty-three and twenty-seven years of age. (The term "serene" in medical terminology is poetic in nuance, but it simply means they were not obvious nervous wrecks.) The other thirteen twins who lacked the gift were not serene. Variously Caucasians and Negroes of various ages and both sexes, they showed great anxiety and apprehension about the test and perhaps seemed to think that something cryptic and unpleasant was about to happen, since they probably associated scientific tests with hypnotism or hexing. The two successful sets of twins happened to have prior knowledge of the biological sciences and were rather nonchalant about the whole procedure.

To my knowledge this extraordinary experiment has not been followed up by others nor has it elicited any discussion or explanation by standard-brand psychologists. It has been swept under the rug, like the directional navigation of animals.[17]

To the parapsychologists, of course, the experiment is regarded as not only unremarkable but primitive, as if one marveled that a dog could be taught to sit up and bark. Yet one must emphasize that this single series of experiments of Duane and Behrendt are the only physical tests conducted under scientifically pure conditions by conservative neurologists that indicate that a signal of an unknown kind can be physically transferred through space from one brain to another.

I should emphasize in the last sentence the key word "*conservative*." Even cultivated people are faced with an abyss more profound than the obvious one popularized by C. P. Snow in dividing people into (1) scientifically minded and (2) artistically minded or merely simple-minded. The point is that parapsychology is not a discipline populated only by quacks and people wearing conical hats covered with the signs of the zodiac. Among a large and growing group are truly dedicated scientists, such as Dr. Thelma Moss, who know how to plan critical experiments, controlled statistically, and who frankly admit the difficulty of choosing between a valid and a questionable response from animals as complicated and goofy as human beings. We are not concerned with a war between science and superstition. The scientific war involved here is more like the dispute in the Middle Ages between Platonists and Aristotelians. It is a matter of point of view and of *breadth of welcome to unexpected data*. The conservative psychologists admit only data, so to speak, that are obtained from observing the behavior

[17] Dr. Thelma Moss calls my attention, however, to the fact that the electrical engineer Douglas Dean (previously referred to as having successfully repeated some of Backster's work) has also duplicated the Duane-Behrendt experiment.

of imprisoned rats. Yet even here they may find themselves tripped up because of a peculiarity in the nature of communication itself. In examining this illusory aspect of communication, let us return to the alpha-rhythm experiment.

We must realize that, although this induction of alpha rhythm was a signal, it was not a communication of the sort that humans regard as such. We must realize time after time that the invention of language greatly complicated human signals. To convey the idea of a thing, one must describe it in a symbolic way (in words that take the place of direct senses), and to communicate longer distances we convert signal and sound into electromagnetic wave forms that are reconverted into sights and sounds. In order to use telepathy, we must imagine again in symbols, and the symbols must presumably go through the same conversion into wave forms and a reconversion into sensory impressions that still represent symbols. Thus telepathy is a different and more complicated task for a symbol-thinking animal than it is for a bird or a dog or perhaps (if Backster is right) for a plant or an amoeba.

The professional parapsychologists take this in stride like a slick hurdler. Admittedly some of them are a rather reckless and arcane bunch and are avoided by prudent scientists such as are (for far better reasons) the hordes of astrologists that now infest modern cities, east and west. Yet some of the parapsychologists skirt the edges of practical applied science and seem to have accomplished something. Take the case of Dr. Henry K. Puharich, president and medical director of a company characteristically named the Intelectron Corporation of New York. Much of Puharich's research has been in finding the solution to permanent deafness. Justifiably he points to the intrinsic strangeness of sensory perceptions. The human ear accepts air impulses and converts them to data pulses in the nerves for processing in the brain. Yet we do not really understand the encoding process nor the nerve conduction process nor how the impulses in the digital form in the nerves give rise to particular "qualities" associated with the original sound input. We would be utterly helpless in trying to understand why we find the music of Mozart singularly pleasing to the nervous system. (We do not even know neurologically what pleasure itself consists of.) In 1961 various investigators reported the human recognition of low-energy pulse-modulated radar beams through an auditory system of "clicks." This indication that electromagnetic waves far outside the visual spectrum can be somehow captured by humans is the approach now being exploited by Intelectron's research program. Is the response to wave frequency due to acoustic sense perception or is there a direct channel to the brain?[18] Puharich tested thirty-two totally deaf people (their cochleas completely destroyed), using low-frequency pulse-modulated radio-frequency energy as a "hearing" stimulus. All thirty-two, he claims, experienced pure tone hearing, speech hearing and music hearing. Puharich believes this proves the existence of a pulse-modulated RF-energy-receiving channel somewhere in the human brain. Puharich's group, perhaps more significantly, claims to have showed the capability of using radio frequencies to provide the normal sensations of color and pattern in the blind.

In playing around with an ESP subject, Puharich put the man in a soundproof chamber, screened him against radio frequency transmission or reception and alleges to have confirmed telepathy over a distance of 200 miles.

Some parapsychologists are not so modest. Dr. I. M. Kogan of the Popov Institute for the Study of Radio Electronics and Communication in Moscow reported at a recent symposium in Los Angeles that his experiments in 1966–67 showed that thought may be conveyed by electromagnetic waves of extremely long wave lengths, with wave crests ranging from 16 to 600 miles apart. By some rather baffling mathematical acrobatics Kogan calculates that the human body generates from four to five times the electrical current needed for long-dis-

[18] When dogs are subjected experimentally to strong microwave radio waves they develop blood defects and may retch and vomit. In the long term the blood marrow is affected. If they are simultaneously exposed to microwaves and X-rays, all dogs die. People working with ultra-high-frequency generators commonly suffer enlargement of the thyroid gland.

tance telepathy, with human "transmitters" and "receivers" up to 1,800 miles apart. Kogan does not describe how the human body might act as an antenna for transmitting or receiving thought, but intimated that such antennae have evolved from biocurrents generated from the neuron networks of the body. (There is a rather hazy persuasiveness embodied in the idea that the carrying waves are of very long wave length, since much less energy is required for the generation of very long waves than short ones.) In one long-distance test between Moscow and Novosibirsk a transmitter tried to project the images of six objects. The receiver correctly described four. Not to be outdone, Dr. Thelma Moss, at the same symposium, reported telepathic ties between subjects in Los Angeles and the University of Sussex, England, more than 5,000 miles away. Since it is impossible, as far as I know, to screen against hypothetical electromagnetic wave lengths of hundreds of miles, the Kogan theory is reasonably safe from physical disproof for a while.

Let us review more closely some of the things that have to be explained. Among other spooky phenomena we shall see that the ancient part of the human brain devoted to non-symbolic sight (as discussed in Chapter 1) is more apt to transmit images than language. If, as I believe, telepathy is one of our forgotten senses, this should have been expected.

Item: In the experiments of Drs. Moss and J. A. Gengeralli of UCLA, professional *artists* showed greater efficiency in receiving the visual messages than even professional "sensitives" ("mediums" largely, though not necessarily quacks in a profitable racket especially in the Southern California area).

Item: In the group telepathic experiments of Moss, Alice E. Chang and Marc Levitt, the transmitting people in Los Angeles looked upon visual scenes classified as "water sports," "Van Gogh," "space," "wild animals," "war pictures," "love." The control messages were letters of the alphabet, numbers and geometrical lines. The receiving groups were in Los Angeles, New York and Sussex, England. The control messages had no effect, but the images were received and described with accuracy far above the laws of chance, yet this "accuracy" must itself be scrutinized.

We are faced here with the difficulty on the part of the receivers in translating images to language. For example, during the transmission of the visual love scene (the famous Rodin sculpture of lovers, *The Kiss*), was one English answer, "Thank God for the mini-skirt!" a reliable response?

In this particular experiment Sussex, England, performed better than New York. In a subsequent, more elaborate set-up that included Edinburgh among six other cities, the results were completely disappointing.

(If we accept Kogan's theory that the electromagnetic waves that carry these messages are of very low frequency, such inconsistencies might be expected. If long waves are being detected, the success should depend not only on the precise location of the receivers in relation to the transmitters, but also on obscure effects of atmospheric interference. It is interesting along this line that electronic scientists have recently detected electromagnetic waves from outer space in which the wave length is nearly *20 million miles*. The source is absolutely unknown. Maybe it is the voice of an angel.)

Item: Dr. Moss, in following up the remarkable difference in telepathic capability of artists compared with, say, engineers, also found that the best receivers could not themselves distinguish between genuine reception and fantasy. Those who confessed they had "made it all up" were usually the most accurate. What this finding seems to indicate is that the process of "making it all up" under these conditions is itself a mental phenomenon of complex and research-worthy strangeness.

Item: The Russians in general have more seriously regarded telepathic studies than has the "Establishment" of American scientists. The Russians are willing even to pay government money on it as a branch of *military* research. In the work at the Bioinformation Institute in Moscow a very definite bias in telepathy toward *visual* rather than linguistic transmission has also been noted. For example, one of the most easily identifiable messages was that of a piece of candy twisted up in brown paper. In general when a message was attempted, it was what Kogan called the "attributes" (the visual peculiarities) that were received rather than the symbolic meaning. A screw driver was received as "a long blackish-handle sort of thing," not as a specific tool. The telepathic sense quite evidently is a survivor of prehistoric eye-mindedness rather than a symbol-sensing development of modern man.

Item: In addition to images, emotions are telepathically easy to receive, assuming that the transmitter is sincerely moved rather than pretending to be. This is probably the basis of the innumerable amateur reports of strange, theatrical perceptions. A man feels a stab of horror; he finds out later that at precisely that moment his wife was dying of an accident in another city. We cannot ignore all these happenings. In many cases the moment of death is merely a gradual slide from coma into death. One should not expect telepathy under such circumstances. But in other cases the moment of death is the most brilliant emotional experience a human being has ever undergone. If someone (a relative or a close friend) is tuned to the same wave length, it is not inconceivable that this awful emotional jolt should find a receiver.

Item: Work at the Maimonides Medical Center in Brooklyn has shown the possibility of influencing a person's dreams by means of telepathy, the non-sleeping agent concentrating, for example, on famous art prints. In this case the external image will often insert itself suddenly and, so to speak, without welcome into the normal rather idiotic flow that the dreaming brain indulges in.

Robert Van de Castle of the University of Virginia Medical School, not only a distinguished expert in ESP but also an engagingly frank person, has found that even more primitive transmissions are possible, such as the postures of fighting and physical gestures. While he was asleep, he found himself going through the pummeling actions of a professor who was (one hopes soberly) shadow-boxing in the same room as an imaginary Cassius Clay. Dr. Van de Castle furthermore found that, beyond the standard dream technique first studied at Maimonides, one person's dreams can affect another's. In an experiment at Maimonides the agent, who was supposed to be awake and concentrating upon a work of art, fell asleep momentarily and dreamed of a Royal Canadian Mounted policeman. Dr. Van de Castle, who was the subject (and has a mild prejudice against the Mounties because he detests Nelson Eddy's singing) found himself suddenly dreaming not of Michelangelo's David but of a Royal Canadian Mounted policeman. (The unpleasant appearance of Nelson Eddy in full halloo is serenading Jeanette MacDonald.) However, again it is significant that the auditory association (la-la-la-la-*la*-la-la-*la*-la-la-*la*) did not, to the relief of Dr. Van de Castle, intrude and this phenomenon was therefore not a complete ESP nightmare. It was simply a ham actor's mercifully short optical appearance.

Item: The newest, perhaps most exciting approach is the combination of hypnosis and telepathy. Here we are in a double mystery. The Svengalian theory as applied in early movies regarded the hypnotist as exerting a dreadful mental tyranny over his subject. Psychiatrists from the Menninger Clinic of Topeka do not regard this as a good theory and, in fact, hypnosis has spiraled down from a fearful, theatrical action to the now accepted hypothesis (quoting from a standard-brand psychologist) that "the relationship between the hypnotist and the subject is one of interpersonal co-operation based upon mutually acceptable and reasonable considerations."

What this bland statement adds up to is that if you don't want to be hypnotized, you cannot be. The hypnotic state involves a rather tender relationship, almost resembling the final passiveness of a woman to her lover. It is worth noting that, of all professional hypnotists, either in the entertainment business or in psychiatry, about 95 per cent are men. There are also some rather shaky statistics showing that male homosexuals of the passive type are three times as susceptible to hypnosis by male psychiatrists as heterosexual men.

Nevertheless, it has been found at the Maimonides Dream Laboratory that hypnotically induced sleep or somnolence is even more susceptible than normal sleep to ESP transmission.

The data are impressive, but I can only confess that there is some element of phoniness about all this. The state of hypnosis is quite different from the dreaming state. It is more akin to the "sleep-walking" condition of which we know very little except that it does not correspond to true dreams in which the dreamer's eyes move incessantly (rapid eye movement, or REM) and in which his brain waves show the normal dreaming rhythm.

Here we are at the crucial crossroads in ESP.

Dr. Thelma Moss, a truly scientific worker in this field, has made a strong statement: "In ESP work first you have to find a volcano, then you have to wait until it explodes." The validity of ESP responses (including the historical ones of Swedenborg, Saint Joan and the biblical hero Joseph) should not be merely vacuumed into a reception-device called "superstition." We are at the verge of a delicate, shimmering, illusive science which perhaps cannot be called a science until we know more not only about electronics but also about life. The time is past, Dr. Moss believes, when you test the human mind by firing a gun behind the subject's head or get him to sit down in a chair which immediately collapses. This "Keystone Comedy" school of psychology is gone, along with the idea that as a woman you suffer from "penis envy."

If I should try to sum up the status of ESP from my point of view, it would be this:

1. Because of modern man's overdevelopment of the linguistic (symbolic) parts of his brain, he has all but forgotten the ESP potentialities that would have made him a true "sensitive" in the way that innumerable animals are sensitive—sensitive, that is, to means of communication that we cannot understand. Along with this has gone a "sense of the world," which we have lost, to our great detriment.

2. However, since man is a phylogenetically young animal, this tremendous, recent drive toward "language-thinking" has not entirely eliminated man's capacity for regaining the "forgotten senses" that reside in more primitive modes—those connected with the most ancient channels such as imagery and emotion—but not language.

3. It still seems possible (although not within the hardened prisons of conventional Western psychology) to reconcile the parapsychologists with "established" science. The most hopeful sign is the remarkable, independent work of electrical engineers in checking phenomena that standard-brand psychologists prissily refuse to acknowledge. As the British author Arthur Koestler has so powerfully emphasized, American psychologists are obsessed with "ratology"—the behavior of inbred rodents in special cages that allow them to behave only like moron prisoners whose only creative outlet is to press a bar and to gnaw or not to gnaw on a morsel of food.

Even within this restricted field of the Skinner Box, the standard-brand psychologists could discover more novelties if they worked with more brilliant animals. Apparently this is not a way to any easy Ph.D. thesis, since wild rodents in comparison with the fat, inbred, guaranteed strains available to universities around the world do not behave according to the rules. They are unacceptably brilliant, fast, and dangerously upsetting to expected data.

4. As a completely American person, I regard it as foolish that the standard-brand psychologists should automatically guarantee our being jolted by our ideological adversaries in a surprise break-through even more devastating to us than that of Sputnik in 1957. I count myself as a conservative scientist of thirty-five years experience, but I do not want to face a 1980 Sputnik that can use brain waves more effectively than nuclear bombs.

Let us return for a moment to our own parapsychologists.

J. B. Rhine and his numerous students and devotees do not insist upon wave lengths or electromagnetic radiation at all. If he had stuck to telepathic experiments with symbol-bearing cards, Rhine might have attained complete respectability as well as fame. The mathematical analysis of his results was well conceived, and in fact was defended by professional mathematicians against the early outcries of horror from standard-brand psychologists. But he was also interested in more muscular feats of the mind, such as raising blisters by hypnosis, curing warts by psychology, the psychokinetic rolling of dice and the power of mind over matter exhibited by the mystics of India. The only really thorough scientific study of yoga tricks was reported in early 1969 by Professor B. K. Anand and Dr. G. S. Chhina, Indians themselves. One of the spectacular things that yogis can do is to stop their own hearts from beating. The Indian savants measured what happened when such a yogi in a trance was studied with an electrocardiograph. It was found that instead of stopping their hearts, they were in fact increasing the heart movements to a fibrillation or flutter. What they do is to build up pressure in the chest cavity. The thin veins returning blood to the heart collapse. Since little or no blood reaches the heart and therefore no blood is pumped out, both the pulse and the regular heart beat disappear. Heart valves have nothing to do, so there are no valve sounds. Yet the electrocardiograph indicates a tremendous acceleration of heart movement. The yogis can maintain the fibrillation state for only a short time before the brain is permanently damaged.

Some yogis let themselves be buried alive and do not escape like Houdini. Anand and Chhina put one in a special airtight box to measure the bodily functions and gas contents. While in a trance, it was found, the yogis could reduce their body requirements for oxygen by 50 per cent of normal. Some yogis can slow their heart beat from a normal of about 72 per minute to 30 per minute. This is a much more important achievement than the "heart-stopping" trick and warrants further study. It indicates a willful control of the sympathetic nervous system, which may be what Kogan is getting at in telepathy via the whole body's nervous network. Some yogis can discipline the central nervous system to ignore painful stimuli, such as placing the hands in freezing water for twenty minutes or walking on hot coals. It has been found that in such a painless trance the yogi's brain is in an advanced state of alpha rhythm. He is not asleep, but he is not really aware of the pain centers. (This is not unreasonable in view of what we had to say of pain in Chapter 4.) On the other hand, some exceptionally talented yogis can focus such complete concentration on one part of the body that the sympathetic nerves that channel into it are under control of the brain, just as was the heart in the heart beat control feat. One very ancient mystic from the Himalayas used meditation to protect the uncovered parts of his body from subzero temperatures in his mountain cave. Sweat would break out on any area on which he was concentrating. He could do this at will at any time.

To go from this kind of body control to Rhine's precognition, clairvoyance and psychokinesis is to transcend the superhuman and embrace the supernatural. Rhine reports that *without* telepathy, the extrasensory subject can identify an unseen card (clairvoyance). He can tell what card is going to be turned next (precognition). Further, by psychokinesis he can influence the roll of dice and can even affect the shuffling of cards to the extent that automatic randomizing card-shuffling devices had to be invented to prevent the "psychic shuffle." (But why couldn't the wondrous one also put the whammy on the mechanical shuffling device?)

There is a simple but overwhelming proof against the general validity of all of these phenomena save telepathy. It resides in the fact that the human race is a race of inveterate gamblers. If anyone could guess beforehand which horse would win, could at will make the dice roll favorably, make cards shuffle themselves in a desired sequence, make the roulette ball settle on the right number (or even if he could do such things a small per cent of times above the dictates of chance and the "house percentage"), he would be a fantastically wealthy man. The very fact that nobody regularly breaks the bank at Monte Carlo or anywhere else, that nobody has ever become a permanently rich man by gambling against statistical odds, is itself a statistical proof that these *psi* capabilities are mythical. We do not need elaborate scientific rebuttal. The rebuttal is at hand in overpoweringly persuasive statistical form throughout the vast world of gambling.

This is not the case with telepathy. The best hypothesis seems to be that direct communication is possible between more-primitive creatures such as birds and lower mammals and that in man this means of communication, although greatly handicapped by the development of massive parts of the cortex now devoted to symbolic thinking, may under favorable circumstances still make itself known, even *by way* of symbolic signals arrowing through space by some as yet undiscovered wave form.

At the present stage of human evolution, it is lucky that we do not have universal telepathy. Whether one communicates telepathically or by telephone or TV, one should (as Thoreau emphasized) have something worth communicating. Certainly this is not now the case. It has, in fact, become less and less the case as the whole world of humans becomes increasingly vulgar and standardized. We would all die of a kind of exponential frenzy of boredom if we knew simultaneously and constantly what everybody else was thinking. The real goal is the reverse of the vulgarization of all thought which Ortega y Gasset so prophetically saw before World War II in his *The Revolt of the Masses*. The real goal is to exalt the total mind by multiplying the *kinds* of sensing and the *kinds* of thinking. The mass mind should be greater, not, as now, less, than the sum of its parts. This does not mean a colossal committee to run a world of slaves or robots, but rather a gigantic, single, many-faceted organism. This is politically the *reverse* of communism, and in another book we shall examine further this goal of a wiser animal, a superanimal, far beyond man, perhaps far beyond any acceptable definition of the animal kingdom itself.

Bibliography

SCIENTIFIC AND TECHNICAL JOURNALS AND SERIALS

Acta Ophthalomologica, Acta Protozoologica, Acta Psychologica, Aerospace Medicine, American Journal of Anatomy, American Journal of Ophthalmology, American Journal of Physiology, American Journal of Psychology, American Journal of Psychosomatic Dentistry and Medicine, American Naturalist, American Scientist, Animal Behavior, Annals of Biochemistry, Annals of the Entomological Society of America, Annals of Entomology and Zoology, Annals of the New York Academy of Science, Annual Review of Psychiatry, Arctic, Ardea, Asia, Auk, Aviation Week, Behavior, Biochemische Zeitschrift, Biological Reviews, Bionica, British Journal of Psychology, Brain, Chemical and Engineering News, Chemical Week, Condor, Copeia, Corrective Psychiatry, Deep Sea Research, Ecology, Economist, Experimental Brain Research, Geo-Marine Technology, International Journal of Neuropsychiatry, International Journal of Parapsychology, International Journal of Psychoanalysis, International Science and Technology, Japanese Journal of Physiology, Journal of Abnormal and Social Psychology, Journal of the Acoustical Society of America, Journal of the American Medical Association, Journal of the American Psychoanalytical Association, Journal of Anatomy, Journal of Animal Behavior, Journal of Aviation Medicine, Journal of Bacteriology, Journal of Biological Chemistry, Journal of Biosocial Sciences, Journal of the British Society of Psychic Research, Journal of Comparative Endocrinology, Journal of Consulting Psychology, Journal of Educational Research, Journal of General Microbiology,

Journal of General Physiology, Journal of Insect Physiology, Journal of Neurophysiology, Journal of the Optical Society of America, Journal of Ornithology, Journal of Parapsychology, Journal of Physiology, Journal of Psychology, Journal of Public Health, Journal of Theoretical Biology, Language, Life Sciences, Limnology and Oceanography, Missiles and Rockets, National Wildlife, Natural History, Nature, Naturwissenschaften, Optometrist Weekly, Ostrich, Perceptual and Motive Skills, Physiological Reviews, Primates, Proceedings of the California Academy of Science, Proceedings of the Association of Experimental Biological Medicine, Proceedings of the National Academy of Science of the United States, Proceedings of the Society of Social Experimental Biological Medicine, Proceedings of the Zoological Society of London, Progress in Brain Research, Psychic, Psychoanalytic Quarterly, Psychological Bulletin, Psychological Review, Psychology Today, Psychophysiology, Quarterly Journal of Experimental Psychology, Quarterly Review of Biology, Science, Science Digest, Scientific American, Smithsonian, Skin Diver, Technology Week, Vision Research, Vision Review, Zeitschrift für Flugwissenschaft, Zeitschrift für Vergleichende Physiologie, Zeitschrift für Tierpsychologie

BOOKS

Andersen, Harold T., ed. *Biology of Marine Animals*. New York: Academic Press, 1969.

Aschoff, J., ed. *Circadian Rhythms*. Amsterdam: Noord-Hollandsche, 1965.

Autori, M., ed. *L'Instinct dans le comportement des animaux*. Paris: Masson, 1956.

Back, F., and R. T. Harms, eds. *Universals in Linguistic Theory*. New York: Holt, Rinehart and Winston, 1968.

Barenboim, G. N., et al. *Luminescence of Biopolymers and Cells*. New York: Plenum, 1969.

Bassler, Ray S., et al. *Shelled Invertebrates of the Past and Present*. Washington, D.C.: Smithsonian, 1938.

Beranek, L. L. *Acoustics*. New York: McGraw-Hill, 1954.

Bliss, E. L., ed. *Roots of Behavior*. New York: Harper & Row, 1962.

Brown, M. E., ed. *Physiology of Fishes*. New York: Academic Press, 1957.

Bühler, K. *Sprachtheorie*. Jena: Fischer, 1934.

Bullock, T. H., and G. H. Horridge. *Structure and Function in the Nervous Systems of Invertebrates*. San Francisco: Freeman, 1965.

Bünning, E. *The Physiological Clock*. Berlin: Springer, 1964.

Busnel, R. G., ed. *Acoustic Behavior in Animals*. New York: Elsevier, 1964.

Cahalane, Victor H. *Mammals of North America*. New York: Macmillan, 1961.

Cahn, P. H., ed. *Lateral Line Detectors*. Bloomington, Ind.: Indiana Univ. Press, 1967.

Campbell, B. A., and R. M. Church, eds. *Punishment and Aversion Behavior*. New York: Appleton-Century-Crofts, 1969.

Carr, Archie. *So Excellent a Fishe—A Natural History of Turtles*. Garden City, N.Y.: Natural History Press, 1967.

Carr, Donald E. *The Deadly Feast of Life*. Garden City, N.Y.: Doubleday, 1971.

——. *The Eternal Return*. Garden City, N.Y.: Doubleday, 1969.

——. *The Sexes*. Garden City, N.Y.: Doubleday, 1970.

Chiba, T., and Kajiyama, M. *The Vowel, Its Nature and Structure*. Tokyo: Phonetic Society of Japan, 1958.

Chomsky, N., and M. Halle. *The Sound Pattern of English*. New York: Harper & Row, 1968.

Clark, L. L., ed. *Proceedings of the International Congress on Technology and Blindness*. New York: American Foundation for the Blind, 1963.

Dailey, F. C., and C. H., Milikan, eds. *Brain Mechanisms Underlying Speech and Language*. New York: Grune & Stratton, 1967.

David, E. E., Jr., and P. B. Denes, eds. *Human Communication: A Unified View*. New York: McGraw-Hill, 1969.

Devereux, G., ed. *Psychoanalysis and the Occult*. New York: International Univ. Press, 1953.

Dorst, J. *The Migrations of Birds*. Boston: Houghton Mifflin, 1967.

Eff, W. D., ed. *Contributions to a Sensory Physiology*. New York: Academic Press, 1969.

Epstein, W. F. *Varieties of Perceptual Learning*. New York: McGraw-Hill, 1967.

Fabre, J. Henri. *The Life of the Spider*. New York: Dodd, Mead, 1929.

Fant, G. *Acoustic Theory of Speech Production*. The Hague: Mouton, 1960.

Fodor, J. A., and J. J. Katz, eds. *The Structure of Language*. Englewood Cliffs, N.J.: Prentice-Hall, 1964.

Freedman, S. J. *The Neuropsychology of Spatially Oriented Behavior*. Homewood, Ill.: Dorsey, 1968.

Frings, H. and M. *Animal Communication*. Boston: Blaisdell, 1964.

Gavan, J., ed. *The Non-Human Primates and Human Evolution.* Detroit: Wayne Univ. Press, 1955.

Gay, W. F., ed. *Methods of Animal Experimentation.* New York: Academic Press, 1968.

Gibert, P. W., et al., eds. *Sharks, Skates and Rays.* Baltimore: Johns Hopkins Univ. Press, 1967.

Gibson, Eleanor J. *Principles of Perceptual Learning.* New York: Appleton-Century-Crofts, 1969.

Gibson, James J. *Perception of the Visual World.* Boston: Houghton Mifflin, 1956.

———. *The Senses Considered as Perceptual Systems.* Boston: Houghton Mifflin, 1966.

Giese, A. C., ed. *Photophysiology.* New York: Academic Press, 1964.

Giese, A. D. *Cell Physiology.* Philadelphia: Saunders, 1962.

Glaser, G. H., ed. *EEG and Behavior.* New York: Basic Books, 1963.

Granit, R. *Sensory Mechanism of the Retina.* London: Oxford Univ. Press, 1945.

Greenewalt, C. H. *Bird Song: Acoustics and Physiology.* Washington, D.C.: Smithsonian, 1968.

Gregory, R. L. *Eye and Brain: The Psychology of Seeing.* New York: McGraw-Hill, 1966.

Greenberg, J., ed. *Universals of Language.* Cambridge, Mass.: M.I.T. Press, 1966.

Griffin, D. R. *Listening in the Dark.* New Haven: Yale Univ. Press, 1958.

Harker, J. *The Physiology of Diurnal Rhythms.* Cambridge, Eng.: Cambridge Univ. Press, 1964.

Hayes, Cathy H. *The Ape in Our House.* New York: Harper, 1951.

Hayes, S. P. *Facial Vision in the Sense of Obstacles.* Watertown, Md.: Perkins, 1935.

Helson, H. *Adaptation-Level Theory.* New York: Harper & Row, 1964.

Herrick, C. J. *The Brain of the Tiger Salamander.* Chicago: Univ. of Chicago Press, 1949.

Hinde, R. A., ed. *Bird Vocalization.* London: Cambridge Univ. Press, 1969.

Howard, I. P., and W. B. Templeton. *Human Spatial Orientation.* New York: Wiley, 1966.

Hulse, Frederick S. *The Human Species.* New York: Random House, 1963.

Hutchins, Ross E. *Insects.* Englewood Cliffs, N.J.: Prentice-Hall, 1966.

Innes, W. T. *Exotic Aquarium Fishes.* Philadelphia: Innes, 1966.

Jay, P. C., ed. *Primates: Studies in Adaptation and Variability.* New York: Holt, Rinehart and Winston, 1968.

Johnston, J. W., et al., eds. *Advances in Chemoreception*. New York: Appleton-Century-Crofts, 1969.

Kellogg, W. N. *Porpoises and Sonar*. Chicago: Univ. of Chicago Press, 1961.

Kellogg, W. N. and L. A. *The Ape and the Child*. New York: Hafner, 1967.

Kerput, G. A., ed. *Problems in Biology*. New York: Macmillan, 1963.

Kleerekoper, Herman, *Olfaction in Fishes*. Bloomington, Ind.: Indiana Univ. Press, 1967.

Lanyon, W. E., and W. N. Tavolga, eds. *Animal Sounds and Communication*. Washington, D.C.: Inst. of Biological Sciences, 1960.

Latil, Pierre de. *The Underwater Naturalist*. Boston: Houghton Mifflin, 1958.

Lenneberg, E. H. *Biological Foundations of Language*. New York: Wiley, 1967.

Lenneberg, E. H., ed. *New Directions in the Study of Languages*. Cambridge, Mass.: M.I.T. Press, 1964.

Marteka, Vincent. *Bionics*. Philadelphia: Lippincott, 1965.

Menaker, M., ed. *Biochromometry*. Washington, D.C.: Nat. Acad. of Sciences, 1970.

Middleton, W. E. K. *Vision Through the Atmosphere*. Toronto: Univ. of Toronto Press, 1952.

Morris, Desmond, ed. *Primate Ethology*. London: Weidenfeld, 1967.

Myers, F. W. H. *Human Personality and its Survival of Bodily Death*. London: Longmans, Green, 1903.

Nastuk, W. L., ed. *Physical Techniques in Biological Research*. New York: Academic Press, 1964.

Needham, Joseph. *The Grand Titration: Science and Society in East and West*. London: Allen & Unwin, 1969.

Neff, W. D., ed. *Contributions to Sensory Physiology*. New York: Academic Press, 1965.

Negus, V. E. *The Comparative Anatomy and Physiology of the Larynx*. New York: Hafner, 1949.

Ochs, S. *Elements of Neurophysiology*. New York: Wiley, 1965.

Pestle, F., and J. G. Greene. *Learning, Perception and Choice*. Reading, Mass.: Addison-Wesley, 1970.

Pope, Clifford H. *The Reptile World*. New York: Knopf, 1960.

Post, Wiley, and Harold Gatty. *Around the World in Eight Days*. London: Hamish Hamilton, 1937.

Pratt, J. G. *Parapsychology: An Insider's View of ESP*. Garden City, N.Y.: Doubleday, 1964.

Racker, E. *Mechanisms in Bioenergetics*. New York: Academic Press, 1965.

Ramsay, J. A., and V. B. Wiggles, eds. *The Cell and the Organism.* Cambridge, Eng.: Cambridge Univ. Press, 1961.

Rasmussen, G. L., and W. F. Windle, eds. *Neural Mechanisms of the Auditory and Vestibular System.* Springfield, Ill.: Thomas, 1959.

Rhine, J. B. *New World of the Mind.* New York: Sloane, 1953.

Rhine, L. E. *ESP in Life and Laboratory.* New York: Collier Books, 1969.

——. *Hidden Channels of the Mind.* New York: Sloane, 1961.

Rock, I. *The Nature of Perceptual Adaptation.* New York: Basic Books, 1966.

Rockstein, M., ed. *The Physiology of Insects.* New York: Academic Press, 1964.

Schaefer, K. E., ed. *Man's Dependence on the Earthly Atmosphere.* New York: Macmillan, 1962.

Schaller, G. B. *The Mountain Gorilla.* Chicago: Univ. of Chicago Press, 1963.

Schneider, G., and R. H. McConnell. *ESP and Personality Patterns.* New Haven: Yale Univ. Press, 1958.

Schröder, C., ed. *Handbuch der Entomologie.* Jena: Fischer, 1929.

Sebeok, T. A., et al. *Approaches to Semiotics.* The Hague: Mouton, 1964.

Sleigh, M. A. *The Biology of Cilia and Flagella.* New York: Macmillan, 1962.

Sliper, E. J. *Whales.* New York: Basic Books, 1962.

Smith, K. V. and W. K. *Perception and Motion.* Philadelphia: Saunders, 1969.

Soal, S. G., and F. Bateman. *Modern Experiments in Telepathy.* New Haven: Yale Univ. Press, 1957.

Sollberger, A. *Biological Rhythm Research.* Amsterdam: Elsevier, 1965.

Spencer, J. L. *The Electrogenetics of Alberto Pirovano.* New York: Hafner, 1965.

Stevens, S. S., ed. *Handbook of Experimental Psychology.* New York: Wiley, 1952.

Stokoe, W. C., et al. *A Dictionary of American Sign Language.* Washington, D.C.: Gallaudet College Press, 1965.

Tavalga, W. N., ed. *Marine Bio-Acoustics.* Oxford, Eng.: Pergamon, 1964.

Taylor, J. G. *The Behavioral Basis of Perception.* New Haven: Yale Univ. Press, 1962.

Thorpe, W. H. *Bird Song.* Cambridge, Eng.: Cambridge Univ. Press, 1967.

——. *Learning and Instinct in Animals.* Cambridge, Eng.: Cambridge Univ. Press, 1963.

Thorpe, W. H., and R. A. Linde, eds. *Bird Vocalization*. New York: Cambridge Univ. Press, 1969.

Turner, V. C. *General Endocrinology*. Philadelphia: Saunders, 1966.

Vasiliev, L. *Experiments in Mental Suggestion*. Church Crookham, Hants, Eng.: Gally Hall Press, 1964.

Walker, E. P. *Mammals of the World*. Baltimore: Johns Hopkins Press, 1964.

Welty, Joel Carl. *Life of Birds*. New York: Knopf, 1963.

Willems, E. P., and H. L. Raush, eds. *Naturalistic Viewpoints in Psychological Research*. New York: Holt, Rinehart and Winston, 1969.

Wolff, E. *Anatomy of the Eye and Orbit*. London: H. K. Lewis, 1968.

Wurtman, R. J., et al. *The Pineal*. New York: Academic Press, 1968.

Yerkes, R. M. *Chimpanzees*. New Haven: Yale Univ. Press, 1943.

Zubeck, John P., ed. *Sensory Deprivation*. New York: Appleton-Century-Crofts, 1969.

Index

340INDEX